Photography
in Dentistry

Theory and Techniques in Modern Documentation

Pasquale Loiacono, DDS
Private Practice, Tropea, Italy

Luca Pascoletti, DDS
Private Practice, Udine, Italy

Translated from Italian by
Rosemary Barber Meligrana

Qe

Q_e

Copyright © 2012 by Quintessenza Edizioni S.r.l.
via Ciro Menotti, 65 - 20017 Rho (MI) Italy
Tel.: +39.02.93.18.08.21 - Fax: +39.02.93.18.61.59
E-mail: info@quintessenzaedizioni.it
www.quintessenzaedizioni.com

ISBN 88-7492-169-1
     978-88-7492-169-0

Graphic designer Valentina Avogadro

Printed in Italy

Contents

Contents

Contents

Chapter 13
Photographic Documentation 309

Dedication

To my two wonderful daughters, Martina
and Nicoletta. May they always believe in
the beauty of their dreams and have the
strength to realize them.

Pasquale Loiacono

To my beloved daughter, Alice, an
irreplaceable source of energy, and
to my great friend and master of life,
Sandro Rodaro.

Luca Pascoletti

Foreword

Writing the foreword to a text requires a great moral and ethical commitment and, I would add, is an important responsibility toward both the authors and the readers. When my friends, Pasquale Loiacono and Luca Pascoletti, the authors of *Photography in Dentistry*, asked me to write the foreword to their book, I was pleased and honored to give a brief introduction to this work for two reasons. First, I have known the authors for several years and have followed the path of their professional growth; second, they are dear friends, and I feel a particular bond of affection toward them.

The major innovation represented by this text is the formation of the team of the two authors, who possess extraordinary qualities and gifts. This fine union of distinct talents has resulted in a work that is scientific and, at the same time, practical. The authors have interacted well together to create a text that is cohesive and extremely useful from a didactic point of view. It provides the reader—the novice or expert dentist-photographer—with a complete guide for obtaining excellent photographic documentation.

I can only express my most sincere compliments to the two authors for achieving a work in which the content and form is well rounded, complete, and supported by excellent illustrations—in other words, a work that I would have been pleased to have written myself. I am, therefore, convinced that this book will be greatly appreciated and put to good use by both novice dentists, aiming to acquire the techniques of photography, and skilled clinicians, who will certainly find theories and ideas to put into practice straightaway.

With my most sincere compliments,

Domenico Massironi, MD, DMD
Private Practice
Milan, Italy

Preface

The idea of creating a manual of photography for dentists originated from a specific cultural frame of reference, the Massironi Study Club, which is based upon the philosophy and teachings of Dr Domenico Massironi. We consider this work to be one of the many fruits borne from the tireless and visionary work of our "Maestro." We are aware that he is not keen on being defined in this manner; however, the influence of his teachings and his scientific rigor leads us to consider him with such profound affection and respect that we are unable to express ourselves in any other way. Thus, a warm thank you goes to him and to all friends of the Massironi Study Club with whom we share an exciting journey of personal and professional growth.

Why a book on photography?

First, we love and strongly believe in photography as a fundamental means toward our professional evolution. On a daily basis, it allows us to verify the path of our learning and to relate, in a positive way, to patients and colleagues alike. Our love of photography, together with our love of our profession, has always led us to wonder how so many competent professionals consider themselves unable to take photographs that are comparable to the quality of their own work. This false conviction deprives them of the opportunity to be appreciated by a wider audience or, more simply, to record their own professional path.

Our second fundamental motivation is an awareness that the current approach toward dental photography is totally lacking in standardized procedures or agreed-upon rules, which are present in all other traditional dental disciplines. Many colleagues turn to nonspecialized photographers to obtain information or to learn how to take dental photographs. However, the answers they receive are vague and often based on strictly commercial interests rather than the outcome of rigorous scientific reasoning.

We believe that any dentist can quickly acquire the rudimentary skills needed to take more-than-adequate photographs or, with very little extra effort, even excellent ones. The real problem is that there are very few comprehensive books on photography designed and written by dentists for dentists. Because we believe that only an insider can be aware of the day-to-day problems that we face in our profession, we were keen to put our knowledge at the disposal of our colleagues, in the hopes of spreading the use of this valuable instrument.

Pasquale Loiacono and Luca Pascoletti

Acknowledgments

My thoughts of gratitude and immense affection go first to my family: to my wife, Marianna, and my daughters, Martina and Nicoletta, for all the time I have taken away from them and, in particular, to my daughters for their contribution as models in this book.

I would also like to thank Dr Domenico Massironi for the great affection with which he has always supported, guided, and motivated me in both my personal and professional growth; my friend, Dr Bruno Alia, for his competent advice on medicolegal matters; Professors Luciano Meligrana and Aurelio Piserà, for their masterly stylistic advice; my dental technicians, Marcello Aiello, Gianluca and Francesco Barbagallo, and Evio Sirianni, for the professional passion and friendship that we share; Rosemary Barber, for her valuable collaboration in the translation of the text; Marco Forelli, for the skills that he has put at my disposal; Fabio Rodaro, for the attention he has devoted to my ideas and the care and skill with which he has executed the illustrations; my friend, Salvatore Accorinti, for the long and valuable conversations about computing and various methodologic and technical details. Another thank you goes to my close friend, Nando Ricciardi, the first person to believe in this project, for the support and affection he has always shown toward me.

Pasquale Loiacono

I would like to thank my great friend and Maestro, Dr Domenico Massironi, who has proved to be an invaluable guide both in my life and my profession. He has believed in and supported this project, providing us from the outset with important and essential advice. I would also like to thank my model, Sara Lirussi, who has willingly and patiently sat for numerous photographic sessions.

Other thanks go to expert professional photographer Alberto Cuoco, for the simplicity with which he has performed the often tricky photographic sequences and the skill with which he has demonstrated the positioning of the operators and the photographic equipment; to our illustrator and friend Fabio Rodaro, who, with wisdom and intuition, has managed to transform often ultratechnical images into pleasing and original drawings.

A heartfelt thanks goes to our orthodontist friend Luca Conoscenti, for his valuable collaboration, which has always proved helpful in developing and achieving often ambitious projects; to Piero Corsi, an irreplaceable friend with whom I share much of my free time, for his visual ideas for teaching and the unconditional friendship that he has always shown toward me.

A particular thank you to my assistants, Silvia Della Ricca, who has actively collaborated in the realization of this book as assistant photographer, and Daniela Baiutti, with whom I have shared my entire professional life and growth, for her help and patience.

Luca Pascoletti

Pasquale Loiacono

Part One

Theory

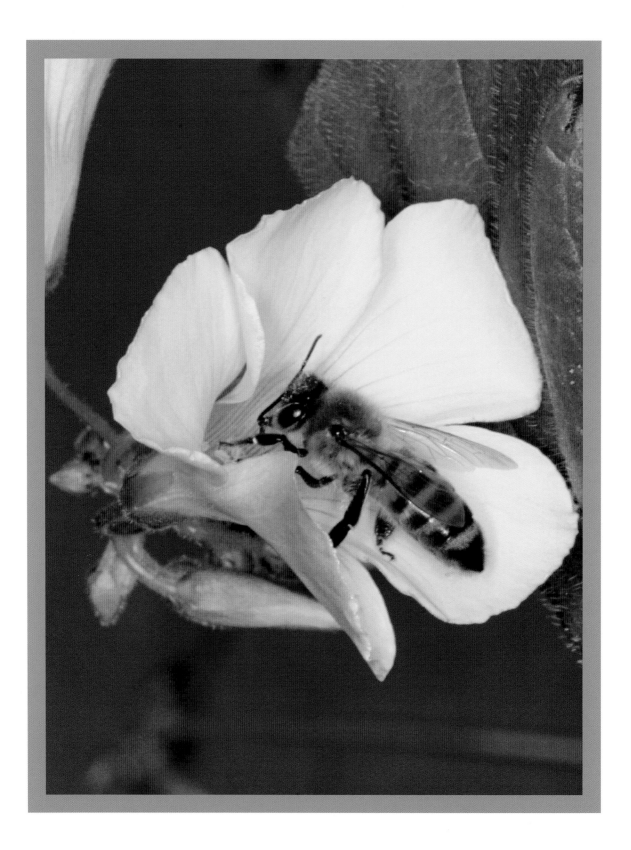

Chapter 1

General Principles
of Photography

[
Scientific communication can only take place if supporting documents are created using universally accepted standards, which enable them to be easily and readily understood and compared over time. A photographic image is a visual document and, as such, must be taken following precise rules, which render it accessible to the entire scientific community.
]

There has been a radical evolution over the past few decades in our manner of thinking, living, and relating to others; notably, these changes have been taking place—and are continuing to do so—ever more rapidly with respect to the past. Setting aside all moral or ethical considerations as to the compatibility of these innovations with an actual improvement in the quality of life, it is obvious that the possibility of communicating rapidly and effectively—for example, by means of mobile phones or the Internet—is transforming our way of life. Although these changes offer extraordinary possibilities, they create problems in understanding and handling new techniques. The rapid exchange of data is dependent upon the presumption that it does, in fact, exist and is written in a language that is, hopefully, accessible to the majority of users.

In the scientific world, this need is even more pressing. Therefore, data that the scientific community uses to spread knowledge and stimulate debate must be of a documentary nature: easily legible, certifiable, comparable, and written in a clear language with universally shared procedures. Data that is documentary in nature is useful internationally and over the course of time and thus becomes a heritage of knowledge for mankind. *The Vocabulary of the Italian Language* by Aldo Gabrielli defines a document as "a medium—generally written—which attests and confirms the reality of a fact." A surprising comment in the marvelous book by S. Chu, *Fundamentals of Color: Shade Matching and Communication in Esthetic Dentistry*, led to a reflection on the status of photography; in discussing the value of digital cameras in communicating color, the author states, "At present, the use of digital photography in dentistry has no set nomenclature, procedure codes, standards, or continuity." This statement regarding the lack of shared rules and procedures in the field of photography effectively sums up a widespread and not unfounded feeling among operators. I believe, and aim to demonstrate with my arguments and work, that this view of photography belongs in the past, and that today dental photography can, and indeed must, be granted the dignity of a technique with its own codified and reproducible rules, universally accepted by the scientific community. While the written word is obviously used to produce documents, medicine is the result of the observation of living structures and their phenomena; we are bound to admit that the power of an image is an irreplaceable means of communication in the field of medicine.

The word *photography* comes from two Greek words meaning, "to write with light." Learning to write with light is no longer the privilege of a few experts, but instead is a necessity for all those who are passionate about their profession and keen to continue to reap greater satisfaction from it. It is absolutely indispensable for the practitioner to master the fundamental principles of photography to fully understand the problems linked to clinical practice and, subsequently, to become independent in handling the photographic medium. As always, the ability to judge both the means being used and the results obtained is the key to professional growth.

The rules concerning specialized dental photography are based on general techniques. It is necessary to have a basic understanding of general photographic principles and techniques to obtain excellent results in a deliberate manner that is neither random nor accidental.

Photography can be defined as the detection and conservation of the light reflected from a particular scene at a given moment. This process requires a light-impervious container fitted with a mechanism that regulates both the quantity of light allowed to penetrate the device and impress the sensor, and the precise moment at which it does so. This device can be defined generically as a *camera*. The first few chapters of this book are dedicated to familiarizing the operator with this instrument and to purely technical aspects, which will be illustrated in detail for the sake of completeness. This technical information will be approached with clarity, focusing only on clinically useful material.

Chapters 5 through 13 deal specifically with clinical aspects of photography. This book attempts to explain and emphasize how light—the real protagonist of esthetic restorations—interacts with the dental substrate to create the phenomenon known as *tooth shade*.

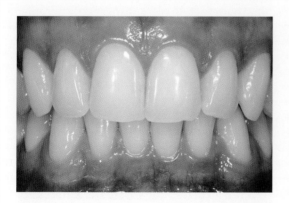

Fig 1-1a
First visit: this image allows the practitioner to assess the condition of the soft tissues, the teeth, and the patient's general health.

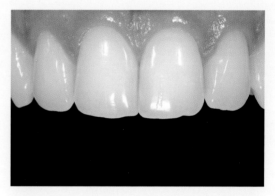

Fig 1-1b
Detail of maxillary anterior teeth shows the power of expression as highlighted by the harmonious proportion between the length and width of the teeth.

> *Close-up photography, or macrophotography, is a specialized dental technique. The closeness of the subject necessitates special photographic equipment and devices to obtain appropriate images and documentation suitable for clinical needs and scientific communication.*

Close-up Photography

It is important to emphasize that dental photography is, without doubt, a highly specialized field, with specific requirements that necessitate a different approach than that of conventional photography. Dental photography belongs to the field of close-up photography, or macrophotography (Figs 1-1 and 1-2).

It is quite possible to master the correct technique for taking excellent photographs of sporting events, ceremonies, scenery, or portraits and not be capable of obtaining comparable results in the field of close-up photography. Similarly, a specialist in implant surgery, who has only worked in this discipline, could not be expected to perform excellent endodontic therapy.

Briefly, in a macrophotograph or close-up photograph, the dimensions of the subject are reproduced onto a sensor with a magnification ratio ranging from 10:1 to 1:10. This definition requires further explanation, because an understanding of the magnification ratio is absolutely essential to complete comprehension of dental photography; chapter 2 clearly explains this concept.

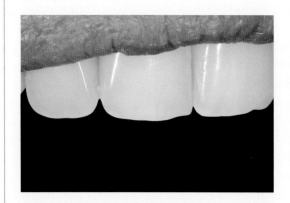

Fig 1-1c
A detail of the relationship between upper lip and incisors.

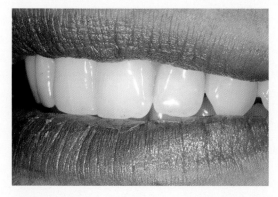

Fig 1-1d
Harmony between teeth and lips.

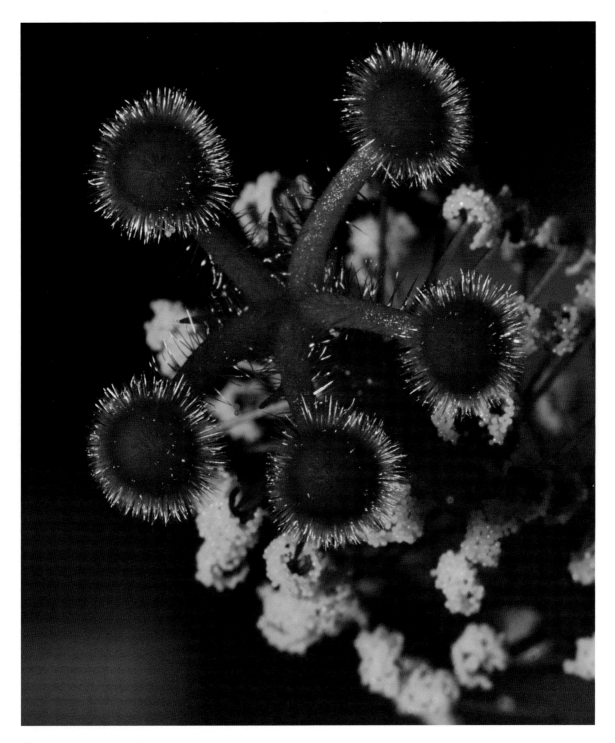

Fig 1-2
Close-up view of the pistils of a typical Mediterranean plant, the hibiscus.

[
All cameras have at least five essential components in common: a sensor, a diaphragm or aperture, a shutter, a system of lenses, and a viewfinder. Most modern cameras also have a built-in light meter. We can distinguish between the various types of cameras by the characteristics of these fundamental components.
]

Basic Components of the Camera

Apart from the hermetically light-sealed rigid outer case, called the *body*, a camera consists of five essential elements: sensor, diaphragm or aperture, shutter, lens system, and viewfinder. All modern cameras also have a sixth component, the light meter, which is now considered an integral part of the camera.

These components will be analyzed in detail to arrive at an overall understanding of their function and importance within the discipline of dental photography.

Compact and Reflex Cameras

First we must distinguish between cameras for general use, which are used in dentistry, and cameras for special use, such as those designed for aerial photography and used for cartographical and topographical studies. For reasons relating to cost and use, the latter have characteristics and require films and sensors of a completely different nature than those of the amateur or professional photographer. In fact, there are cameras that use 200 × 250–mm film to achieve maximum detail in large frames. Digital sensors are available in special formats as well. Kodak produces 51 × 39–mm sensors, which are capable of greater than 50 megapixels and approximately 360 MB per photograph.

Cameras for general use can be divided into two large families: compact cameras and single-lens reflex (SLR) cameras (Figs 1-3 and 1-4). Compact cameras were developed in response to technical demands for simplification and cost reduction. They are characterized by special automatic devices that perform various tasks for the operator, thus making them suitable for inexpert users; even a child can take a wonderful photograph!

This advantage of compact cameras is also a drawback, because it prevents the expert operator from employing optional settings that, as we will see later, are essential to the requirements of the practitioner. SLR cameras are more costly and complex to handle but allow the operator a virtually unlimited choice of parameters, including lens choice. In fact, one of the fundamental characteristics of SLR cameras is the possibility of selecting lenses of various focal lengths, which provide different angles of view and thus different magnification ratios.

Dentists often ask, "Which equipment do I need to take a good dental photograph?" The correct response is that the operator must choose each instrument with the final result in mind. To answer this question accurately and thoroughly requires a detailed analysis of the components and the functions of the two types of cameras.

For a complete understanding of available equipment, the operator should be aware that an intermediate category exists between compact and SLR cameras: the professional-consumer or so-called prosumer type. *Prosumer cameras*, also called *SRL-like cameras*, have hybrid characteristics; they allow greater control over the procedures for acquiring the image, but lack interchangeability of the lens. At present, some manufacturing companies are launching a new type of hybrid

[*To choose an appropriate camera for a particular task, it is necessary to analyze the modes of function and characteristics of the various types of cameras and their usefulness in relation to clinical needs. The categories from which to choose the most suitable camera for dental photography are compact and single-lens reflex (SLR).*]

camera onto the market, based on a format developed by Olympus and Panasonic, called *Micro Four Thirds* in reference to its sensor format and its smaller bayonet lens attachment, which is built without a mirror or the pentaprism that typifies SLR cameras. These components have been replaced by an electronic viewfinder. As in other SLR cameras, the lenses of Micro Four Thirds cameras are interchangeable. The same manufacturers are also marketing adapter rings to allow the use of preexisting SLR lenses

by the new generation of cameras. The Micro Four Thirds system came into existence, therefore, with the intention of reducing the encumbrance and weight of SLR cameras while maintaining the option of lens substitution. All innovations that the market currently offers, and will offer in the future, should be judged on their basic usefulness for the peculiar needs of the dental field and its clearly defined equipment needs and correlated techniques.

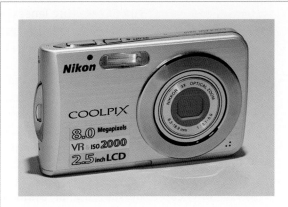

Fig 1-3
The modern compact Nikon Coolpix S210 camera, without Galilean viewfinder, is equipped with a liquid crystal display (LCD) panel for live view mode.

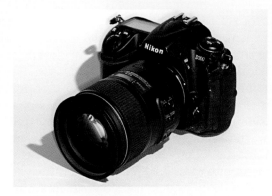

Fig 1-4
A digital Nikon D300 camera equipped with a complementary metal-oxide semiconductor (CMOS) sensor in a classic Advanced Photo System (APS-C) format.

[
The sensor of a camera is the device that instantly registers the brightness of the scene to be photographed. The sensor can be analog, a coating of silver halide placed onto celluloid film, or digital, a specialized electronic device. There are various types of digital sensors; compact cameras are generally fitted with the 4:3 sensor format and are therefore less expensive.
]

Components of a Digital Camera

Analog and digital sensors

An analysis of the components of the camera should begin with what is commonly called the sensor, the sensitive device that registers the light conditions of a scene at a particular moment. The *sensor* is equivalent to the retina of the eye. Originally, the sensitive element consisted of layers of silver halide emulsion on glass or thin celluloid strips, hence the term *film*. However, over the past few years the use of digital sensor technology has become widespread. One advantage of digital technology is instant visualization of the image. It is important to point out that the principles and techniques of photography did not change upon the introduction of digital sensors; however, the immediate availability of and ease in handling the image were significant changes. If one should choose to photograph using film, splendid results definitely can be obtained, and this medium still maintains all its original fascination and usefulness. However, given the versatility of digital photography as applied to dentistry, it is advisable to expand one's knowledge of this technology.

The structural and functional characteristics of the digital sensor will be illustrated in chapter 4. At this point, however, it is necessary to emphasize certain concepts concerning the differences between digital sensors in compact and SLR cameras.

A main difference between the two, given equal megapixels, is the general dimensions of the sensor and of the individual light-sensitive elements. To economize space, a smaller-format sensor is used in compact digital cameras than in SLR digital cameras. The photodiodes or photodetectors, the light-sensitive elements, are also smaller in compact cameras: approximately 1.8 to 2 μm, as compared to 6.8 to 7 μm in the SLR camera sensor. This variation in size does not affect the nominal resolution of the photograph as expressed in megapixels. It does, however, affect the final overall quality of the photograph; in fact, smaller light-sensitive elements require greater amplification of the electrical signal and thus result in the appearance of undesired visual effects, called *electronic noise*. It should also be noted that few compact cameras allow the recording of image files in the raw image format, which, as we will see later, is the only format that is considered to have medicolegal value.

[*The light-sensitive elements of compact camera sensors are smaller and of poorer quality than those of SLR cameras. The nominal resolution of a sensor is not, in itself, sufficient to express overall picture quality; the ultimate quality of an image is the combined result of the characteristics of the sensor, the lenses, and other components of the camera.*]

Sensor format

The term *sensor format* refers to both the general size of the sensitive element, indicated by the product of the measurement of the horizontal and vertical sides of the sensor, and the shape or proportion between the sides, known as the *aspect ratio* (Figs 1-5 to 1-7). A precise definition of sensor format, whether in film or electronic devices, is essential because it has important conceptual and practical implications.

For film, the format can be expressed in numbers or letters. For example, the designation 135 refers to 24 × 36-mm film; 126 refers to 30 × 30-mm film; Advanced Photo System (APS) identifies a 17 × 30-mm film (Table 1-1).

The sensor format can also be described by the aspect ratio, which is the proportion between the two sides. In a 1:1 format, the two sides are equal; other formats include 4:3 and 2:3. Generally, a 2:3 format is considered standard, because it represents the proportions of the 24 × 36-mm format, which is the most common format for amateur and professional use. A 4:3 format is typically used in compact cameras.

Digital sensor formats are described in the same way as traditional film sensors, although they may vary slightly from the established measurements for film standards. The most commonly used format in digital SLR cameras is the classic APS (APS-C) sensor. The classic 2:3 format measures about 16 × 24 mm. Manufacturers may install sensors that vary slightly from this measurement, while still being classifiable as APS-C. For example, Nikon makes a 15.6 × 23.6-mm APS-C sensor that they call DX format, and Canon produces a 14.8 × 22.2-mm APS-C sensor (see Fig 1-6).

Table 1-1 *Various film formats*

Film acronym	Format (mm)	Actual measurement (mm)	Ratio between sides
APS–C (classic)	17 x 25	25.1 x 16.7	3:2
APS–H (high definition)	17 x 30	30.2 x 16.7	16:9
APS–P (panoramic)	9 x 30	9.5 x 30.2	3:1
135 (35 mm)	24 x 36	24 x 36	2:3
126	30 x 30	27 x 28	1:1
120	45 x 60	45 x 57	3:4
70	60 x 60	57 x 57	1:1
Flat sheet	8 x 10 inches	20.3 x 25.4	4:5

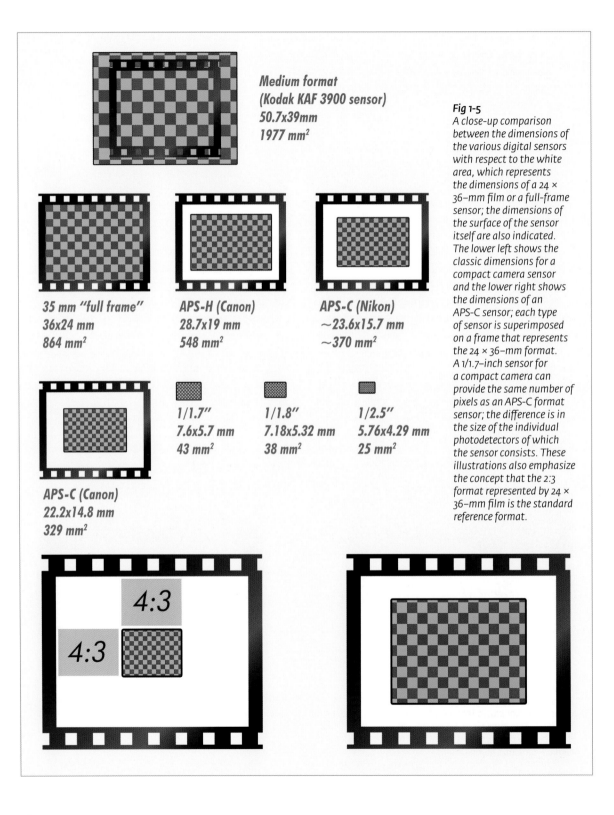

**Medium format
(Kodak KAF 3900 sensor)
50.7x39mm
1977 mm²**

**35 mm "full frame"
36x24 mm
864 mm²**

**APS-H (Canon)
28.7x19 mm
548 mm²**

**APS-C (Nikon)
~23.6x15.7 mm
~370 mm²**

**APS-C (Canon)
22.2x14.8 mm
329 mm²**

**1/1.7″
7.6x5.7 mm
43 mm²**

**1/1.8″
7.18x5.32 mm
38 mm²**

**1/2.5″
5.76x4.29 mm
25 mm²**

4:3

4:3

Fig 1-5
A close-up comparison between the dimensions of the various digital sensors with respect to the white area, which represents the dimensions of a 24 × 36–mm film or a full-frame sensor; the dimensions of the surface of the sensor itself are also indicated. The lower left shows the classic dimensions for a compact camera sensor and the lower right shows the dimensions of an APS-C sensor; each type of sensor is superimposed on a frame that represents the 24 × 36–mm format. A 1/1.7-inch sensor for a compact camera can provide the same number of pixels as an APS-C format sensor; the difference is in the size of the individual photodetectors of which the sensor consists. These illustrations also emphasize the concept that the 2:3 format represented by 24 × 36–mm film is the standard reference format.

The term format *indicates the product of the linear measurements of the two sides of the sensor and the ratio between them.*

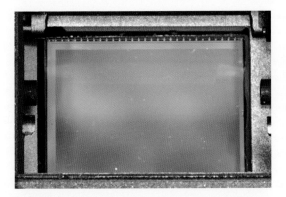

Fig 1-6a
A Canon CMOS digital sensor, observed from the point of view of the lens, with the mirror raised and the shutter open. This allows the sensor's surface to be cleaned. It is normal for specks of dust or other minute material to settle on the sensor; these appear as black spots on images with a light background. Modern cameras are equipped with automatic devices for cleaning the sensor, which are extremely useful and highly recommended.

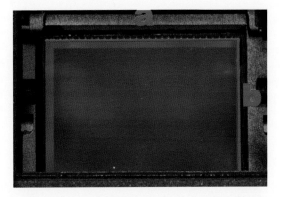

Fig 1-6b
The format of this Canon CMOS sensor can be expressed as the product of the linear measurements of the two sides (14.8 × 22.2 mm), or as the ratio between two sides, 2:3 (the ratio between 14.8 and 22.2).

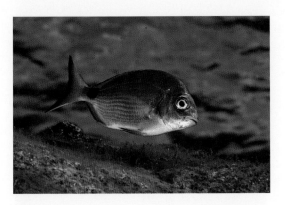

Fig 1-7a
An underwater photograph taken with a Nikon D80 camera, Nikkor macro lens with f = 60 mm (Nikon), f/13, t = 1/65 s. This image is in 2:3 format, which expresses great beauty and harmony, and it won the 2008 Isola del Giglio Photosub Championship.

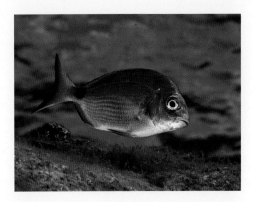

Fig 1-7b
The same image, cropped in 4:3 format, clearly offers less impressive visual impact because of the different proportions of the sides.

> The diaphragm, commonly referred to as the **aperture**, is represented by the symbol f/ followed by a numeric value. The aperture is a device with a variable opening that regulates the amount of light that reaches the sensor. The higher the numeric value or f-stop, the more closed the aperture and the less light that reaches the sensor. On the contrary, lower f-stop values reflect greater aperture and a greater amount of light reaching the sensor.

Aperture or diaphragm

The aperture, also called the *diaphragm*, is a mechanism of thin plates built into the lens that regulates the amount of light reaching the sensor according to its degree of opening.

It can be compared to the pupil of the eye, which regulates its degree of aperture in response to varying light conditions (Fig 1-8). In SLR cameras, the aperture is always set on maximum to allow the image on the viewfinder to be as clear as possible. It adjusts to a selected value only at the moment of taking the shot.

In the field of photography, the degree of aperture is indicated by the symbol f/ followed by a number that represents the relative aperture. Relative aperture is the focal length of a lens divided by the diameter of a particular aperture (Fig 1-9). Relative aperture is also called the *f-number* or the *f-stop value*.

Thus, if an aperture is listed as f/8, the aperture value goes into the focal length of that particular lens eight times; stated differently, the aperture corresponds to one-eighth of the focal length. Relative aperture is a fractional concept; the higher the numeric value of an f-stop, the smaller, or more closed, the aperture. Similarly, a smaller numeric f-stop value corresponds to a larger or wider aperture (Fig 1-10).

The maximum aperture value, generally inscribed on the front rim of the lens, indicates the lens speed. A lens marked f/2 will have a maximum aperture diameter corresponding to exactly half the focal length. It is interesting to note that the fastest lenses in the world are the 50-mm Noctilux (Leica) and the 50-mm Dream

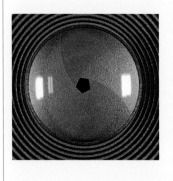

Fig 1-8
Detail of the thin blades that form the aperture. The aperture is on maximum closure. Note that upon close observation of the image, the sides of the photograph appear to be curved and distorted rather than straight; this is a well-known optical illusion.

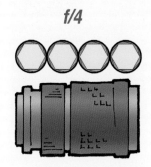

f/4

Fig 1-9
The f-stop value is focal length of the lens divided by a particular aperture value.

[
The value, or number, of the aperture represents the number of times a particular linear measurement of aperture goes into the focal length of the lens. A particular amount of light corresponds to the numeric value of the aperture. Each lower or preceding aperture value corresponds to a doubling of the amount of light reaching the sensor; each higher or subsequent aperture value reduces the amount of light by half.
]

Lens (Canon), which have maximum apertures of f/0.95. For an optical engineer to achieve such a level of brightness represents a true technological achievement, and any further improvement in brightness in the future will prove extremely difficult.

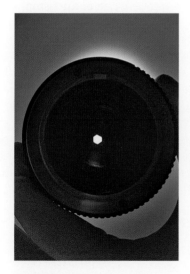

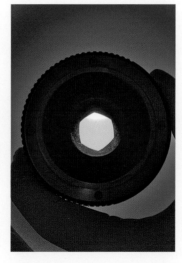

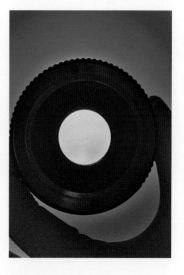

Fig 1-10a
Minimum aperture: the focal length of the lens is divided by this measurement many times, and therefore the aperture will have a high numeric value.

Fig 1-10b
Intermediate aperture.

Fig 1-10c
Maximum aperture, which corresponds to the lens speed. If this measurement is 25 mm, and the lens has a focal length of 50 mm, the lens speed will be equal to 50 ÷ 25 = 2; f/2 or, more simply, 2. Note that the numeric value is low, indicating a greater aperture.

The shutter, which is normally in a closed position, exposes the sensor to the light coming from the lens. The shutter-release button controls its opening and closing, and its speed is inversely proportional to the exposure time of the sensor. Each shutter speed corresponds to a specific exposure time and thus to a particular amount of light reaching the sensor. The exposure time is inversely proportional to the shutter speed.

Shutter and shutter speed

The shutter is a device for exposing the sensor, directly related to the aperture. It is mobile and built into the body of the camera in front of the sensor. Normally, the shutter is closed, but when it opens, as controlled by the shutter-release button, light coming from the lens is allowed to reach the sensor (Fig 1-11). Exposure time is the length of time that the shutter stays open and the sensor remains exposed to the light coming from the lens. Shutter speed is the term commonly used to describe exposure time. It is inversely proportional to the exposure time; halving the shutter speed doubles the exposure.

An important characteristic of the shutter is that its speed can be selected by the operator and can range from a few seconds to hundredths or thousandths of a second. An average- to high-quality SLR camera can achieve a shutter speed of 1/8000 s. Some cameras are equipped with a *B setting*, or *bulb exposure*, which allows the shutter to stay open indefinitely. This option is useful for nighttime photographs requiring a very long exposure time.

Each shutter speed value determines the amount of light that strikes the sensor. When the length of exposure time is doubled, the amount of light that reaches the sensitive element also doubles. Similarly, when the exposure time is halved, the light reaching the sensor is halved (Fig 1-12).

A time value of 125 means that the shutter will stay open for 1/125 s. The next time value will be 1/250 s, meaning that the shutter speed doubles and the exposure time is halved. The time value that precedes 1/125 s will indicate a halving of the shutter speed and, consequently, a doubling of the exposure time, corresponding to 1/62.5 s; by convention, this speed is rounded to 1/60 s. Each increment represents a halving or doubling of the exposure.

The same concept applies to the aperture: each f-stop, or aperture value, indicates a halving or a doubling of the amount of light that passes through it. If we compare light reaching the sensor to a liquid, the aperture is the device that regulates the rate of flow of that liquid within a duct (the lens), while the shutter represents the tap that opens or closes the duct itself at a precise moment.

Reciprocity law

The diaphragm and the shutter work together in strict synergy to produce exposure combinations that effectively determine the total amount of light that strikes the sensor. The exposure combinations are regulated by the *reciprocity law*, which states that various combinations of shutter speed and aperture will provide the same total amount of light (Fig 1-13). If the shutter speed is doubled, the time that the shutter remains open is halved, and the amount of light that reaches the sensor is also reduced by half. To maintain the original amount of light reaching the sensor, the degree of aperture must be increased by one stop (or value). In the same way, if the aperture is decreased by two stops, the amount of light reaching the sensor can be maintained by increasing the exposure time by two values.

The criteria by which the exposure pair is selected depends on the subject. A rapidly moving object needs a very short exposure time, so the aperture is sacrificed to allow the necessary amount of light to impress the sensor. This condition is called *shutter priority mode* (Fig 1-14).

If the aperture must be reduced, the exposure time must be lengthened, a condition called *aperture priority mode*. If the total amount of light resulting from the combination of these factors is insufficient for correct exposure, additional sources of light, such as the flash, are needed. The concept of the synergy between the shutter and the aperture forms the basis of the automatic devices of the camera, which can be either shutter priority or aperture priority mode.

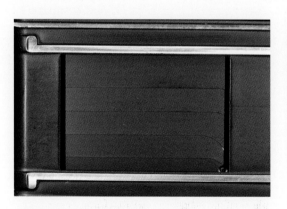

Fig 1-11a
The back of a shutter, observed from the point of view of the sensor, in its normal closed position. The speed of opening of the curtain, and thus the length of time it offers light to the sensor, represents the exposure time.

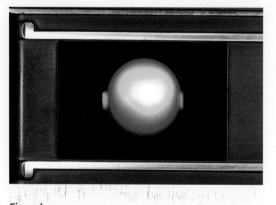

Fig 1-11b
The open shutter reveals the light coming from the diaphragm of the lens. To achieve this image, the shutter-release button was held down in B setting, or bulb exposure. In this mode, the shutter stays open as long as the shutter-release button is held down by the operator, which may be necessary in very poor lighting conditions.

Fig 1-12
Fluids can be used to illustrate the relationship between shutter speed and exposure time. A tap left open for a very short time, 1/500 s (represented by the stopwatch), corresponds to a high speed for closure of the tap (represented by the tachymeter). The quantity of fluid that reaches the container is minimal. If the aperture time is doubled, thus halving the speed, the quantity of water is doubled. The role of the shutter in exposure is identical. Doubling the speed means that the aperture time is exactly halved, as is the quantity of light which reaches the sensor.

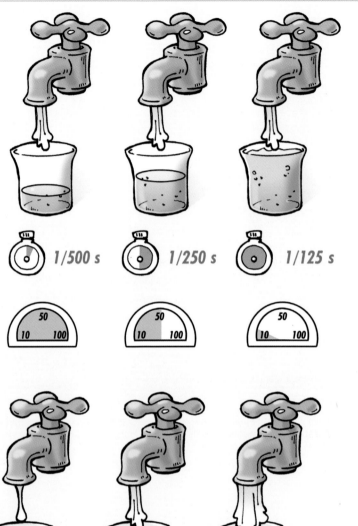

Fig 1-13
Fluids can be used to illustrate the reciprocity law. To fill a glass with an identical quantity of water, the rate of flow from the faucet can be varied by means of the degree of aperture of the tap or by modifying the length of time the tap is opened. Various combinations of tap aperture and opening time give identical results in terms of the quantity of fluid supplied. With a camera, the same conditions exist; the total quantity of light that reaches the sensor is regulated by the aperture and the shutter.

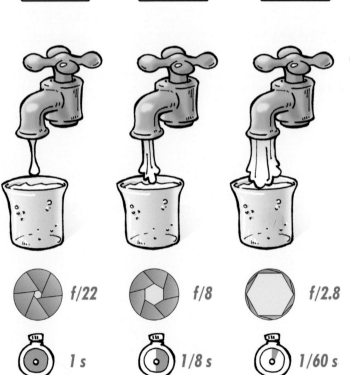

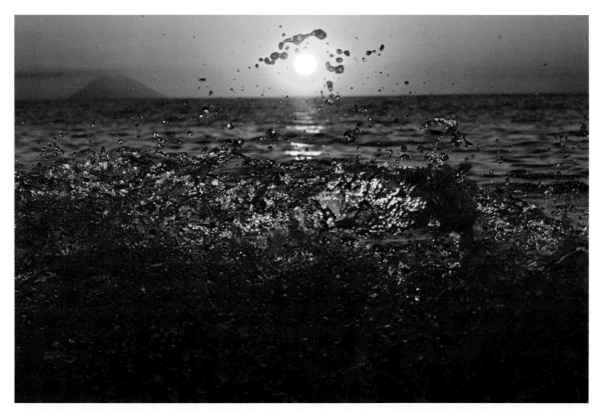

Fig 1-14
An image taken with shutter priority mode at a shutter speed of 1/800 s captures the breaking of a wave and the details of the spray; the volcano of Stromboli at sunset is visible in the background, as seen from a beach in Tropea, Calabria, Italy.

[
The viewfinder of the camera allows the photographer to compose or frame the image. Compact cameras are fitted with a Galilean viewfinder or, more recently, with a liquid crystal display panel, which avoids the problem of parallax. SLR cameras enable the operator to choose the frame by directly observing the scene through the viewfinder, thus obtaining a greater degree of precision and accuracy.
]

Viewfinder

The viewfinder of the camera is the lens through which the photographer observes what the sensor sees at the moment of recording the image. Therefore, it allows the photographer to choose or compose the frame correctly according to his or her requirements or taste. There are two types of viewfinders, Galilean and prismatic; the former is used in compact cameras, and the latter, in SLR cameras.

The Galilean viewfinder is a lens generally located above the shutter of the compact camera. It allows the operator to perceive approximately what the sensor will record at the moment of the aperture of the shutter. This approximation is a result of the substantial difference between what the lens "sees" and what the viewfinder "sees." They have different perspectives because of the different angle from which they view the subject in the frame. This phenomenon is called, in optical terms, *parallax* (Fig 1-15). The problem of parallax has been overcome by the latest generation of compact cameras, which have *live view mode*. In this mode, the frame to be recorded through the lens is previewed on a liquid crystal display (LCD) on the back of the camera.

The prismatic viewfinder contains a pentaprism, or five-sided prism. To understand how a pentaprism works requires knowledge of the manner in which an SLR camera works.

These cameras are called *reflex cameras* because they are fitted with a mirror. After light passes through the lens, a mirror reflects the light, turning the image upside down. The light travels to the pentaprism, which reverses it again to obtain the correctly oriented final image. At the moment of exposure, the mirror rises, offering light to the sensor and at the same time cutting off the vision of the image in the viewfinder; this produces the characteristic click of the release button (Fig 1-16).

The image seen through the prismatic viewfinder is identical to that perceived by the sensor, without parallax error. The image seen through the viewfinder is normally slightly reduced with respect to that perceived by the sensor; the viewfinder has an inferior frame coverage, about 95% of that perceived by the sensor. This problem is not present in the most expensive cameras, whose refined components allow total coverage of the scene in the viewfinder.

SLR cameras usually display important information on the lower part of the viewfinder, such as the time, the f-stop, and the exposure meter readings. This allows the operator to vary the settings without taking his or her eyes off of the viewfinder itself. Some cameras, such as the Nikon D300, display a reference grid in the viewfinder, which can prove extremely useful in avoiding unwanted inclinations of the frame.

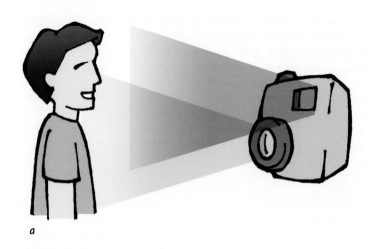
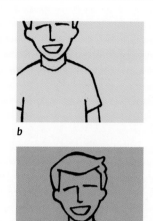

Fig 1-15
(a to c) Parallax error is caused by the different angles of view of the lens and the viewfinder. To avoid this distortion, modern compact cameras have live view mode.

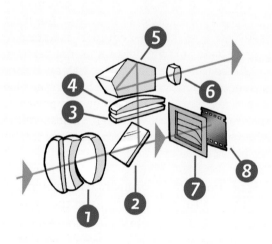

Fig 1-16
Order of functioning of an SLR camera. (1) The light penetrates the lens, (2) is reflected onto the mirror, (3) passes through the focusing lens and (4) a condensation screen, (5) is turned upside down by the pentaprism, and (6) is finally displayed on the viewfinder. Upon pressing the shutter-release button, the mirror will rise and (7) the shutter will open, (8) allowing the sensor to be impressed.

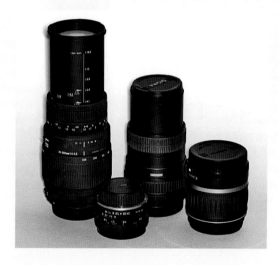

Fig 1-17
The variety of optical lenses available for SLR cameras is a great advantage for their users, especially considering the particular photographic needs of the dental field.

[*The live view mode allows the operator to view the scene being framed on a screen at the back of the camera; it is an alternative to the optical viewfinder, but it can cause difficulty with framing and is therefore inadvisable for use in the dental field. The option of changing lenses, selecting the most appropriate to a particular need, is one of the most advantageous characteristics of the SLR camera.*]

Live view and video modes

In *live view mode*, it is possible to instantly view the scene framed on the display at the back of the camera; this function, which has been present in compact cameras for some time, has recently been added to digital SLR cameras. Viewing the subject on an LCD screen offers several advantages: the operator can compose a scene directly, holding the camera at a distance, with arms stretched out or, in macrophotography, placing the camera at ground level. Technologic evolution has led to the manufacture of mobile display screens with adjustable inclination, which further improve the versatility of the SLR camera while maintaining high-quality results.

In addition to the live view mode, modern cameras also produce high-definition videos that may, in the future, serve as a useful complementary form of documentation. However, they do not seem to be essential for dental needs at present. In fact, the duration of these video sessions is extremely limited, as is the mono sound quality. They are not comparable to high-definition video cameras. Because of the complexity of focusing the camera and for reasons of stability, it is far preferable in the dental field not to use the live view mode; it is more appropriate to support the camera in the classic manner, holding it firmly with both hands and framing the scene through the optic viewfinder.

Lens

Another major difference between compact and SLR cameras is the characteristics of the lenses used to direct light to the sensor. In compact cameras, the lenses are not interchangeable and generally have a short focal length, but they do have a zoom function that enables the operator to vary the focal length to adapt to a variety of situations. However, such options involve making concessions in quality; with so many options, the operator must choose the best compromise for a particular situation, but by so doing, he or she forfeits the opportunity of achieving excellence, which is the exact opposite of our working philosophy.

On the other hand, the lenses are interchangeable in SLR cameras, allowing the operator to maintain the highest quality in various situations. The most up-to-date photographer, whether amateur or professional, can choose the most suitable lens for his or her own requirements (Fig 1-17).

The subject of SLR camera lenses is so important that it warrants in-depth analysis, which is carried out in chapter 2. The choice of the right lens, together with its correct use, is one of the most critical factors in enabling excellence in the photographic field. It is worth mentioning again that a new kind of compact camera, the Micro Four Thirds, has been recently introduced; it lacks the mirror or pentaprism typical of SLR cameras, but allows for the substitution of lenses.

The exposure meter is the electronic device that measures the light present in the framed scene. It is nearly always built into the camera itself. The through-the-lens (TTL) reading is a measurement of light taken through the camera's own lenses.

Exposure meter

The exposure meter is an electronic device or sensor consisting of photosensitive semiconducting elements, typically built into the camera. Such a device measures the *exposure*, or total amount of light present at a precise moment in the area framed by the lens. This measurement enables the camera's processor to calculate the optimal shutter speed–aperture combination, or exposure combination, to obtain a correctly exposed photograph with the right brightness.

Through-the-lens metering

As discussed above, the exposure meter is built into the body of the camera itself, allowing the device to measure light by means of the same lens used by the camera, technically referred to as *through-the-lens* (TTL) metering. The same concept of TTL metering is used in control of the flash. The flash system works in synergy with the exposure meter of the camera to control the amount of light emitted by the flash to achieve optimal exposure (Fig 1-18).

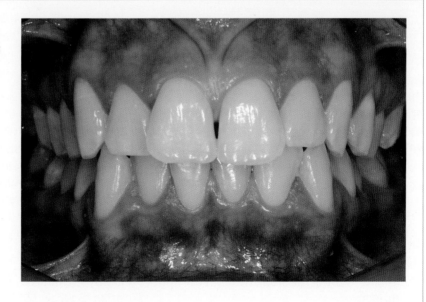

Fig 1-18
A photograph that can be considered a good document is easily legible for depth of field and focus, taken according to correct spatiality rules, and therefore repeatable over time. An image with these characteristics can be presented at any scientific conference without exposing the photographer to any basic criticism.

[

The correct handling of a camera is fundamental to achieving the best results in minimal time and with the least effort. The operator's arms should be kept close to the body to serve as a support. The posture should be such that the center of gravity of the torso can be moved backward or forward without losing the required stability.

]

Correct Handling of the Camera

Ergonomics and optimal management of available resources are equally important in photography and in normal clinical practice. The most precious resources are the practitioner's time and mental and physical energy. In fact, the following practices have been studied with particular care and attention by the author to optimize the time needed to take photographs and to avoid wasting the practitioner's energy. As in other areas of dentistry, the correct handling of the instrument in clinical photography is a decisive aspect for achieving maximum results with minimum effort and time.

The camera must be held firmly in the right hand, which has the fundamental function of supporting and stabilizing it; it is essential to be able to reach the shutter-release button easily and to activate it with the index finger of the same hand (Fig 1-19a). The left hand, facing upwards, supports the lens and, at the same time, with the thumb on the opposite side to the index and middle fingers, rotates the focusing ring to set the focus (Fig 1-19b). Camera handling must be done naturally and smoothly, but also with firmness, so as to be fully in control of the instrument.

The elbows and arms must be close together, pressing lightly against the body for greater stability, to allow composition of the picture with optimal results (Fig 1-19c). The need for stability is why it is not advisable to use the live view function.

The focusing technique particular to dental photography requires the practitioner to make movements toward and away from the subject (see chapter 7), with the feet apart to allow the full range of movement of the torso backward and forward.

The practitioner must place one leg slightly flexed in front of the other, with the feet at an angle of 80 degrees; this increases stability and offers a wide range of back-and-forth movements of the torso. This posture is similar to that of athletes in the sport of wing shooting, who use this technique for the same reason.

The camera should rest firmly against the face during the composition of the picture, which allows the operator to experience the camera as an extension of the body; in the sport of wing shooting, the athlete, having taken up position with the weapon, has only to follow the target with his or her eyes to strike it. The photographer-dentist needs to establish such a close rapport with his camera that it becomes an extension of his or her own eyes, just as practitioners use a periodontal probe as an endoscope in mentally visualizing and mapping the periodontal condition.

The most stable position of the torso can be achieved by placing the lower limbs a certain distance apart, one in front of the other, so that the operator's feet form an angle of 80 degrees. The right hand holds and stabilizes the camera; the left hand, with the palm facing upwards, supports the lens and focuses the image.

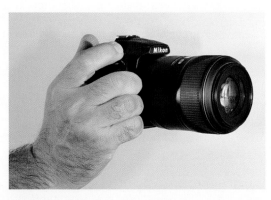

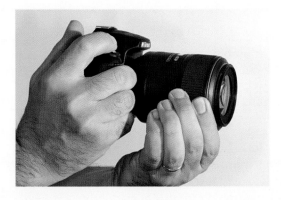

Fig 1-19a
The right hand holds the camera firmly so that the index finger reaches the shutter-release button with ease, while the thumb regulates any adjustments.

Fig 1-19b
The left hand, palm upwards, supports the lens and, with thumb and index and middle fingers, comfortably rotates the focusing ring.

Fig 1-19c
The operator holds the camera correctly, firmly pressing it against the face, being careful to keep the arms close to the body; this position allows the use of the limbs as a natural support or tripod for the camera. One of the operator's legs should be positioned so as to form an 80-degree angle with the feet, allowing the center of gravity of the torso to move back and forth and aiding with correct focusing.

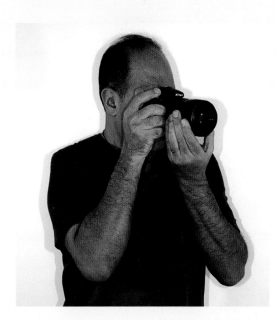

[
Photography is a valid instrument for creating visual scientific documents. Because such documents should be easily understood and compared, they must be created according to certain universally shared and repeatable rules.
]

Camera Choice on the Basis of Documentation

Examination of the components and main functions of the camera (Table 1-2) has answered the question posed at the beginning of this chapter: "What equipment do we need to take a good clinical photograph?" A good working philosophy is that a satisfactory photograph succeeds in representing a certain clinical situation promptly and effectively with the right characteristics to become a universal document.

What does the term *to document* mean?
In the scientific field, documentation refers to the recording and preservation of data that attest or demonstrate the reality of clinical facts and the communication of this data in a clear language, with codified procedures accepted by the entire scientific community. Dental photographs must fulfill certain fundamental requirements: correct exposure, framing, focusing, and depth of field. Furthermore—and this is essential—they must be repeatable and, therefore, comparable over time. The photograph must be taken from a perspective that is superimposable at the beginning and at the end of the treatment and, subsequently, over the course of years, for necessary follow-ups.

A critical examination of a series of images will shed light on the characteristics of the functioning and the performance of compact cameras (Fig 1-20).

Compact cameras are designed so that their various functions are almost totally automatic; it is extremely difficult to formulate criteria for achieving repeatability of an image and a magnification ratio. The largest magnification ratio possible is certainly not adequate to clinical needs and can be achieved only by significantly distorting the perspective. Currently available compact cameras do not have the option of using a ring-type flash; the Nikon Coolpix 4500 camera body and Nikon SB-29 ring flash have been discontinued. Therefore, the lighting of the image to be recorded is not optimal with compact cameras.

Another problem is shot delay, also known as *shutter lag*: the camera, at the moment of pressing the shutter-release button, does not instantly carry out the command, but instead takes fractions of a second or even seconds to calculate the exposure and focus.

Moreover, compact cameras do not allow the operator to effectively decide the focal point and, consequently, the depth of field of an image. The actual dimensions of the minimum aperture in compact cameras allow for good depth of field (see chapter 6).

Compact cameras are fitted with smaller-format sensors and smaller photosensitive elements, which do not create a high-quality image. The sensor has a 4:3 format, which is why compact-camera images appear squarer in comparison to the standard 2:3 format universally used in scientific presentations. Moreover, and most importantly, they do not allow for the substitution and use of specialized lenses.

In conclusion, it is extremely difficult to achieve and control a proper magnification ratio using a compact camera. It is only with great

[*Compact cameras do not respond as effectively as SLR cameras to scientific documentation requirements. The latter are considered the gold standard for dental photography.*]

difficulty that these cameras allow the operator to manually select a focal point; neither do they permit easy depth-of-field control. In practice, they do not allow for reliable and controlled repeatability of an image. These cameras are not suitable for scientific dental photography, although they are useful on many occasions in everyday life.

An analysis of the characteristics of the SLR camera shows that they overcome all the criticisms of the compact camera: precise control of focus, depth of field, and exposure and the opportunity to use an appropriate lens and flash. SLR cameras allow total and repeatable control of the image. In the dental field, the only way to achieve excellent photographs is with an SLR camera, which, to date, represents the gold standard for dentistry.

It has already been mentioned that the fundamental characteristic of these cameras is the interchangeability of the lenses. **Why is it so important to be able to substitute the lenses?**
An in-depth answer to this question is needed to gain complete understanding of the problem and the working logic of lenses, which will help the clinician to consciously and autonomously overcome difficulties related to clinical photography.

Table 1-2 *Comparison of SLR and compact cameras*

	SLR cameras	Compact cameras
Ease of handling and automatism	++--	++++
Repeatability of the image	++++	----
Ability to substitute lenses	Present	Absent
Perspective distortion	++++ None with suitable lenses	+--- Proportional to magnification ratio
Magnification ratio	++++	+---
Choice of focal point	++++	----
Choice of depth of field	++++	----
Exposure control	++++	++--
Depth-of-field range	++--	++++
Shutter control parameters	++++	+---
Uniformity of lighting	++++ With ring flash	---- Ring flash not available
Dimensions of photodetectors	About 7 μm	About 1.8 μm
Dimension of sensor	++++	----
Quality of images	++++	++--
Shutter-release speed	++++	----
Shutter lag	++++	----

Table of comparison between reflex and compact cameras with respect to clinical requirements. The only relative advantages of the compact camera over the SLR camera are ease of handling and depth of field. However, after brief and appropriate training, the use of the SLR camera becomes easier and more intuitive.

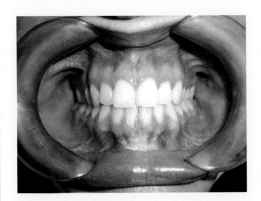

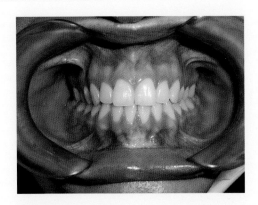

Fig 1-20a
Image taken with a Nikon Coolpix S210 compact camera. Analysis of the photograph shows that, with the macro mode activated to increase the magnification ratio, the closer the operator gets to the subject, the more distorted the perspective becomes. The arch appears deformed; the front teeth are enlarged with respect to the molars, and the arch is overly narrow in the transverse dimension, if compared to the same image taken with an SLR camera. Moreover, the right side of the photograph is lighter because the position of the camera's flash is off-center. The posterior quadrants are also not as well lit as the anterior areas.

Fig 1-20b
Moving away from the subject distorts the perspective slightly less. The lighting appears more even but remains asymmetric from the right to the left and from the anterior to the posterior areas. The operator is forced to use a digital zoom to increase the focal length and thus the magnification ratio, although it remains inadequate.

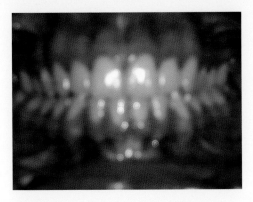

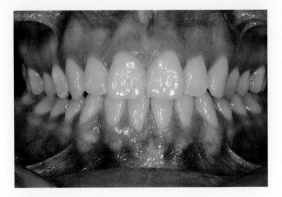

Fig 1-20c
Moving closer to the subject to increase the magnification ratio while maintaining the previous focal length, without using the zoom function, makes focusing impossible. With a compact camera, it is impossible to avoid perspective distortion while maintaining the correct magnification ratio and focus.

Fig 1-20d
The same shot taken with a Nikon D300, Nikkor f = 105 mm macro lens, and a R1C1 flash system (Nikon) with four SB-R200 Speedlights (Nikon). All the faults pointed out in Figs 1-20a to 1-20c have been overcome. The difference between the previous photographs in 4:3 format and this image in 2:3 format is clear.

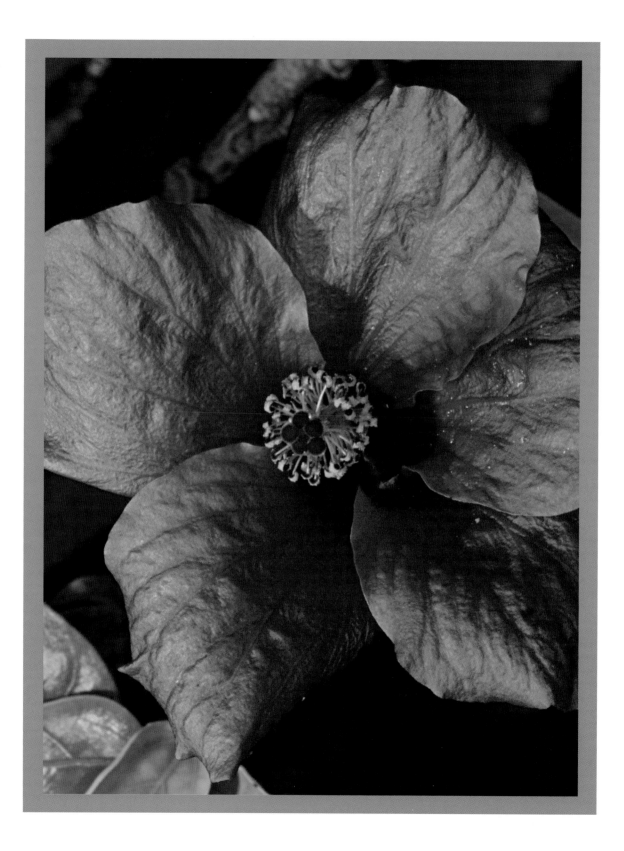

Chapter 2

The Optical System

[
An examination of the general principles of geometric optics gives the operator a basic understanding of the functioning of camera lenses and of the physiology of vision. This knowledge will prove useful when becoming acquainted with the optical phenomena that are directly involved in the practice of dental photography.
]

Principles of Vision

Geometric optics teaches us that certain types of lenses, called *converging* or *positive lenses*, concentrate light rays on a focal point. These light rays are presumed to be parallel to each other as they travel away from the source from which they were generated. This expression, *focal point*, originates from the observation that, because of this principle of convergence, a lens placed in bright sunlight on a summer's day can concentrate light energy to the extent that combustible objects can easily catch fire (from *focus*, Latin, meaning a fireplace or fire) (Fig 2-1).

The focal length of a simple lens is the distance between the center of the lens, called the optical center, and the maximum point of convergence of the light rays, or the focal point (Fig 2-2). The focal point occupies an area and is actually a focal plane.

Because the basic optical and physiologic principles of vision are somewhat analogous to a camera, a discussion of these principles can help in understanding the functioning of the camera. It is important to understand the fundamental phenomenon that **when the distance of an object from the lens varies, the distance between the lens and the focal plane varies reciprocally** (Fig 2-3).

In particular, when the distance between the object and the lens decreases, and the lens moves closer to the object, the distance between the lenses themselves and the focal plane increases. The focal plane therefore tends to move away from the lens and to reassemble itself behind the sensor, whether this be the retina of the eye or the film, resulting in a loss of clarity of the image. The image becomes out of focus. In an optical system consisting of two or more lenses, a *virtual optical center* is created, the result of the interaction of the various lenses. This is similar to the interaction between the lens of the eye and corrective lenses. The movement of the virtual optical center, together with consequent variations in focal length, is the concept behind both the correction of sight defects and the focusing of the camera (Figs 2-4 to 2-8).

In photography, as the camera moves closer to the subject to make it larger, the lenses have a tendency to concentrate the light rays onto a focal plane located behind the sensor plane; therefore, the image that appears on the sensor will not be sharp; it will be out of focus. To focus the image, the optical center of the lenses can be moved away from the sensor plane using the focusing ring, or the object itself can be moved away from the lens. Both methods will result in the aligning of the focal plane and the sensor plane, obtaining an image that is sharp and in focus. The importance of this concept in dental photography will be explained in chapter 7. When attempting to focus perfectly on a detail, this very technique of moving closer to or away from the detail itself will be used so that the focal plane will coincide with the plane of the sensor.

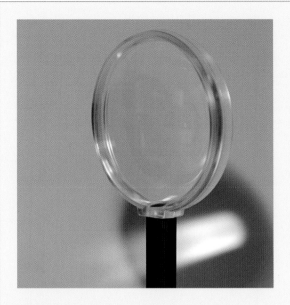

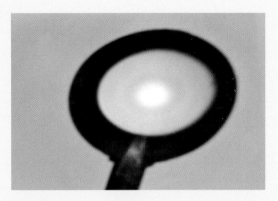

Fig 2-1b
The shadow of the magnifying lens held at a distance from a sheet of paper. At this orientation, the large illuminated area shows that the sun's rays do not reach maximum convergence and are not in focus.

Fig 2-1a
A convergent biconvex magnifying glass.

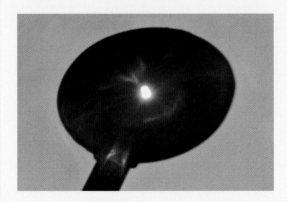

Fig 2-1c
By varying the distance between the lens and the paper, it is possible to focus the sun's rays, so that the rays reach maximum convergence in an area called the focal plane.

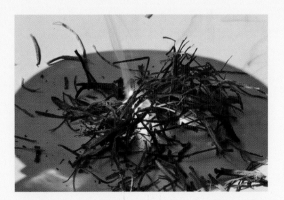

Fig 2-1d
A small amount of dry grass on the focal plane will catch fire within a few seconds because of the energy concentrated by the convergence of the light rays.

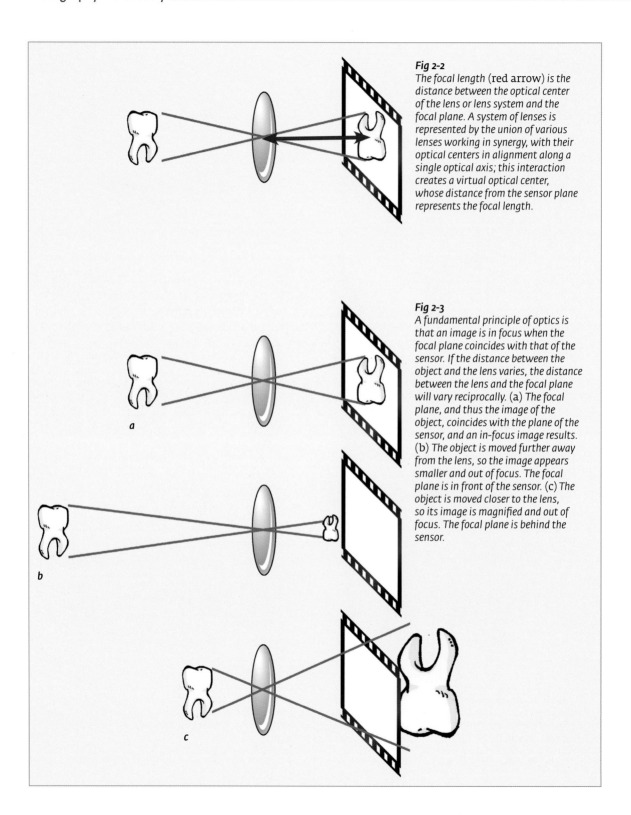

Fig 2-2
The focal length (red arrow) is the distance between the optical center of the lens or lens system and the focal plane. A system of lenses is represented by the union of various lenses working in synergy, with their optical centers in alignment along a single optical axis; this interaction creates a virtual optical center, whose distance from the sensor plane represents the focal length.

Fig 2-3
A fundamental principle of optics is that an image is in focus when the focal plane coincides with that of the sensor. If the distance between the object and the lens varies, the distance between the lens and the focal plane will vary reciprocally. (a) The focal plane, and thus the image of the object, coincides with the plane of the sensor, and an in-focus image results. (b) The object is moved further away from the lens, so the image appears smaller and out of focus. The focal plane is in front of the sensor. (c) The object is moved closer to the lens, so its image is magnified and out of focus. The focal plane is behind the sensor.

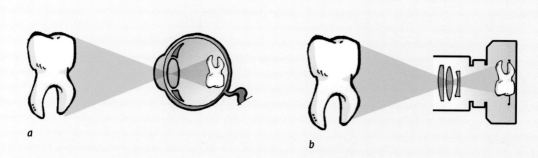

Fig 2-4
(a) In the eye, light rays converge on the retina by means of the lens, bringing objects into focus. (b) The same phenomenon occurs in the camera, in which the lens is artificial and the retina is replaced by film or a digital sensor.

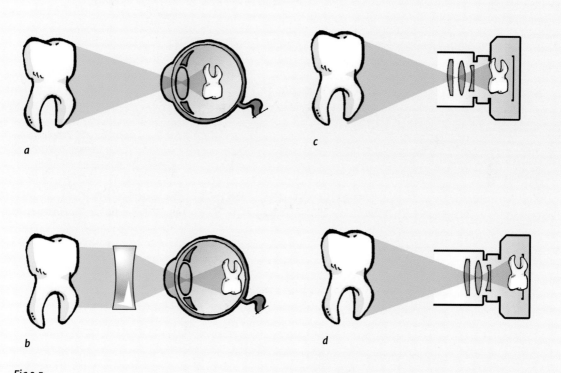

Fig 2-5
(a and b) In the presence of refraction defects such as myopia or nearsightedness, the image forms in front of the retina and will require correction by divergent or negative lenses, which reposition the focal plane further back. The interaction between the lens of the eye and the corrective lens creates a new virtual optical center, which allows the image to be repositioned onto the retina. (c and d) The same phenomenon occurs when cameras frame faraway objects: the image is out of focus because it assembles in front of the sensor. To bring it into focus, it is necessary to adjust the optical center of the lenses by bringing it closer to the sensor.

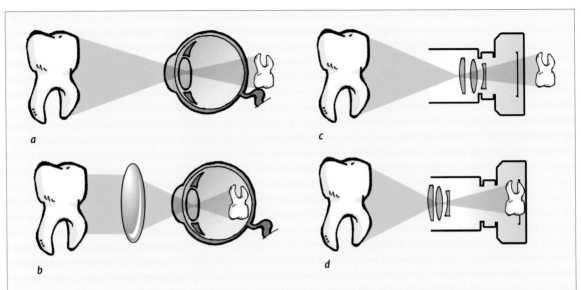

Fig 2-6
(a and b) *In the case of hyperopia or farsightedness, the focal plane is positioned behind the retina, requiring correction with convergent or positive lenses, which bring the focal plane forward onto the retina.* (c and d) *Similarly, when the camera attempts to focus on very close objects, the image appears out of focus because it assembles behind the sensor. To bring it into focus, the lens must be moved further away from the sensor. In macrophotography, if the lens is brought closer to the subject, the image will appear out of focus; to bring the image into focus, the lens must be moved away from the sensor. In both the eye and the camera, it is the optical center that is moved forward, away from the sensor.*

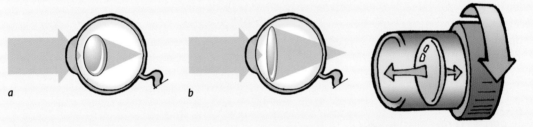

Fig 2-7
(a and b) *Every time we glance quickly from an object in the distance to one nearby, the image is momentarily out of focus because the eye needs time to adjust the curvature of the lens to bring the image into focus onto the retina. This adjustment, called* accommodation, *allows the focal plane to coincide with the retinal plane, creating a sharp image. Presbyopia is a condition in adults in which the lens becomes less flexible, resulting in insufficient accommodation ability. The image that forms behind the retina can only be brought into focus by moving the object away from the lens, which brings the focal plane towards the retina. An alternative is the use of corrective lenses, which interact with the lens to modify the position of the optical center towards the corrective lens, projecting the focal plane correctly onto the retina.*

Fig 2-8
In the camera, the curvature of the lens cannot be adjusted. To focus on a close-up object, the distance between the optical center of the lens and the sensor must be increased by means of the focusing ring, varying the focal length.

[
The focal length is a fundamental parameter of every lens and controls its optical behavior and functional characteristics. The focal length determines the angle of view and magnification factor of the lens. Doubling this length results in a reduction in the angle of view and an increase in magnification of the image by a factor of two.
]

Focal Length

The previous chapter identified the ability to interchange the lenses as the primary advantage of single-lens reflex (SLR) cameras. Camera manufacturers conceived and accomplished production of a camera whose lens could be substituted with other lenses as needed. To fully understand the importance of the focal length of the lens in camera operation, it is essential to analyze the meaning of this concept. The focal length of a lens system has been defined as the distance between the optical center of the system of lenses and the plane of the sensor when the focusing ring is set at infinity. The focal length is conventionally indicated by f = followed by a numeric value expressed in mm.

The optical system of a camera is made up of numerous lenses that work together in synergy to form a central optical apparatus, with the optical center of the various lenses perfectly aligned along a single axis called the *optical axis*. The optical center of the system of lenses is that point along the optical axis at which the optical resultant of the various lenses is concentrated (Fig 2-9). The light ray that travels along the optical axis and passes through the lenses themselves is defined as the central ray. The optical center of the lenses may be virtual, positioned beyond the lens itself. For example, some lenses with f = 300 mm are considerably shorter than their nominal focal length.

When the focus is adjusted, the focal length, or distance between the lens and the sensor, is modified. In some cameras such as disposable cameras, the focal length is fixed and not variable. This means that the focus has been fixed at a position of infinity by the manufacturer.

If the focus is set at infinity using the focusing ring, the camera perceives a range of distances at which the focus is acceptably sharp; this range extends from the minimum focusing distance to infinity. This distance can be increased or decreased by modifying the focal length with the focusing ring.

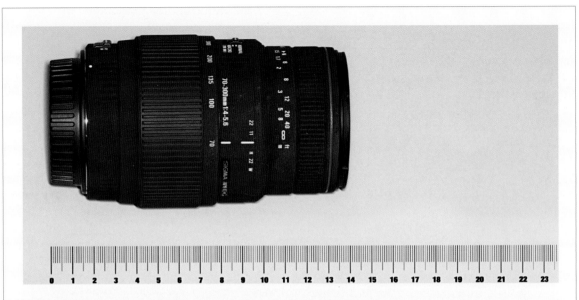

Fig 2-9a
A 70-300–mm zoom lens, set for middle-distance photography with an average magnification ratio. A focal length of 70 mm has been selected, and the focus is set at infinity. The actual total length of the lens is about 140 mm. The optical center lies about halfway along the optical axis of the lens.

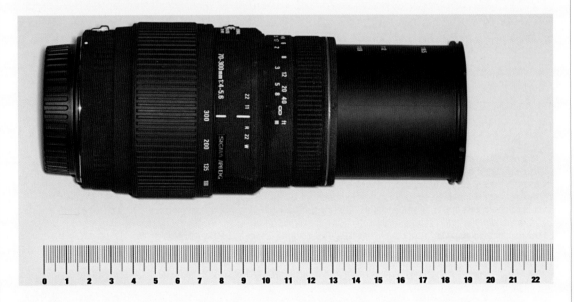

Fig 2-9b
The zoom lens is set for telephoto or long-distance photography, with a high magnification ratio and the subject at a distance. A focal length of 300 mm has been selected, and the focus is set at infinity. The actual total length of the lens is slightly less than 200 mm. The optical center lies beyond and in front of the lens itself.

Angle of View and Magnification Factor

The focal length is the parameter that determines the angle of view, or the area of space, measured in degrees, perceived by the eye or by a specific lens. The natural vision of the human eye is the reference point by which the magnification factor of any optical system is calculated.

By definition, the magnification factor of natural vision is expressed as 1. The object distance is equal to the image distance. When the focal length is doubled, the perceived angle of the field of view is reduced by a factor of two and the magnification is increased by a factor of two; by convention, this magnification factor is written 2×. The × signifies that the magnification factor

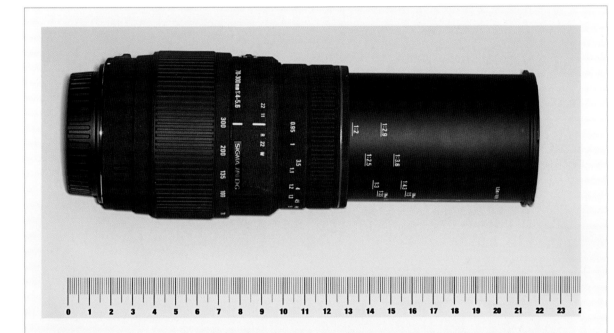

Fig 2-9c
The zoom lens is set for close-up photography with the nominal focal length also set at 300 mm, but with the minimum focusing distance at 95 cm, as visible on the focusing ring. To focus the image, the lens and optical center must be moved away from the sensor, lengthening the lens and the actual focal length. The virtual optical center lies beyond and in front of the lens itself. Zoom lenses are equipped with various focal lengths within a focal range, the two numeric values that indicate the shortest and longest lengths available on that lens. This lens has a focal range of 70 to 300 mm, which can also be indicated as a multiple of the lowest focal length, or 4.3× (300 ÷ 70 = 4.3). The focal range can be nominal, simply referring to the numeric values of the focal length, or actual, reflecting the magnification factors obtained by combining the lens with a particular sensor. The lens in the photo, when combined with a full-frame sensor, has a nominal range of 4.3× but an actual range of 1.4× to 6× (70 ÷ 50 = 1.4; 300 ÷ 50 = 6), in which the image is magnified 6 times with respect to normal vision. A 6× magnification factor, obtained by a 300–mm focal length, corresponds to a 1:2 magnification ratio; the two concepts, although linked, are not identical.

is a multiplicative factor. Each multiple of the focal length corresponds to a multiple of the magnification factor.

If the focal length is multiplied by four, the resulting magnification factor is 4×. Similarly, when the focal length is reduced by half, the magnification factor is 0.5×, creating an image half the size of natural vision. To summarize, reducing the focal length results in an increase in the perceived angle of the field of view and a decrease in the magnification factor. An increase in the focal length results in a decrease in the angle of view and an increase in the magnification factor, or size of the object perceived by the observer (Table 2-1). In this instance, there will be a cropping effect so that a smaller portion of the subject will be included in the photograph, and it will appear magnified (Fig 2-10). The prismatic magnifying system commonly used in clinical practice has a magnification factor of 4.3×, meaning that the practitioner's vision of the scene is magnified 4.3 times with respect to normal vision.

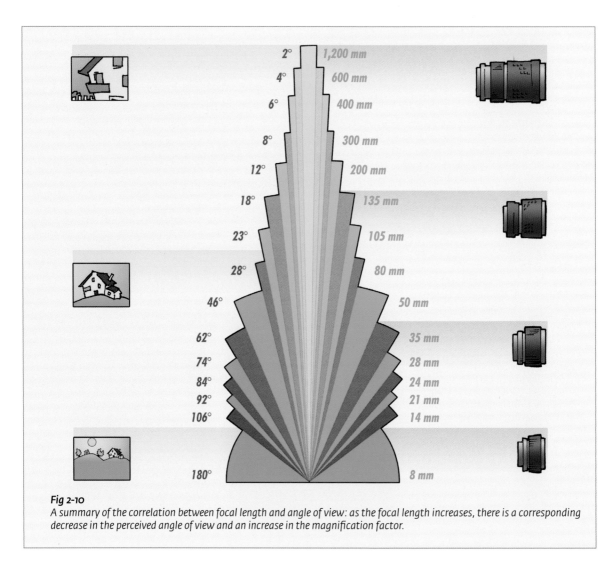

Fig 2-10
A summary of the correlation between focal length and angle of view: as the focal length increases, there is a corresponding decrease in the perceived angle of view and an increase in the magnification factor.

Table 2-1 *Relationship between focal length, angle of view, and magnification factor*

Focal length	Angle of view	Magnification factor
Increases	*Decreases*	*Increases;* *image of object is magnified*
Decreases	*Increases*	*Decreases;* *image of object is reduced*

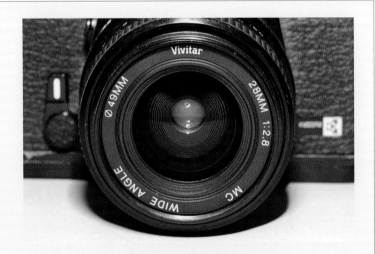

Fig 2-11
The characteristics of a lens are inscribed on the lens itself: 28 mm indicates the focal length; 1:2.8 indicates the lens speed, or maximum aperture; ø 49 mm refers to the diameter of filters or ring accessories that can be attached if required; and the words "wide angle" describe the type of lens. Because the focal length is 28 mm and the lens speed is f/2.8, the maximum aperture is 10 mm (28/10 = 2.8). "MC" indicates that this is a macro lens with a short minimum focusing distance.

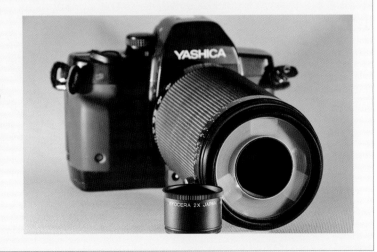

Fig 2-12
The Yashica Dental Eye camera uses a classic 24 × 36–mm film format. Next to the camera is the additional 2× lens required to increase the magnification factor. The additional lens is a focal multiplier. The direct relationship between focal length and magnification ratio is clearly evident.

[
A lens can be referred to as normal or standard when its focal length is equal to the measurement of the diagonal of the sensor onto which the image is projected. In this situation, the angle of view perceived by the lens is similar to that of the human eye and the magnification factor is 1×. Lenses can be classified on the basis of the ratio between their focal length and the size of the diagonal of the sensor.
]

Concept of Normality and Classification of Lenses

Before discussing magnification ratio, which is the fundamental photographic parameter in the field of close-up photography, the most common lenses and their relative focal lengths will be described (Figs 2-11 and 2-12). However, magnification ratio remains the fundamental working and constructive parameter that distinguishes and classifies lenses.

The first lens to be considered as a reference point is the *standard lens* or *normal lens*. It is often assumed that a normal lens has the same angle of view as the human eye; this is true, but only because of a technical point that requires explanation. A normal lens has a focal length that corresponds to the length of the diagonal of the sensor (Fig 2-13). A lens with this characteristic has a very similar angle of view to that of the human eye, so that it neither enlarges nor reduces images with respect to the natural vision of the eye.

Normality of a lens is, therefore, a characteristic that depends on the ratio between the focal length and the diagonal dimension of the sensor and not, intrinsically, on the lens itself. There is no one lens that can be considered, in absolute terms, normal for all film or sensor formats; each sensor format will recognize its own normal lens (Table 2-2). For example, the normal lens for the Nikon DX format sensor (15.6 × 23.6 mm) will have a focal length of 28 mm, which is the approximate value corresponding to the 28.3-mm diagonal length; a lens with f = 50 mm is normal for a 24 × 36–mm sensor format, but this 50-mm

lens is equivalent to a telephoto lens when combined with a DX format sensor. This concept of equivalent focal length is illustrated in chapter 4.

The concept of normality allows lenses to be classified into three categories: standard, wide-angle, and telephoto. If the focal length is decreased with respect to the normal lens, the angle of view is increased, reducing the dimensions of the subject in the frame; a short focal-length lens is referred to as a *wide-angle lens* because it increases the angle of view. If the focal length is increased with respect to the normal lens, the angle of view is decreased and the subject is enlarged, corresponding to an increase in the magnification factor; this lens is classified as a *telephoto lens*, and it allows the details of distant objects to be seen clearly.

A lens with variable focal length is called a zoom lens because the focal length can be rapidly changed (Fig 2-14). A zoom lens is manufactured so that different *focal lengths* are available in a single lens. While versatile, they sometimes result in lower optical quality as compared with lenses with a set focal length. Zoom lenses are characterized by their focal range, the pair of numeric values that indicate the two extremes of focal length available for that particular lens. A 70-300–mm zoom lens has a minimum focal length of 70 mm and a maximum of 300 mm and includes all intermediate focal lengths. The focal range can also be expressed in multiples of the shortest focal length. The nominal focal range of the lens in the above example would be identified as 4.3× (300 ÷ 70 = 4.3). This value is nominal, because it is an intrinsic characteristic of the lens itself and does not take into account

[*If the length of a normal lens is taken as the reference point for a particular sensor, a lens can be defined as wide-angle when its focal length is shorter than that of the normal lens and as telephoto if its focal length is longer than that of the normal lens. Wide-angle lenses tend to make the image smaller, thus diminishing the magnification factor, whereas telephoto lenses have the opposite effect, making the image larger and increasing the magnification factor.*]

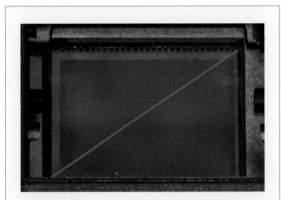

Fig 2-13
The diagonal length of this Canon 14.8 × 22.2–mm CMOS sensor (red line) is slightly less than 28 mm; a normal lens for this sensor will correspond approximately to the same size.

the effect of the sensor format combined with it. For practical purposes, the actual achievable magnification factor is more important than the focal range, so it is useful to calculate the focal range with reference to the specific behavior of the lens-sensor combination. This defines the actual *focal range*, a term that highlights and explains more clearly the concept of the magnification factor linked to the focal length. The 70-300-mm lens (nominal range 4.3×), when combined with a 24 × 36-mm sensor, produces an actual magnification factor from 1.4× to 6× (70 ÷ 50 = 1.4; 300 ÷ 50 = 6). Recall that a lens with f = 50 mm is normal for a 24 × 36–mm sensor. The 70-300-mm lens enlarges the scene framed, with respect to the normal 50-mm lens, by 1.4× to 6×.

Table 2-2 *Relationship between the format of the sensor, its diagonal, and corresponding normal lenses*

Sensor format (mm)	Sensor diagonal (mm)	Normal lens (mm)
15.6 x 23.6	28.3	28
24 x 36	43.26	50
60 x 60	84.85	80
90 x 120	150	150
180 x 240	300	300

An example of normal lenses for different formats: lenses with different focal lengths, when used with a sensor of an appropriate dimension, function normally and have virtually the same angle of view and thus the same image. Notice how a particular lens, which can be wide-angle for one type of sensor, can function as a telephoto lens for a different-sized sensor.

> *The nominal focal range is an intrinsic and set characteristic of a lens with variable focal length; the actual range varies when the lens is combined with a sensor of a particular format. The concept of the actual focal range, linked to the magnification factor, derives from the general principle of the normality of the lenses.*

The same 70-300–mm lens combined with a smaller-format Canon APS-C sensor, whose diagonal length is 26.6 mm, functions like a 110-480–mm lens. It maintains a nominal range of 4.3×, but presents an actual range and magnification factor from 2.6× to 11.3× (70 ÷ 26.6 = 2.6; 300 ÷ 26.6 = 11.3). Therefore, the concept of actual range better expresses the functional characteristics of a lens with variable focal length. Note that the concept of magnification factor linked to the focal length is related to, but different from, the magnification ratio. The magnification factor is a multiplicative factor of the size of the framed scene with respect to normal vision, while the magnification ratio is a very accurate and specific parameter used in close-up photography. The magnification ratio is the result of a numeric division between the dimensions of an image projected and reproduced onto the sensor by the system of lenses and the dimensions of the actual object. The magnification ratio is one of the most important and specific parameters of close-up photography and will be analyzed in depth in the following section.

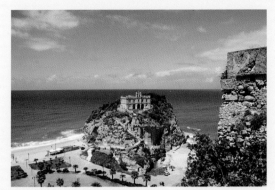

Fig 2-14a f = 30 mm; 0.6× magnification factor.

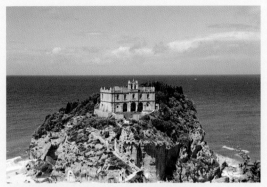

Fig 2-14b f = 50 mm; 1× magnification factor.

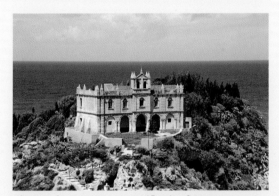

Fig 2-14c f = 100 mm; 2× magnification factor.

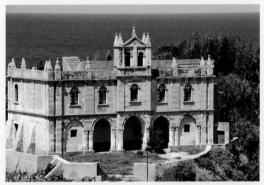

Fig 2-14d f = 200 mm; 4× magnification factor.

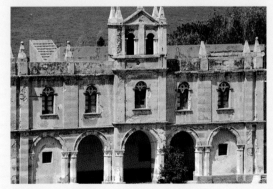

Fig 2-14e f = 350 mm; 7× magnification factor.

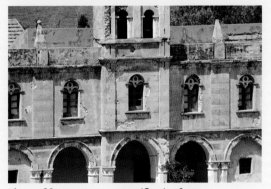

Fig 2-14f f = 450 mm; 9× magnification factor.

Fig 2-14
A series of photographs of the same subject, the Sanctuary of Santa Maria dell'Isola in Tropea, Calabria, Italy, taken with various focal lengths and a full-frame sensor, to show the correlation between the angle of view and the magnification factor.

[
The magnification ratio is a specific parameter of close-up photography that indicates the dimensional representation of the image of the actual object projected onto the sensor. When it increases, the image becomes larger; the opposite occurs when it decreases. The magnification ratio is expressed by means of numeric values on the focusing ring.
]

Meaning and Interpretation of the Magnification Ratio

The magnification ratio is the ratio between the object projected onto the sensor and the actual dimensions of the object itself. It is important to understand that the magnification ratio concerns the dimensional representation of the image of the actual object projected onto the sensor, and the object always maintains its actual dimensions. The virtual dimensions of the object, as processed by the system of lenses, varies, becoming larger or smaller according to the focal length of the lens itself.

If an object is 1 cm tall, and its image as reproduced on the sensor through the lenses is also exactly 1 cm tall, the magnification ratio is 1:1, or life size (Figs 2-15a and 2-15b). If the ratio is 1:2, or half size, the image on the sensor is half as tall as the actual object, or the actual size of the object is twice that of the image projected onto the sensor (Figs 2-15c and 2-15d). If the ratio is 2:1, the image on the sensor is twice as tall as the actual object (Figs 2-15e and 2-15f). A 1:4 ratio indicates that the size of the image on the sensor is one-fourth that of the actual object, and so on. The magnification ratio can also be indicated as 1×, 2×, etc. An increase in the numeric value means that the magnification ratio increases; inversely, fractional values such as ½× and ¼× indicate a reduction of the magnification ratio.

It is important to understand that the magnification ratio and magnification factor can both be indicated by ×. Despite being correlated, these concepts are totally separate.

An increase in the magnification factor always corresponds to an increase in the magnification ratio, but the former refers to the number of times larger the image is perceived with respect to normal vision, and the latter refers to the relationship between the actual size of the object in the frame and its projection onto the sensor. The magnification ratio has great significance in close-up photography. If the ratio increases, the image projected onto the film or digital sensor will appear larger, and vice versa. In practice, if the magnification ratio is increased, the image is enlarged; if the ratio is decreased, the image is reduced. The magnification ratio has an important role in dental photography because it is by means of this ratio that the practitioner is able to create a photograph for documentary purposes.

Documentation with images is the art of bringing to the attention of the observer what one feels is important, or what one wants to show, while excluding everything else that might be a distraction. These distractions, called *visual tension*, are extraneous elements that inhibit the natural and relaxed perception of details. By means of the correct magnification ratio, the operator can exclude everything that creates visual tension and distracts the observer (Fig 2-16). A good photograph can be taken simply by being aware, prior to taking the image, of the comparison between what one would like to see and what one actually does see through the viewfinder.

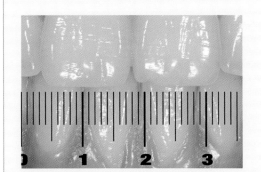

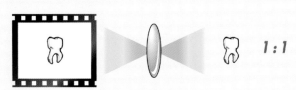

Fig 2-15b *Illustration of the 1:1 ratio.*

Fig 2-15a
A 24 × 36–mm sensor coupled with an f = 100–mm macro lens, photographing in a 1:1 ratio, captures an image with these characteristics: 1 mm on the ruler, or 1 mm of the object, corresponds exactly to 1 mm on the surface of the sensor. This image is referred to as life size.

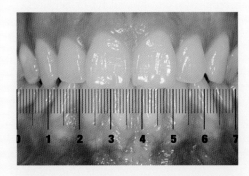

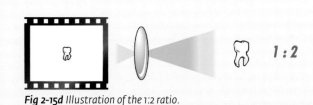

Fig 2-15d *Illustration of the 1:2 ratio.*

Fig 2-15c
The same 24 × 36–mm sensor combined with a 1:2 ratio on the lens captures an image in which 2 mm of the object corresponds exactly to 1 mm on the surface of the sensor. The 36 mm–wide sensor will contain 72 mm of the object.

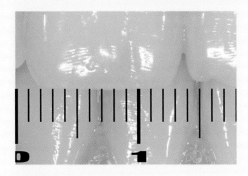

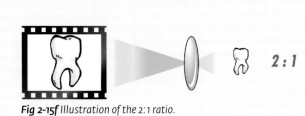

Fig 2-15f *Illustration of the 2:1 ratio.*

Fig 2-15e
Photographing in a 2:1 ratio, each 0.5 mm of the object corresponds exactly to 1 mm on the surface of the sensor, so the 36-mm–wide sensor will contain only 18 mm of the actual object.

[
The magnification ratio is the fundamental instrument in composing the image, eliminating anything that must not be perceived in the framed scene or anything that could interfere with the view of important details. The correct magnification ratio is simply an expression of the will and ability of the operator.
]

It can be said that a photograph is first composed in the mind, by means of analysis and synthesis, which results in visualization of the correct image prior to taking the photograph itself. In light of this idea, a concept must be noted that is so obvious that it may appear banal: the camera is an instrument and, as such, is neutral; it is the operator who, with clear ideas and technical skill, makes the difference. Not to minimize the importance of the quality of the apparatus, which should be excellent, but a device remains simply a device. The true creative strength is the mind; the mind must visualize the image in advance and must be in command of the shutter-release button. The operator's sensitivity, motivation, skill, and experience gives him or her the ability to distinguish that which is important to record and communicate from that which is superfluous or a source of interference. This process of analysis and synthesis, which results in the composition of the correct frame, presumes an excellent knowledge of the subject to be photographed. It is clear that to be able to record visual data and communicate it correctly, the data must be recognized and identified accurately in advance. However, it is not always possible to obtain completely satisfactory results. As in other branches of medicine, there are certain patients who are either not able or not willing to cooperate sufficiently and are therefore not easy subjects to photograph. Moreover, the patient's anatomy is a contributing factor. Particularly wide or long dental arches, insufficient mouth opening, and muscle spasms are all factors that can prevent a good photographic result.

Common terms should be defined to classify the various types of photographs (Table 2-3): the term *telephotography* refers to a magnification ratio from 1:10 to 1:∞ (Fig 2-17); *macrophotography* or close-up photography, from 10:1 to 1:10 (Fig 2-18); and microphotography, from 10:1 to ∞:1 (Fig 2-19).

Table 2-3 *Classification of photography according to the range of the magnification ratios*

Classification	Magnification ratio
Telephotography	From 1:10 to 1:∞
Macrophotography or close-up photography	From 10:1 to 1:10
Microphotography	From 10:1 to ∞:1

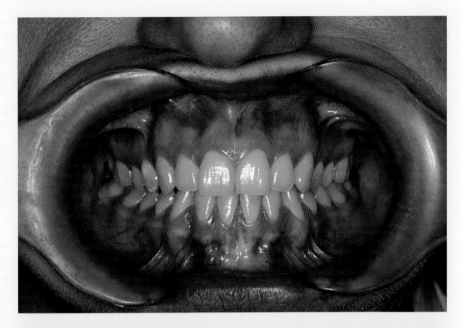

Fig 2-16a
The magnification ratio of this shot appears to be incorrect: the cheek retractors, the nose, and the lips are all elements that cause visual tension and should have been eliminated prior to taking the image.

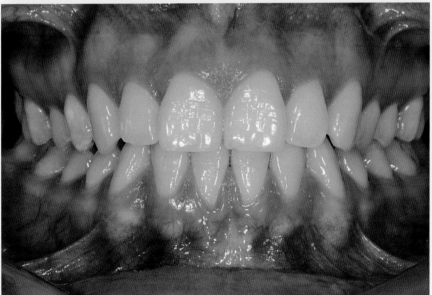

Fig 2-16b
The same image, taken with the correct magnification ratio. The ideal magnification ratio eliminates the sources of visual tension and allows for optimal perception of the patient's dental condition. The magnification ratio of this image is about 1:1.5, within the range defined as macrophotography or close-up photography (10:1 to 1:10).

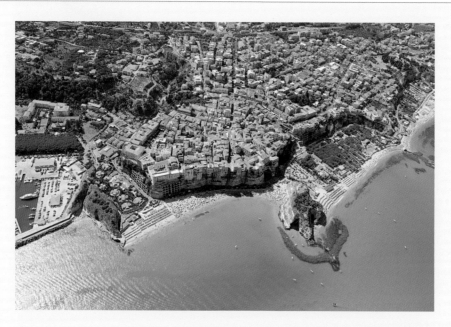

Fig 2-17
This aerial image falls within the definition of telephotography. The magnification ratio of this photograph is 1:∞.

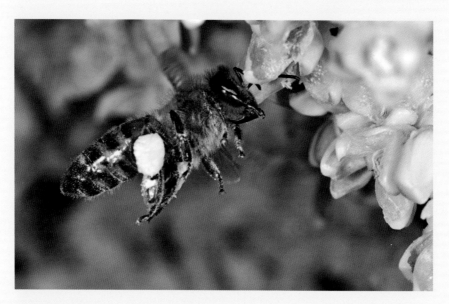

Fig 2-18
This image of a bee is an example of macrophotography.

> *It is absolutely essential that there should be no extraneous elements in the photograph such as saliva, aspirators, cheek retractors, or nonpertinent anatomical parts of the patient or of the operator, such as fingers.*

Elements of Visual Tension

Management of the photographic field includes controlling elements of visual tension, as well as choosing the correct magnification ratio.

The operator must be careful not to include elements such as fingers, mirror edges, cheek retractors, saliva ejectors, teeth of the opposing arch, tongue, lips, or nostrils in the frame (Fig 2-20). Other elements of interference such as halation, residual saliva, or scratches on the surface of the mirror corrupt the image and make all the operator's efforts in vain. Moreover, excessive saliva in the floor of the mouth or residual plaque or food on the surfaces of the teeth are distracting elements, except in initial photos used to document a clinical case. The following practical section explains how to optimize the clinical management and quality of an image.

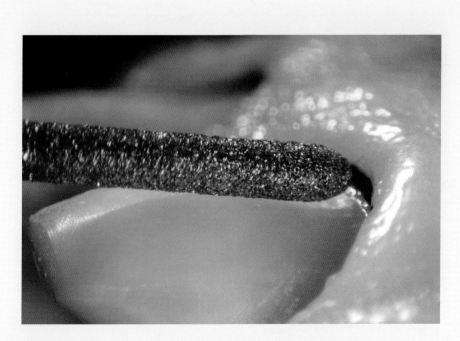

Fig 2-19
A microphotograph with a magnification ratio of about 15:1.

[
Dental photography is a magnification ratio–priority technique, where only what is really useful for documentary purposes is included in the frame. To be able to correctly compose the image, therefore, it is essential to have an excellent knowledge of the subject to be taken: one can only photograph well what one knows well.
]

Golden Questions

The operator must ask and answer two fundamental questions prior to taking the photograph: "Can I see all that interests me in the frame? Can I see anything in the frame that causes visual tension?"

The correct visual tension is born from a dynamic combination of what is framed by the camera and the ideas and intentions of the operator; this leads to the successful capture of an image that is visually pleasing and, most importantly, communicates all the information in a correct and immediate manner (Fig 2-21). The right magnification ratio is the fundamental instrument that controls the composition of the frame and the content of the photo. The understanding of this parameter is the main key to success in dental photography. Dental photography must be a magnification ratio–priority technique.

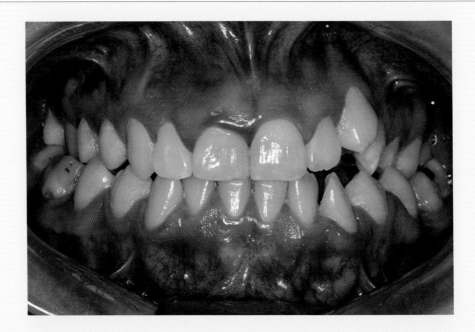

Fig 2-20
To capture the image of this wide mandibular arch, the cheek retractors were included in the frame. Anatomical considerations resulted in a less-than-ideal image.

Dental photography is a magnification ratio–priority technique

As in other types of technology applied to medicine, dental photography requires commonly accepted protocols and rules that give continuity of results and conviction to the operators who use them. The primary rule is the correct use of the magnification ratio. Just as the camera has automatic settings such as shutter priority mode, so must the dentist have an automatic, mental perspective: *photography is a magnification ratio–priority technique.*

It is clear that the correct use of the magnification ratio goes hand in hand with a thorough knowledge and command of the subject to be photographed. The framing of the subject presumes a great familiarity with the details to be shown and communicated by means of the photograph. A logical conclusion from the above rule is that one can only photograph well what one knows well.

Fig 2-21
The perception of the details is fluid and pleasing, without causing visual strain. The natural translucency of the teeth and a defect in the surface of the enamel of the right central incisor can be perceived.

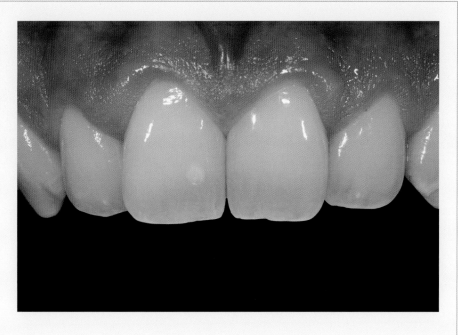

> When the lens is brought very close to the subject, the parts of the subject nearest the lens are magnified, despite correct focusing. This creates perspective distortion, rendering the image not exactly true to life and, thus, not usable for documentary purposes.

Importance of the Distance Between Lens and Subject

All photographers recognize the instinct to bring an object closer to enlarge the image and perceive the details better. This instinct is based on general optical principles concerning the relationship between the lenses, the object, and the focal plane, concepts that have already been discussed in chapter 1.

The distance between the sensor and the object is another decisive factor in varying the magnification ratio, but the potential for errors in perspective sometimes makes this an impractical choice for purposes of scientific documentation.

Perspective Distortion

A problem with normal or wide-angle lenses is that the closer the operator gets to the subject, the more perspective error is created, despite correct focusing. The areas nearest to the lens appear larger than those further away, and the image seems unnaturally distorted (Fig 2-22). Introduction of distortion is exactly contrary to the requirements of documentation, which are to represent reality in a faithful manner.

Normal and wide-angle lenses, which require the operator to get very close to the subject to increase the magnification ratio, should be excluded from the dental photographic armamentarium.

It is therefore necessary to find the right balance between the two factors that control the magnification ratio: focal length and distance from the subject. Hence, it is essential to use lenses with a fairly long focal length, which allow magnification of the image without getting too close to the subject and also avoid perspective distortion.

While it would appear that a lens with a focal length of about 100 mm would be ideal for dental photography, a long focal-length lens has a long minimum focusing distance. The operator is unable to get close to the subject because doing so results in the image being out of focus. The long minimum focusing distance forces the operator to move away from the subject, resulting in an unwanted reduction in the magnification ratio, which is the opposite of the operator's intention. The solution to this problem is macro lenses.

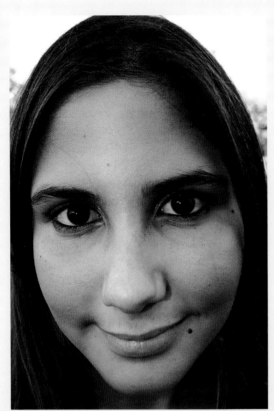

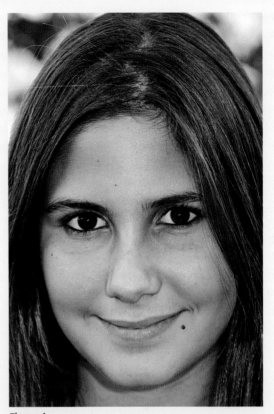

Fig 2-22a
Close-up picture taken with an f = 50–mm macro lens. The appearance of the subject is unnatural because the areas closest to the lens are magnified with respect to those further away, and the photograph appears unnaturally distorted.

Fig 2-22b
The same close-up image taken with an f = 100–mm lens. The magnification ratio is identical but, because of the greater focal length, the image has been taken at a distance, allowing for the correction of perspective errors and faithfully reproducing the model's features.

To avoid perspective distortion, photographers use telephoto lenses with focal lengths of about 100 mm, but these lenses have the disadvantage of a long minimum focusing distance. Macro lenses allow the dentist to reduce the minimum focusing distance to acceptable levels; they are the gold standard for dental macrophotography.

Macro Lenses

Macro lenses have a short minimum focusing distance and a long focal length, so they preserve necessary sharpness of the image (Fig 2-23). They address, at the same time, both factors that determine the magnification ratio, the focal length and the distance from the subject, while maintaining excellent image quality without perspective distortions (see Fig 2-22b). These lenses are more costly than standard lenses.

Other methods of reducing the minimum focusing distance and increasing the magnification ratio exist, such as extension tubes or bellows. These devices are inserted between the body of the camera and the lens to increase the distance between the lens and the sensor, but because they reduce image quality and depth of field, their use is not recommended.

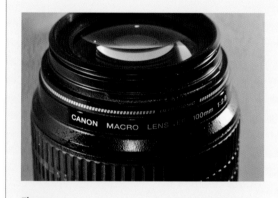

Fig 2-23
Canon f = 100–mm macro lens. Lenses designed to reduce the minimum focusing distance have the word macro *inscribed on them and are generally brighter; this lens has a speed of f/2.8.*

The Gold Standard for Lenses in Dentistry

To summarize, the gold standard for lenses in dental photography is the macro lens with a focal length of 100 mm, which represents the best compromise among the various requirements highlighted. Currently, there are also macro lenses on the market with f = 105 mm. Why exactly 105 mm, and not 90 mm or 120 mm? Lens focal length depends on the preferences of manufacturers, which, for simplification and economy, decide on the standard focal lengths to produce and sell.

> *The various possible magnification ratios and their relative focusing distances are shown on the body of the lens. These reference points allow the operator to take an image at a future date with an identical magnification ratio. The reproducibility of a particular image over time is one of the fundamental prerequisites for scientific documentation.*

Visualization of the Magnification Ratio

To help the photographer and to provide parameters that allow for the reproducibility of an image, the magnification ratio is normally inscribed on the focusing ring of macro lenses. It is important to remember that all lenses refer to a standard sensor, the 24 × 36–mm format. If a different-sized sensor is used, the actual magnification ratio will differ. This situation is linked to the concept of normality of the lens and to equivalent focal length and is fully illustrated in chapter 4.

To become familiar with the macro lens, an in-depth and detailed analysis of its focusing ring is indicated (Fig 2-24). The first figure is a ratio; the number on the left indicates the maximum magnification possible, and the number in the center indicates the relative proportion of the object with respect to the image produced on the sensor. The colon between the two values indicates that this is a mathematical ratio. The two lower figures are the focusing distance in feet and meters corresponding to the magnification ratio selected; this information allows the image to be repeated at a later date using exactly the same magnification conditions. By noting the precise distance from the subject for that particular image, it can be reproduced in a virtually identical manner at any given moment. It is essential to be aware that the reproducibility of an image at a different time or place is one of the essential prerequisites for scientific documentation because it allows for the comparison of homogenous data.

Fig 2-24a
A view of the magnification ratio in a 100-mm macro lens paired with a 24 × 36–mm full-frame sensor. The yellow figure in the top left-hand corner indicates the relative proportion of the image of the object projected onto the sensor; the figure in the top center indicates the actual proportion of the object. In this case, the proportion is 1:1. The two figures underneath indicate the distance, both in feet and in meters, between lens and correctly focused object, relative to this magnification condition. To focus an object correctly and represent it with a 1:1 magnification ratio, the operator must stand at a distance of 31 cm. This value corresponds to the minimum focusing distance.

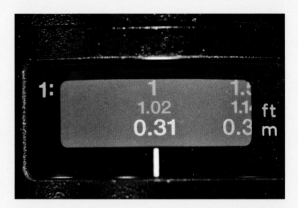

Fig 2-24b
The lens is set at a 1:2 magnification ratio and a focusing distance of 39 cm. Moving only 8 cm away from the object results in a halving of the magnification ratio; the object will be reproduced onto the sensor at half the size of its actual dimensions. This shows how the proximity of the lenses to the object is a fundamental parameter in controlling the magnification ratio.

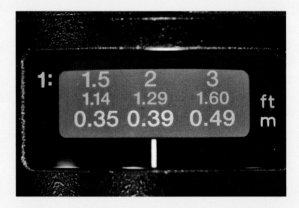

Fig 2-24c
At a distance of about 50 cm, the operator can achieve a magnification ratio of about 1:3. Thus, if the operator moves only 18 cm away from the minimum focusing distance (31 cm), the magnification ratio changes from 1:1 to 1:3.

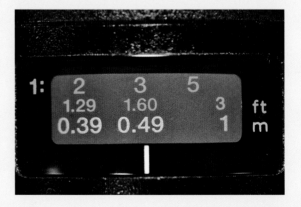

Fig 2-24d
1:6 magnification ratio. As the operator gradually moves away from the object, the magnification ratio decreases rapidly, and the focusing distance, together with the depth of field, increases proportionally.

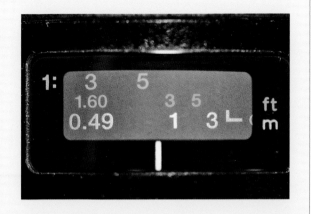

Fig 2-24e
At about 3 m away from the object, up to a focusing distance set at infinity, the magnification ratio range is no longer definable as macrophotography. Because the lens does not have to be moved away from the sensor plane to focus, the focusing ring is set on infinity, and the actual focal length corresponds to the nominal length. The macro function of the lens is no longer used.

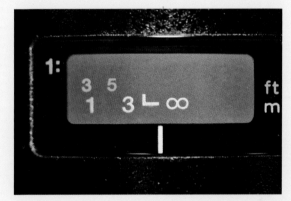

Fig 2-24f
The lenses allow the focusing distance to be blocked to limit the magnification ratio. In this case, the minimum focusing distance is brought to 48 cm, which corresponds to a maximum magnification ratio of 1:3.

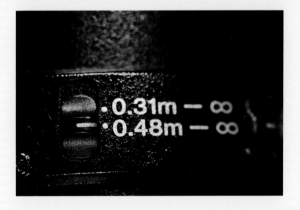

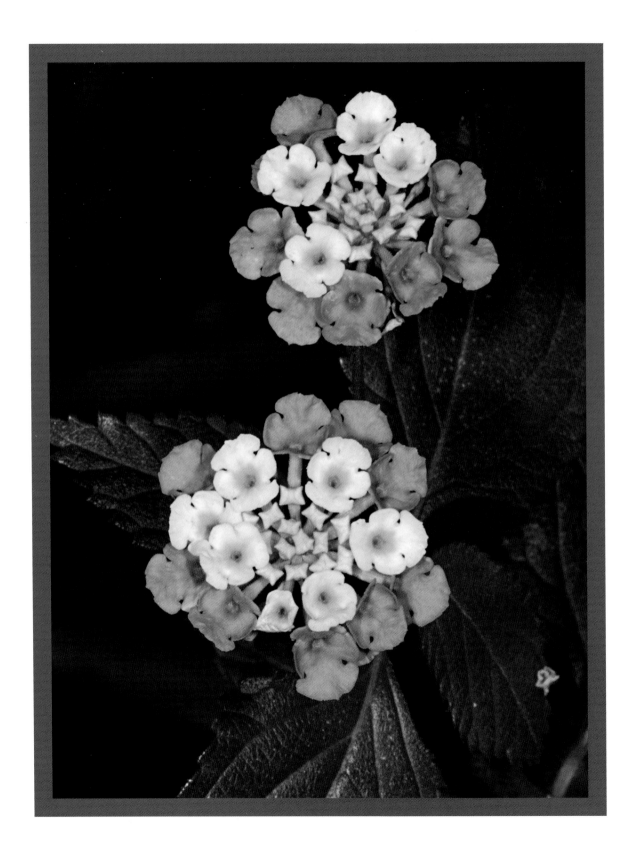

Chapter 3

The Concept
of Exposure

Exposure is the expression of the brightness of an image; in general and artistic photography, it is possible to achieve particular effects by varying the exposure, often by underexposing the subject. In scientific and dental photography, the correct exposure of the image is of highest importance in obtaining the correct reading of the visual document.

Definition of Exposure

Exposure is a basic photographic concept that was introduced during the description of the exposure meter, the instrument that measures the total amount of light reflected in the frame.

Exposure is the product of the intensity of the light passing through the aperture multiplied by the time the shutter remains open. The interaction of shutter speed and aperture determines the total amount of light that strikes the sensor.

Various aperture–shutter speed combinations supply the same amount of light, or exposure, according to the law of reciprocity. Exposure is a calculation of the amount of light present in a photo; in dentistry, a photograph is correctly exposed if the amount of light is suitable for an optimal reading of the image (Fig 3-1a).

The term *overexposure* means that excessive light prevents an optimal reading of the image (Fig 3-1b), and *underexposure* means that the total amount of light is insufficient for an optimal reading (Fig 3-1c).

In the fields of creative and artistic photography, the same parameters are not applicable; for example, underexposure can create pleasing or interesting effects (Fig 3-2). However, for the creation of scientific documents, correct exposure is an indispensable prerequisite to achieving a photograph that is acceptable for documentation purposes.

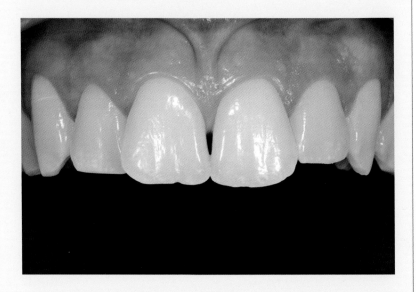

Fig 3-1a
This image has been correctly exposed.

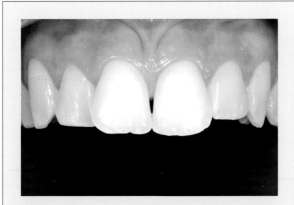

Fig 3-1b
This image has been overexposed.

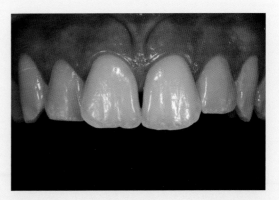

Fig 3-1c
This image has been underexposed.

Fig 3-2
In this photograph of a night landscape during a full moon, the image has been underexposed, but it still conveys emotions and is clearly readable. Image taken with a Canon EOS 20D at f = 50 mm, f/5.6, ISO 800, t = ½ s.

> *The exposure meter is the device that measures the brightness in the frame, allowing the camera to calculate the optimal amount of light needed to achieve a good image with the aperture–shutter speed combination. The through the lens (TTL) meter is a type of built-in exposure meter that assesses the brightness directly through the camera lens.*

Role of the Exposure Meter

The exposure meter is the device that measures the light present in the frame and transmits this information to the camera's processor.

This information is used by the camera's processor to select the most suitable aperture–shutter speed combination for each image. The two types of exposure meters are *reflected-light meters* and *incident-light meters*. Reflected-light meters have the same viewpoint as the observer and measure the *reflectance*, or the amount of light reflected, in the frame.

Incident-light meters are placed directly on the scene to be recorded, and they assess the amount of light that illuminates the scene itself. Reflected-light devices can be either autonomous or built into the camera itself, but incident-light meters are separate from the camera and must be positioned apart from the operator. Modern single-lens reflex (SLR) cameras allow the operator to vary the aperture–shutter speed combination while maintaining the exposure or to override the exposure meter and force the exposure.

Through-the-Lens Reading

Cameras with a built-in exposure meter are used in dental practice. For greater precision, they measure the intensity of the light passing through the camera's own lens to strike the sensor. TTL exposure-meter readings can be affected by various factors, such as strong background illumination, called *backlighting*, which occurs when the light reflected from the main subject is less than the light coming from the background. In this situation, the exposure meter will give an incorrect reading based on the light from the entire scene. When this happens, the main subject of the photograph, which should have been emphasized, will be unpleasingly underexposed.

The exposure meter reading is a fundamental piece of information for the camera's processor. However, to obtain the best results, this reading will often need to be interpreted and integrated by the operator. For this reason, constant practice is recommended so that the operator can effectively evaluate the results of his or her photographic work.

The exposure lock allows the operator to obtain the correct exposure even in the presence of strong differences in the brightness in the frame. However, this situation does not occur very frequently in dental practice. More often, the need arises to vary the area where the brightness is measured, especially in the presence of strong differences caused by the use of contrastors.

Exposure Lock and Measuring Procedures

All cameras have two built-in functions that allow the operator to work around undesirable light readings. The operator can select the frame of the main subject, read the light reflected from it, and then set this reading using the exposure lock function. This reading is maintained even when the frame is widened to include a strongly lit background (Fig 3-3). The second function allows the operator to select the area of the scene where the light measurement is to be taken. He can choose to calculate the average light of the entire scene, or to measure only the light in the center of the scene itself.

This problem typically does not arise in dental photography, because most dental images are taken in a close-up field with the use of a flash, in the total absence of backlighting. However, a procedure in which the average light measurement is weighted towards the center is apropriate for all situations of interest to the dentist. The light reading is calculated on the entire scene in the frame, with a slight preference for the central area, called the *matrix.*

Different cameras of the same model may behave slightly differently and may need small adjustments to correctly expose the image. In particular, the use of contrastors affects the exposure (see chapter 7), and it is useful to be aware of the camera's functions to find the best settings for one's requirements.

These aspects must be examined more closely in an effort to understand how to correct the exposure. A thorough knowledge of the working principles will allow practitioners to explore all the possibilities of photographic equipment. These splendid devices, however, remain inanimate objects, only made valuable by the skill and sensibility of the operator.

Fig 3-3
(a) This image was taken with backlighting and no adjustment.
(b) The same image is taken with exposure lock set on the lower part of the image and then repositioned onto the whole scene. This technical adjustment produces a better exposure of the areas that are not well lit.

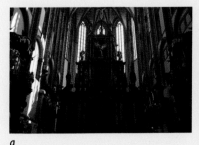

a

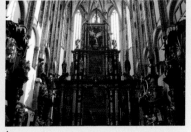

b

[
The exposure meter is calibrated so that it measures the brightness in the frame using, as a benchmark, an average brightness value represented by a gray card with 18% reflectance. This can lead the exposure meter itself into error in the presence of very light or very dark objects. It is, therefore, necessary to control the exposure with appropriate adjustments.
]

Reflectance and the Standard 18% Gray Card

Exposure meter errors may also appear when very light or very dark subjects are photographed because the exposure meter has been designed to estimate the average brightness in the frame and to compare it against a standard scene. The meter tends to adjust all situations of brightness to this set parameter. Built-in exposure meters measure reflectance, the amount of light reflected in the frame. The light that strikes an object can be totally or partially reflected or even be completely absorbed. The reflectance of an object can be expressed as a percentage. A totally white object will have 100% reflectance of the light rays that strike it; a totally black object will have 0% reflectance and absorb all of the light rays without allowing any reflection. Objects that are neither completely white nor completely black have a theoretical reflectance, which varies from 1% to 99% according to the degree of gray present.

Reflectance is a fundamental parameter of esthetic dentistry because it allows us to define the value, or the brightness, of a tooth. Some teeth appear very white because they have a high value or a high reflectance and appear pleasingly luminous; dark teeth have a low reflectance value and appear gray and dull. From a photographic point of view, it has been observed that a degree of gray midway between white and black, recorded on film, does not, as might be expected, have a 50% reflectance; the actual figure is 18%. The gray corresponding to this value is used as a benchmark for the brightness of a photograph.

All exposure meters are calibrated to calculate the brightness of a scene and compare it against the brightness of an 18% gray card, also called *mid-tone gray*. This creates a problem, because the exposure meter tends to force the brightness of a scene to adjust it to this standard degree of reflectance; therefore, when the operator frames a white object with high brightness, the exposure meter will assign it a measurement that tends to make the object itself less bright and will underexpose the image. The opposite occurs when very dark or black objects are framed; the exposure meter will tend to overexpose the image to render it as similar as possible to mid-tone gray (Figs 3-4a to 3-4c). This circumstance means that the operator must correct the exposure when dealing with extremely light objects, such as teeth, or extremely dark objects. In the physiology of vision, this is called *value contrast*.

Exposure-meter readings must be interpreted and, if necessary, integrated. The operator is able to correct the exposure of an image, both at the time of image acquisition using the camera's specific functions and later, at the processing stage.

IN THE PRESENCE OF WHITE OBJECTS, THE CAMERA TENDS TO UNDEREXPOSE; IN THE PRESENCE OF BLACK OBJECTS, THE CAMERA TENDS TO OVEREXPOSE

Exposure Correction

The camera's automatic devices have been designed to simplify procedures to ensure satisfactory image results, and it is undeniable that they enable the taking of excellent photographs with minimum effort in most cases. In particular, automatic settings based on exposure-meter measurements allow the camera to decide the amount of light needed for correct exposure on the basis of parameters chosen by the operator and environmental light conditions. In some situations, the exposure calculated by the built-in exposure meter does not satisfy the operator's requirements or taste. For this reason, the camera allows the exposure to be modified by the operator.

It is possible to override a particular exposure meter reading and to force the camera to overexpose or underexpose the image (Figs 3-4d to 3-4i). The practitioner should not be afraid of exploring and making use of this option, because the clear aim is to write, by means of light, clearly legible documents, free from flaws. Similarly, a document written with faded ink or with ink smudges such as to render it illegible should not be acceptable. The practitioner must become expert in carefully judging the exposure of all photographs taken, so as to make corrections when necessary.

In intraoral images, the whiteness of the teeth results in a high reflectance, which is further enhanced by the shininess of the tooth surface. The exposure meter tends to overestimate the brightness in the frame, and the camera underexposes the photograph. This underexposure implies a greater brightness of the image than actually exists.

The quality of a scientific document must be judged by its degree of correspondence to reality, and correct exposure is an essential prerequisite for dental documentation. For this reason, it is advisable to set an exposure correction on the camera of roughly +⅔ or +1 exposure value (EV), a slight overexposure (Figs 3-4j to 3-4l). A whole exposure value number corresponds to an aperture of one stop higher or lower or to a shutter speed that is halved or doubled.

Exposure may also need to be corrected in the presence of metallic accessories such as rubber dam clamps or base supports for shade guides. These can cause reflections that can deceive the exposure meter, resulting in an extremely underexposed image. Even objects placed onto a black or dark background can deceive the exposure meter, resulting in an overexposed image. This is common when photographing prostheses or orthodontic appliances.

Every camera is fitted with an exposure correction button that allows the operator to achieve excellent results by means of rapid consecutive adjustments (Figs 3-5a to 3-5c). There is a similar button for the flash, giving the operator two methods to correct the exposure (Figs 3-5d and 3-5e). The result of using either button is the same, because they both affect the duration of the flash as determined by the camera–exposure meter synergy.

The exposure can be corrected after recording the image by means of special programs at the processing or postproduction stage. However, a photograph should be excellent at the stage of image acquisition; it is unacceptable to manipulate an image to make it appear suitable for a particular purpose, even if software allows it. The basic aim is to faithfully document reality, not to manipulate it to make it appear better than it is. It is neither ethical nor scientifically correct to manipulate images beyond slight corrections of exposure, contrast, or color; minor modifications, such as slight cropping or rotating of the image, are admissible to correct the magnification ratio or the orientation of the image.

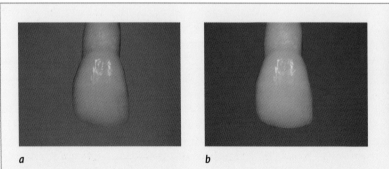 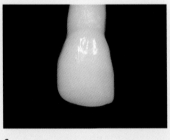

a   b   c

Figs 3-4a to 3-4c
A tooth is photographed against three different backgrounds, with no exposure correction. The tooth against the white background appears less bright, while the white background itself looks gray. Against the black background, the tooth appears much whiter and more luminous than in the other images, and it appears more natural in its brightness against the gray background. The exposure meter has interpreted the white background as standard gray, and the camera has greatly underexposed the image. The opposite has occurred against the black background, resulting in overexposure. The different brightness or value of the tooth is the primary parameter perceived by the human eye, much more so than the difference in color of the tooth. This is a fundamental concept in esthetic restorations. This series of photos effectively demonstrates the physiologic phenomenon of simultaneous value contrast.

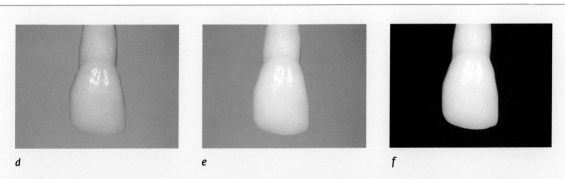

d   e   f

Figs 3-4d to 3-4f
The series of three photographs is repeated with an exposure correction of +1 exposure value (EV). Against the white background, the tooth is represented more realistically, but against the black background, overexposure has created a decidedly poorer-quality image.

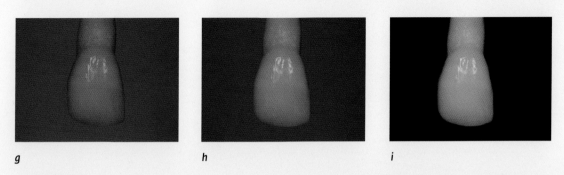

g   h   i

Figs 3-4g to 3-4i
The series of three photographs is repeated with an exposure correction of -1 EV. Against the white background, the image of the tooth is poorly lit, but the image is much better exposed against the black background. Different exposure settings result in considerable variation in the perception of the brightness of the tooth. A simple photograph is not a reliable method to transmit information related to the brightness of the tooth. To convey the value of the tooth more effectively, it should be photographed with appropriate exposure corrections alongside an object of known brightness to which it can be compared, such as a shade guide.

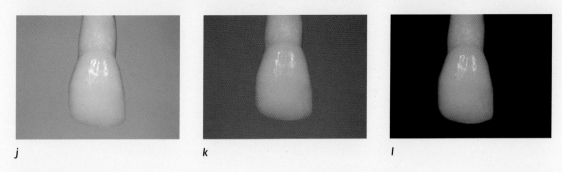

j   k   l

Figs 3-4j to 3-4l
This series of photographs shows the influence of background brightness on the exposure. To convey the correct brightness of the tooth itself against different backgrounds, the following corrections were made: +1 EV against the white background, -1 EV against the black, and no change in EV against the mid-tone gray. The perceived differences in brightness depend on the physiologic phenomenon of value contrast.

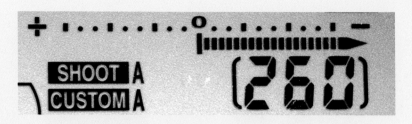

Fig 3-5a
The exposure scale of a Nikon D300 is in gradations of ⅓ EV. The reading indicates an underexposure equivalent to 3 EV, corresponding to three aperture or shutter-speed stops. This scale only provides information about the brightness in the frame. The number underneath the exposure scale indicates the number of shots remaining.

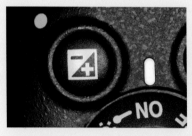

Fig 3-5b
The exposure of this Nikon D300 can be modified by manually setting it higher or lower with this button.

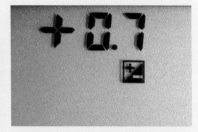

Fig 3-5c
An overexposure of about + ⅔ EV has been selected to obtain the correct exposure of a light subject such as a dental arch. The exposure meter will supply its own measurements, but the camera's processor will assume control to achieve a slight overexposure. The symbol at the bottom of the display shows that a correction to the exposure has been activated.

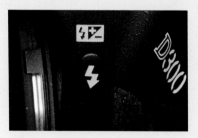

Fig 3-5d
The flash exposure of the Nikon D300 can be modified with this button.

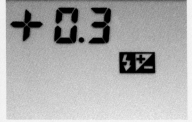

Fig 3-5e
The correction to the flash exposure is shown on the display. The symbol at the bottom of the display shows that this correction has been activated.

[
Just as background conditions may affect the accurate perception of the brightness and color of an object by the exposure meter, so also can surrounding conditions affect human vision. These phenomena are called contrast effects, *and they can be simultaneous or successive and affect perception of the value, hue, or chroma.*
]

Physiology of Vision: Contrast Effects

The working logic of the exposure meter, which tends to standardize the brightness level in the frame, is very similar to that of the combined eye-brain system. The cerebral cortex tends to process and harmonize visual perceptions, often resulting in phenomena that are defined as *optical illusions*. Other phenomena are connected to the functional breakdown of the retinal photoreceptors. When the retina is stimulated for a prolonged period of time, rhodopsin in the receptors for the perception of a particular color is temporarily depleted. This leads to sensitization of the inactive cones, a process that is the basis of the physiologic phenomenon known as *contrast*.

Contrast can be simultaneous or successive and can relate to *value* (brightness), *hue* (color), or *chroma* (degree of saturation). Successive contrast effects can be positive, by analogy, or negative, by contrast. These phenomena are caused by the physiology of the visual receptors and subsequent cortical processing.

Moreover, they are related to the composition of the hue. The effect of combined hues differs in the presence of an *additive synthesis,* as in the case of colored lights, or a *subtractive synthesis*, as in colored pigments.

Simultaneous *value contrast* causes a tooth to be perceived as whiter if observed on a dark background and vice versa, similar to the exposure errors of the camera (see Fig 3-4). Simultaneous *hue contrast* affects the perception of a particular nuance of hue in an object in the presence of a background of a complementary shade. Every color recognizes its own particular complement; red is complementary to green, blue to orange, yellow to purple. A characteristic of complementary colors is that they become gray when mixed. Simultaneous hue contrast is very important in discriminating tooth shades. For example, in the presence of bright red lipstick, a greenish nuance will be perceived in the color of the teeth; if the furniture in a photography studio is bright navy blue, the teeth will appear to have an orange hue (Figs 3-6a to 3-6f).

[

Chroma contrast affects the perception of brightness of an object when placed on two different backgrounds of the same hue with different saturations such as light pink and bright red. Value contrast affects the perception of the brightness of an object placed on two backgrounds of differing brightness such as white and black.

]

Chroma contrast affects the perception of color intensity, so the same object against two backgrounds of the same color but different saturation will appear less chromatic on the more intense background and vice versa (Figs 3-6g and 3-6h). For example, in the presence of very inflamed gingiva, a red of high chroma, the teeth will appear less chromatic and therefore whiter. Successive chroma contrast occurs after observing a very chromatic object. The effect will be positive after a brief viewing of the object; after looking away from the object, new objects will be perceived as the same color as the previous one, because of sensitization of the specific photoreceptors for that hue. Successive chroma contrast will be negative after long observation of an object of a particular hue; objects viewed immediately afterwards will be perceived in the color complementary to the previous one, because photoreceptors for the original color have been desensitized.

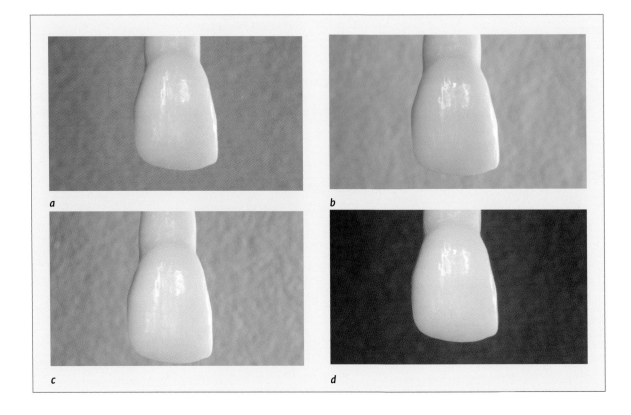

a

b

c

d

Hue contrast is the perception of different hues when viewing the same object placed on two backgrounds of a complementary hue such as red and green. This phenomenon is very important in dentistry because it alters the correct perception of hues and can therefore interfere with the acquisition of data relating to colors for the creation of esthetic restorations.

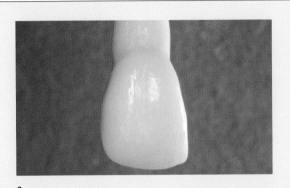

e

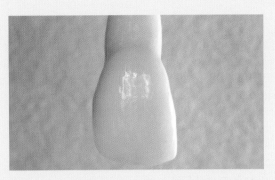

f

Fig 3-6a to 3-6f
This series of photographs shows the phenomenon of simultaneous hue contrast. The same tooth placed side by side onto two backgrounds of complementary hue will be perceived with nuances of the color complementary to the background. Orange is complementary to blue, green to red, and violet to yellow.

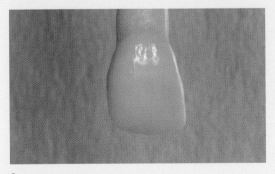

g

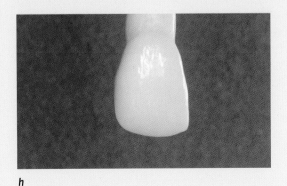

h

Fig 3-6g and 3-6h
Chroma contrast causes the same object, photographed with identical camera settings, to appear less chromatic on a more intense background and vice versa.

The International Standards Organization (ISO) speed is the parameter that measures the sensitivity of the device to be exposed. The higher the ISO value, the less the amount of light needed to obtain correct exposure. Because high ISO values result in less sharpness, altering the image, low ISO values are necessary in the presence of a flash. If the use of a flash is not possible, high ISO values may be chosen.

ISO Speed

The ISO system was established to unify two standardization scales, the American Standards Association (ASA) and the Deutsches Institut für Normung (DIN). The ISO scale defines the degree of sensitivity of a sensor to light. *Sensitivity* is defined by the speed at which the sensor is exposed: the faster the sensor, the less the amount of light needed to obtain correct exposure. An ISO speed of 100 represents average sensitivity. Each successively larger number on the scale, 200, 400, 800, etc, indicates a doubling of the sensitivity of the previous number. Successively smaller values, 50, 25, etc, indicate a halving of the sensitivity of the previous number.

This is true for both films and digital sensors. For film, the sensitivity or ISO speed is chosen by the manufacturer during the production process, and the composition of the sensitive emulsion cannot be modified. The sensitivity of a digital sensor can be rapidly adjusted because the camera's software can modify the amplification of electrical signals from the sensor itself. An ISO 100–speed sensor, standard sensitivity, needs a particular amount of light to achieve optimal exposure. If the ISO setting is changed to 200, the same exposure can be achieved with half the amount of light,

as if the value of the aperture were increased by one stop or the shutter time was doubled. A negative aspect of an increase in sensitivity, common to both kinds of sensors, is its effect on the graininess of the image. Faster films require the use of larger silver halide grains that modify more rapidly when struck by light, with the end result being a loss of image detail and an appearance of graininess upon image enlargement.

Increasing the ISO speed of the digital sensor requires amplification of the electrical signals coming from the sensor, causing artifacts called *background electronic noise* that resemble film graininess (Fig 3-7). Electronic signal amplification and fluctuation cause a variation in brightness among the pixels that is not present on the object itself.

Increasing the ISO speed is not ideal in optimal light conditions or in the presence of a flash, but it is an indispensible option when a lack of light risks serious underexposure of the photograph or a blurred image because of an excessively long shutter time in combination with a rapidly moving subject. Moreover, increasing the ISO speed is useful when photographing radiographs on illuminated view boxes.

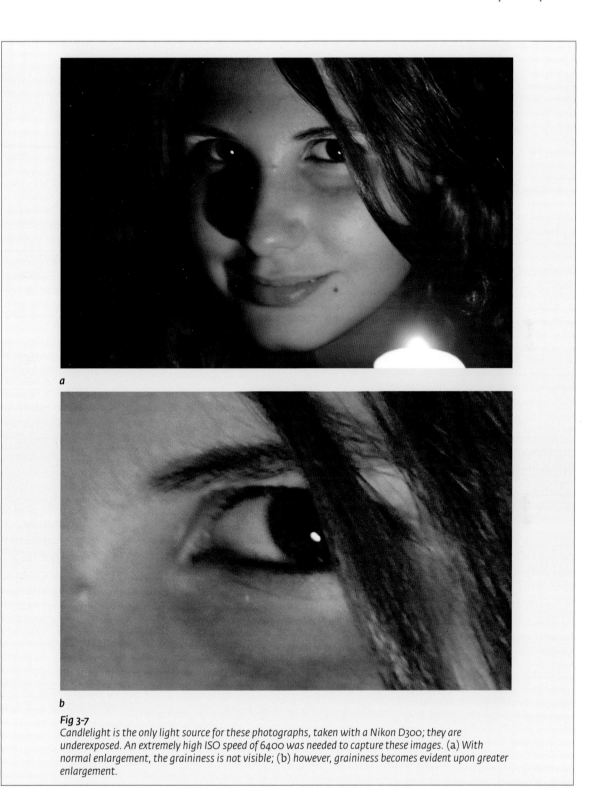

a

b

Fig 3-7
Candlelight is the only light source for these photographs, taken with a Nikon D300; they are underexposed. An extremely high ISO speed of 6400 was needed to capture these images. (a) With normal enlargement, the graininess is not visible; (b) however, graininess becomes evident upon greater enlargement.

[
White light is the sum of electromagnetic waves of different lengths, each of which has its own chromatic characteristic. The prevalence of a particular wavelength is shown by the chromatic quality of the light perceived, also called color temperature. *Orange-red long waves correspond to low temperatures, and violet-blue short waves correspond to high temperatures.*
]

Perception of Color and Color Temperature

A general principle of optics is that perceived light is the synthesis of electromagnetic waves of different lengths, which manifest themselves in a particular color. The human eye perceives light waves 480 to 760 nm in length; the interval between these two values is known as the *visible light spectrum*. In nature, this is represented by the rainbow, which is the result of the refraction of white light into the spectrum of electromagnetic waves that compose it, through minute drops of water suspended in the atmosphere (Fig 3-8).

Each wavelength of visible light corresponds to a color. Long wavelengths are seen as orange or red and short ones as violet or blue. Color vision is based on the perception of wavelengths reflected by an object after the object has been struck by light (Fig 3-9). Color is not, therefore, a property of matter, but is instead linked to the behavior of light in relation to an object with peculiar intrinsic characteristics such as opacity, transparency, and translucency, and extrinsic or surface characteristics (see chapter 7).

The intrinsic properties of the object can determine total reflection of light, regardless of wavelength, making the object appear completely white. The total absorption of light will make an object appear completely black. The reflectance or degree of reflection of an incident light ray can be measured quantitatively and, importantly, qualitatively. Partial and selective reflection of specific wavelengths from the object gives rise to the physiologic phenomenon of color perception. The extrinsic or surface characteristics are important with regard to the angle of reflection of light, which can be mirrorlike, called *specular* or *diffuse*. Diffuse reflection of light reduces the degree of translucency because it increases the degree of reflectance (Fig 3-10). The effect of surface characteristics on the reflectance of an object has a great impact on the perception of light and color; dental laboratory technicians, who put much care and effort into creating the ideal surface texture for restorations, know this only too well.

Light sources can emit a spectrum of waves in which some wavelengths are more prevalent than others; these wavelengths are called *dominant*. For example, the common incandescent light bulb primarily emits waves in the orange-red part of the spectrum, and xenon light sources primarily emit blue waves.

[
The phenomenon of color is the expression of a specific wave reflected off an object. A white object reflects all the waves of various lengths, and a black object absorbs them completely; a colored object reflects the specific wavelength that is perceived by the observer as color, resulting in a phenomenon of selective reflection of the light rays.
]

Fig 3-8
A double rainbow shows the natural refraction of light into its individual light-wave components. Image taken with a Canon EOS 300D at f = 40 mm, f/10, ISO 200, t = 1/250 s.

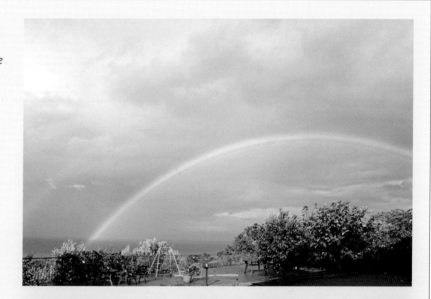

Fig 3-9
A typical, brightly colored sweets stall in the ancient market of Boqueria in Barcelona, Spain.

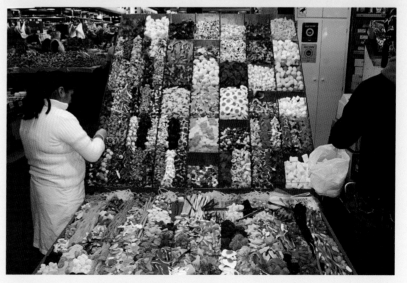

For constructive reasons, every artificial source of light has its own particular color temperature. In natural light, depending on the time of day or atmospheric conditions, one specific type of light wave corresponding to a characteristic color temperature will be prevalent and will appear in the photograph as dominant.

Color temperature is a way to characterize various light sources. This numeric value, expressed in degrees kelvin (°K), after the physicist who developed the absolute temperature scale, is the temperature at which a black object must be heated to become incandescent and radiate light of the same hue as the light source. The higher the color temperature, the more prevalent the blue-violet short waves; the lower the color temperature, the more prevalent the red-orange long waves.

All light sources have their own color temperature based on the spectral composition of the light emitted from that source. The light from an ordinary candle has a color temperature of about 1,500°K, and a common tungsten light bulb emits light at about 3,000°K. Daylight at midday on a partially cloudy day has a color temperature of about 5,500°K to 6,000°K; its components are balanced, and lighting engineers describe it as natural light.

The composition of light is extremely important in photography because a particularly prevalent wavelength in light can appear as a dominant in a photograph. This effect is not always negative or undesirable; a photograph of a beautiful sunset will show a pleasing, warm orange dominant, which will render the photograph particularly evocative (Fig 3-11).

A photograph taken in full daylight, with a clear sky, will have a very high color temperature, with a prevalence of azure waves, and is described as cold light (Fig 3-12).

It is clear that the term *color temperature* does not refer to the intrinsic heat of the object that reflects it; it is the temperature to which a black object must be heated to emit the same hue of light as the light source.

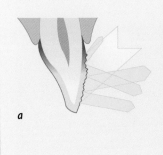
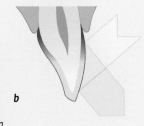

Fig 3-10
(a) *The diffuse reflection of light results from the morphologic characteristics of the tooth surface. The characteristics of the tooth surface can be divided into horizontal (microtexture created by the striae of Retzius) and vertical (macrotexture created by lobes and development grooves) aspects. The texture of the surface, with its microscopic concavities and convexities, causes an irregular reflection of light, which greatly contributes to the perception of a natural tooth. This diffuse reflection increases the degree of reflectance of the surface and thus diminishes the translucency of the tooth. (b) Progressive loss of surface texture results in specular reflection of light, which reduces the natural and youthful appearance of the teeth and also contributes to the lowering of their value.*

a

b

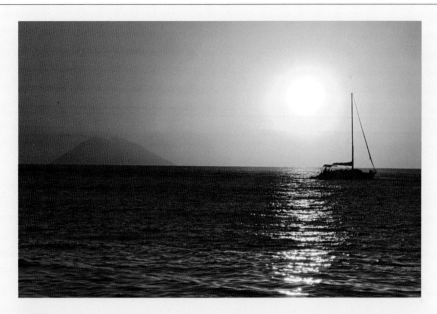

Fig 3-11
The volcano of Stromboli is seen at sunset from a beach in Tropea; the orange dominant is present because of the prevalence of red-orange long waves. Image taken with a Canon EOS 20D, f = 120 mm, f/22, ISO 400, t = 1/500 s, manual exposure mode.

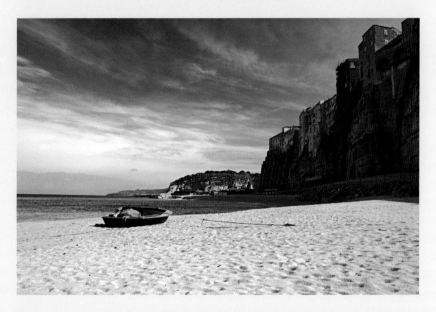

Fig 3-12
An image taken in the morning shows a prevalence of azure short waves. Image taken with a Canon EOS 300D, f = 35 mm, f/8, ISO 100, t = 1/200 s. To enhance color saturation and to eliminate reflections, a polarizing filter has been used.

[*White balance is the function on cameras that allows us to correct the color temperature present in the frame, or to select the quality as required.*]

White Balance

Reflected light perceived by the human eye and by the camera has a certain color temperature. The human eye is always able to perceive white as white, even in different color-temperature conditions. Because of the interaction between the eye and information provided by experience and memory, humans are able to contextualize color data.

The digital sensor has difficulty discriminating the correct white in the presence of a particular color temperature, and this difficulty is manifested by the appearance of undesired chromatic dominants. To avoid or lessen the appearance of undesired dominants, part of the sensor's photosensitive elements are entirely devoted to the correct calculation of the color temperature, and thus to the color white. Alternatively, a separate sensor can be added, dedicated exclusively to this function. In addition to these manufactured devices, the software of the camera can be set to correct the dominants using the *white balance* command. Predefined options can be set for the most frequent color-temperature situations. For example, in the presence of an incandescent light, fluorescent light, or flashbulb light, the camera can be set to adequately compensate for the color temperature in advance. Another camera option called *auto white balance* analyzes the color temperature and automatically corrects the dominants. This is the option that generally meets most photographers' requirements. In the camera's menu (Fig 3-13), various situations are listed: bright sun, cloudy sky, or shade, and incandescent, neon, or flash lighting. It is also possible to select the color temperature within a range from about 3,000°K to 10,000°K for greater accuracy or to insert particular dominants.

A fourth option is to set the camera at a particular type of white, chosen by the operator as a benchmark.

Moreover, correction of the chromatic dominants can be performed after recording the image, with image-processing programs (Fig 3-14). However, only unprocessed raw image formats have medicolegal value, so any subsequent processing in a different format will have no value from a legal-documentation point of view. This problem is avoided by keeping an original raw image file and only processing copies of the image.

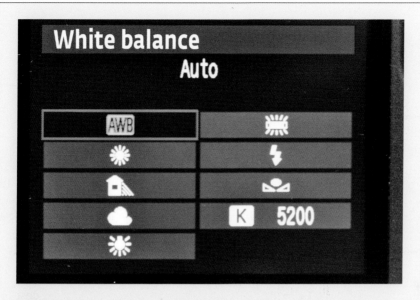

Fig 3-13
The white balance menu of a Canon 40D camera shows that the auto white balance function has been selected. Other options on the menu are bright sun, long shadows, cloudy sky, artificial light, fluorescent light, flash, customized white-balance settings, and color temperature.

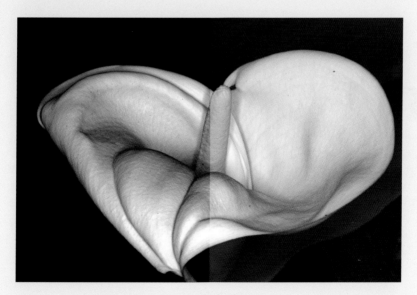

Fig 3-14
This image of a white flower illustrates the concept of exposure meter correction. The right half of the photograph has been corrected by a photograph-retouching program to show the natural brightness of the flower; the left half shows the original image as captured with the exposure-meter settings.

[
The photograph is a precious instrument for understanding and communicating surface characteristics and translucency, parameters of dental anatomy that contribute to determining the color of teeth. Color can only be determined precisely and repeatedly with appropriate spectrophotometers for clinical use. These two techniques may eventually be integrated so that we are able to obtain optimal results in the communication of color.
]

Photography for the Communication of Color

The phenomenon of color, regardless of the observer's emotional experience and contrast effects, is the result of a complex interaction between numerous parameters, which those who perform esthetic dentistry know only too well. It is a difficult subject and requires an in-depth approach. Color is not to be chosen or taken, nor can it be transmitted by means of simple numeric formulas. It requires a precise diagnostic and strictly scientific path to be determined with accuracy.

To make a correct diagnosis of color, the operator must be aware of all parameters that contribute to its definition. The most important are hue, chroma, and value (the three dimensions of color according to Munsell) and pigmentation (the fourth dimension according to Muia). Equally important are the intrinsic optical properties of the object, opacity and translucency, and the extrinsic optical properties of the tooth surface, such as texture and microscopic concavities and convexities. The operator must understand that some parameters can be measured and documented in a rigorously objective manner, and some can only be represented and documented photographically in a more or less effective and subjective way. Because of the problems related to exposure variables and the functioning of the camera itself, it is impossible to measure and document the hue, chroma, and value of a tooth with absolute objectivity with the camera; this can only be achieved with a certain degree of approximation.

The camera is not a measuring device, because it only creates a representation of reality; the process of acquiring the image is influenced by numerous parameters that are not entirely controllable, including the amount and quality of the lighting, the shooting angle, and general and intrinsic manufacturing characteristics of all types of cameras. Opacity and translucency can be effectively documented, mainly by using contrastors, as can the optical properties connected with surface characteristics (Fig 3-15). The difficulty in perceiving the three main dimensions of color can be partly overcome by the use of contextual benchmarks with a known hue, chroma, and degree of value. By comparing the characteristics of the chroma of the teeth on the photographic image itself with the sample benchmark represented, for example, by an element on the shade guide, the correct hue and brightness can be determined with some accuracy.

The spectrophotometer is the most scientific and accurate method to determine and document the main color dimensions. This device measures the specific length of the visible electromagnetic waves. Portable polarized-light spectrophotometers, specially designed and particularly suitable for dentistry, already exist on the market. These devices allow for effective registration and communication of data concerning color to the laboratory. However, all data should be supported by good photographic images.

Photographs complete the color diagnosis by recording characteristics of the surface and structure of teeth, general facial features, and oral cavity tissues, giving the dentist detailed information about the overall context of the patient. Photographs capture nuances, details, emotions, and impressions relating to a particular clinical situation and patient, which no other device, however sophisticated, can. In conclusion, the two devices, the spectrophotometer and the camera, should be complementary in achieving excellence in esthetic dentistry; while technology is a fundamental aid, the sensitivity, taste, and experience of the operator must be considered of primary importance.

Fig 3-15
Surface texture is very important in the perception of color. The complexity of the surface of these natural teeth greatly contributes to the perception of the beauty and harmony of the teeth themselves. This image highlights how studying a photograph allows the practitioner to arrive at a diagnosis and to understand the patient's actual dental situation; study of photographs also improves the practitioner's powers of discernment of an image's most minute details. The surface texture determines the type of light-wave reflection from the tooth's surface. When the tooth surface has a flat and regular nature, the light rays are reflected from the surface in a parallel fashion, resulting in specular reflection. If the light rays are reflected in a disorderly way because of the surface's irregularities or complexities, an observer will perceive a diffused reflection and less translucency of the tooth. A pronounced surface texture, typical of young teeth, is gradually lost over time or as a result of aggressive brushing.

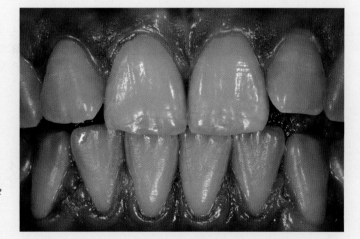

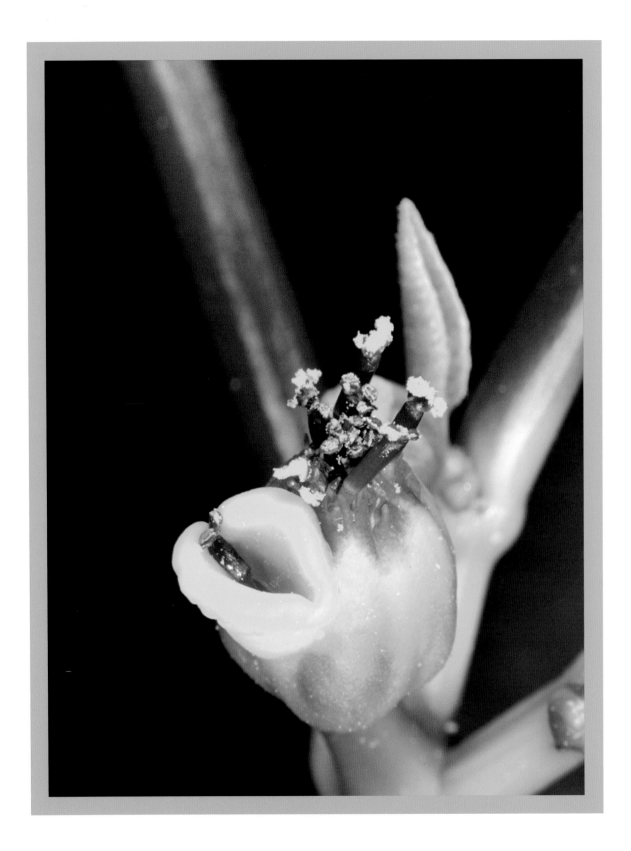

Chapter 4

Principles of
Digital Photography

While the fundamental principles of photography do not vary whether analog or digital equipment is used, only digital technology allows the operator to view and quickly manage the image in a versatile manner. It allows for rapid correction of any errors and thus helps the operator to improve his or her personal technique. Digital technology also enables the storage of large quantities of visual documents.

The difference between analog and digital photography lies in the characteristics of the sensor, the device that is struck by the light. In analog photography, the sensor is the film, but in digital photography, an electronic device replaces the film and can be thought of as an "electronic film." This basic difference is separate from and does not preclude the general principles of photography, such as composition of the frame, lighting, and the use of lenses.

The ease and versatility with which a digital image can be used, however, represents a significant departure from film-based photography. This aspect, together with continual and rapid improvement in the technology itself, is the key to the success of this form of photography. In particular, a decisive factor is the huge advantage of instant viewing and analysis of the image and the option to immediately retake the photograph if it is judged to be unsatisfactory.

This advantage is somewhat of a double-edged sword; an awareness that retaking an image costs nothing, and that it can be retaken innumerable times, can lead the operator, in error, to photograph with only cursory attention, rather than the level of care required to take an adequate photograph the first time. Because time is a precious commodity in dentistry, and to do something well takes the same time as to do it badly, the dentist must always photograph with the same level of attention that would be used if the work were being presented at an important scientific conference. Every visual document acquired could be precious for legal or scientific purposes, and the most important photographs might turn out to be those not taken.

Another advantage of digital photography is acceleration of the learning curve. The option to instantly assess the image taken using a basic knowledge of photography allows us to understand and consequently correct mistakes. As a result, photographic techniques can be rapidly and effectively refined. Moreover, large quantities of digital images can be easily stored, contributing to the creation of a valuable personal data bank.

For these reasons, a photographic handbook for dentistry should explain clearly and thoroughly both general photographic techniques and, in particular, digital techniques. To understand and use the extraordinary capabilities of digital photography equipment, it is necessary to analyze their characteristics and working logic. Although the text that follows may seem technical and weighty in nature, the information will be very beneficial to aspiring photographers.

[*Traditional analog or film-based photography retains its fascination and vitality; it is a mistake to consider it an outdated technique or to think that it should be completely replaced by digital technology.*]

Sensors in Analog Photography

Analog photography uses photosensitive film. The sensitive element and the source of the term *film* is the silver halide emulsion on a very thin transparent support.

When the silver halide crystals come into contact with light, they undergo an irreversible change, becoming denser in direct proportion to the intensity of the light that strikes them. After exposing the film, it is necessary to soak it in suitable chemical reagents to remove the unmodified crystals and to stabilize those that remain behind. This procedure is known as film *developing and fixing*, and it creates a *negative*. After appropriate processing in a darkroom, the image exposed on the film is printed onto sensitive paper; the result is the classic photograph.

Film for slides can be manipulated to directly create a positive image on the transparency. These images can be projected without being first printed onto paper, although they may be printed if desired. Slide film is called *reversible film*, because the image can be converted from negative to positive (Fig 4-1).

Fig 4-1
A photograph of the Stromboli volcano, a plume of smoke visible on the summit; intermittent explosions are typical of this volcano. The image was taken with Fujichrome Sensia ISO 100 daylight-type film and a Yashica FX 2000 at f = 500 mm, f/9, t = 1/200 s.

[
The digital sensor transforms luminous energy into electric energy via the photovoltaic effect; this process does not involve irreversible physical or chemical variations in the sensor, which can therefore be exposed indefinitely.
]

Digital Sensors

The digital sensor, an electronic version of film, functions in a completely different manner than analog film. Light, or more specifically, luminous flux is directed onto photosensitive semiconductor elements, which produce very weak electric currents in direct proportion to the number of lumens present; this is the photoelectric effect. A very similar principle, called the *photovoltaic effect*, applies to the functioning of solar panels, which produce electric energy by exploiting the sun's rays. The man who discovered the photoelectric effect was the famous scientist Albert Einstein, who in 1905 published his work on the particle nature of light, in which he proposed and explained the existence of the photoelectric effect. It is not common knowledge that the 1921 Nobel Prize in Physics was not conferred on him for his fundamental work on the theory of relativity, published the previous year, but was awarded for his work concerning the nature of light and the photoelectric effect. The prize was awarded, according to the citation, "for his services to Theoretical Physics, and especially for his discovery of the law of the photoelectric effect."

The photosensitive elements, photodiodes or photodetectors, are applied to a silicon wafer. The electric signals coming from the photodetectors are extremely weak, so they must be suitably amplified before being digitalized, or transformed into a series of numeric binary-code values. The exposure of the sensor is reversible, which means that, theoretically, it can be repeated indefinitely, unlike traditional film, which is irreversibly exposed to light and cannot be reused.

Thus, the digital sensor can be considered the heart of the camera; for this reason, it is useful to become familiar with its basic workings. Two types of sensors are used in digital cameras. The first one to be created in 1969 was the charge-coupled device (CCD), the result of the work of two American scientists, William S. Boyle and George E. Smith. For their labor, they were awarded the Nobel Prize in Physics on October 6, 2009, "for the invention of an imaging semiconductor circuit—the CCD sensor."

The sensitive elements of a CCD sensor are arranged in a line, and each element transfers the charge produced by the photovoltaic effect to the next one; the timed sequence of impulses generates an electric signal, which can be used to create digital data (Fig 4-2a). The sensor consists of numerous lines of photosensitive elements, each with its own supply for the amplification of the signal. This arrangement creates uniform amplification and low background noise. A drawback of CCD sensors is the need to construct a complex amplification system, which is costly for the manufacture of larger sensors.

To overcome this disadvantage, the complementary metal-oxide semiconductor (CMOS) was developed (Fig 4-2b). In this type of sensor, each photosensitive element has its own signal-amplification system, so large CMOS sensors are less expensive to manufacture than CCD sensors. A drawback of CMOS sensors is their tendency to create background noise and color dominants. These problems can generally be overcome by the camera's sophisticated software.

Currently, the only major manufacturers of average- to high-priced cameras, including those used in dentistry, are oriented toward the production and marketing of CMOS-type sensors. Manufacturers have found that the cost of producing a CCD-type sensor with the same dimensions as 24 × 36–mm film is prohibitive. Sensors with 24 × 36–mm dimensions are also called *35-mm* or *Leica format*, after the German optics manufacturer who first marketed it; this is considered the standard for common use today.

Digital sensors that correspond to the 24 × 36–mm format are also called *full-frame sensors* and, given their cost, are mainly found in high-priced cameras. For cameras in the average- to high-priced bracket, manufacturers install smaller, cheaper CMOS sensors such as the classic Advanced Photo System (APS-C) sensor, which measures 15.8 × 23.6 mm in the Nikon D300 camera and 14.8 × 22.2 mm in the Canon EOS 40D camera.

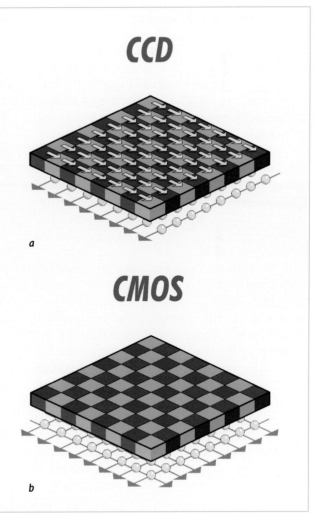

Fig 4-2a
In the CCD-type sensor, electric charges travel in a linear fashion, and the signal is amplified for an entire linear sector. This promotes amplification conformity and low background noise. Each colored sector corresponds to one photosite, which can contain one or more photodetectors according to the technology being used. The color array represents the Bayer filter, which separates the various wavelengths and correctly recomposes the colors. Each sector corresponds to a pixel on the final image. The resolution of the photograph is represented by the total number of pixels. The retina's photoreceptors, responsible for color vision, work in a similar manner, because they are specialized for the discrimination of the same primary colors: red, green, and blue. The recomposition and final visualization of color takes place during subsequent cerebral processing of the peripheral information.

Fig 4-2b
In the CMOS-type sensor, each sensitive element is amplified, allowing the dimensions of the sensor to be enlarged while minimizing costs, with the disadvantage that there is a tendency toward the creation of background noise and color dominants. However, the sophisticated software of the camera can compensate for these errors.

[
The two types of digital sensors, CCD and CMOS, are distinguished by their design and manner of operation. For the practitioner, the most important characteristic of the sensor is its format, or the dimension of its two sides and the proportion between them.
]

The manufacture and marketing of digital cameras is in such rapid evolution that it is foolish to even think of keeping up with the constant changes in equipment, which tend to confuse rather than facilitate the task of the photographer. For example, Leica is introducing a new format of digital sensor, 30 × 45 mm with a capacity of 37 megapixels, with the intention of replacing the classic format they established in the past. However, a good APS-C–format camera of average or average-to-high quality and price can easily satisfy the most conscientious practitioner's needs for several years. Moreover, it should not be forgotten that outstanding photographs and irreproachable documents can be taken with a traditional film-based camera.

Rapid technologic development has cut production costs so that today full-frame–sensor cameras are available at accessible prices. However, the quality attained by smaller-frame sensors is such that we can confidently rely on them to achieve splendid photos. On the basis of working characteristics and the practitioner's needs, the difference between the two is not fundamental, because distinguishing between a photograph taken with an APS-C–type sensor and one taken with a full-frame–type sensor would require much experience and technical skill in reading the image (Figs 4-3 and 4-4).

A photograph for dental purposes should be judged by other parameters. The spatiality, the magnification ratio, and the correct depth of field are the best criteria with which to evaluate the beauty of a photograph in the field of dentistry.

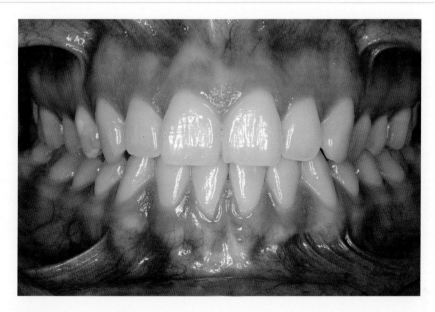

Fig 4-3a
An image taken with a Canon EOS 5D digital single–lens reflex camera equipped with a full-frame CMOS sensor, Canon 100-mm macro lens, and Canon MR-14EX ring flash.

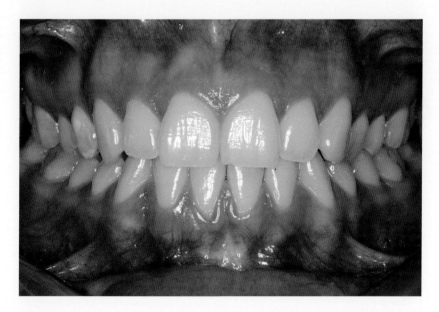

Fig 4-3b
The same image taken with a Canon EOS 40D camera fitted with an APS-C sensor, Canon 100-mm macro lens, and MR-14EX ring flash. The particular behavior of each camera is the reason for the slight differences in exposure, which are correctable.

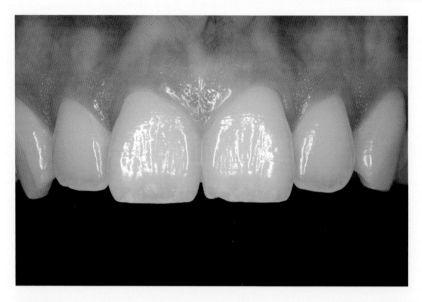

Fig 4-4a
An image taken with a Canon EOS 3D camera fitted with a full-frame CMOS sensor, Canon 100-mm macro lens, and MR-14EX ring flash.

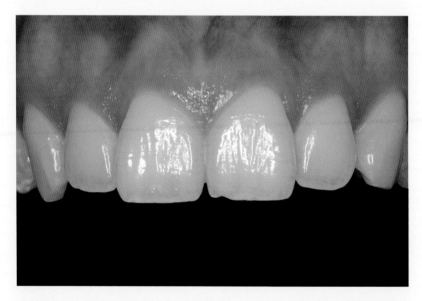

Fig 4-4b
The same image, taken with the Canon EOS 40D, Canon 100-mm macro lens, and MR-14EX ring flash. Photographs for dental purposes should be judged on parameters of spatiality, correct magnification ratio, and correct depth of field, rather than minute details of photographic technique, which are imperceptible to most users.

[
The terminology and concepts relating to digital sensors must be explained so that the operator can better understand the working logic of the sensor itself and can use these terms with the propriety and accuracy that scientific documentation requires.
]

Photosites, Photodetectors, and Pixels

The light information coming from the specific portion of physical space occupied by the framed object is recomposed by the lenses onto a specific physical space on the sensor called a *photosite*, which contains one or more miniature photosensitive electronic devices called *photodetectors*. The photosite is the physical place where the tiniest details of the image are captured. Thus, the surface of the sensor is subdivided into numerous microscopic spatial sectors, each of which contain one or more photodetectors, also called *photodiodes*, which are semiconducting elements with the function of transforming luminous energy into proportional electric currents. These extremely weak electric currents are sent to a processor inside the camera called an *analog-to-digital converter*, which transforms the electric signals into numeric data, executing the digitalization of the data.

Each photosite corresponds to a matrix of elementary visual information or an element of the image called a *pixel* (a contraction of the words *picture* and *element*). It is strange to think that these elements, the pixels, were invented thousands of years ago by ancient artists, who, with tesserae of various colors, learned to compose complex images such as mosaics (Fig 4-5). Similar to an antique mosaic, the final image of a digital photograph is made up of thousands of pixels, as if it were a visual mosaic composed of minute tesserae. Each pixel shows one, and only one, color and one intensity of brightness, but together many pixels make up a complete mosaic of innumerable nuances of brightness and hues. The single or multiple photodetectors present on a photosite provide the necessary information to produce a single element of the image, one pixel.

The photodetectors cannot distinguish between the different wavelengths that produce various colors because they only perceive the intensity of the luminous flux. For this reason, each photosite is covered by a selective filter, called a *Bayer filter* or a *color filter array*, which allows the photosite to acquire the light intensity relative to only one of the three primary colors, red, green, or blue. A Bayer filter consists of a mosaic of filters for each of the three primary colors and is positioned on the photodetector grid according to a particular and precise pattern (see Fig 4-2).

The photoreceptors of the human eye work together in a similar way. One type of photoreceptor, the cone, is specialized in discriminating between the three primary colors, while the other type, the rod, perceives only the degree of brightness in absolute terms. The cones for the detection of color function best in bright light (photopic vision), but the rods are activated by even very weak light (scotopic vision).

In classic digital sensors, because each photosite is filtered for one of the three primary colors, the data from a single photodetector cannot fully determine on its own the color present on the pixels. Color information must be completed by a mathematic procedure known as *interpolation*, which calculates missing or insufficient data by exploiting the information from nearby photodetectors.

DIGITAL CAMERA TERMINOLOGY
- **PHOTOSITE:** Spatial area that contains the photosensitive element of the sensor
- **PHOTODETECTOR:** Photosensitive electronic device
- **PIXEL:** A single visual element of an image
- **BYTES:** The computing elements necessary to describe a pixel

Other types of sensors have been designed to improve the definition and quality of the image. For example, the Foveon X3 sensor (National Semiconductor) is constructed so that the three photodetectors needed to obtain a complete color description of the pixels are superimposed onto a sole photosite; thus, there is no need for reconstruction of the missing chromatic components by interpolation. According to the manufacturers, this sensor provides better color accuracy.

To summarize the concept of the pixel, light strikes one or more photodetectors present on a sensor's photosite; through the photovoltaic effect, proportional currents are generated and transformed into numerical data by the analog-to-digital converter, obtaining the number of bytes that are needed to describe a pixel.

Although even prestigious photography magazines may state that a particular sensor "has" or "is made up of" a certain number of megapixels, it would be more correct to say that a sensor *supplies* the megapixels. For example, the Foveon X3 sensor has about 10.2 million photodiodes laid out on 3.4 million photosites, supplying 3.4 megapixels. The number of pixels does not coincide with the number of bytes needed to describe it. In fact, the number of bytes required to describe a pixel is directly proportional to the color space and to the intrinsic quality of the pixel itself. Fewer bytes are required to describe a completely white pixel than to describe a pixel of a particular shade of violet.

The photosite is a spatial concept that describes an area of the sensor where light is captured; the photodetector is a functional concept, describing a microscopic electronic device. Byte is a computing concept, and a pixel is a visual concept or the elementary part of an image. Although these concepts are interdependent, each has its own specificity and must not be confused.

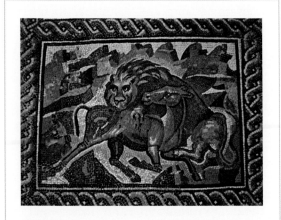

Fig 4-5
This ancient Roman mosaic is composed of tesserae, just as a digital image is made up of pixels. (Courtesy of the Archaeological Museum, Taranto, Italy.)

Because of the strict relationship between sensor format, focal length, and lens behavior, an f = 50-mm lens (normal for a full-frame sensor) used with a smaller-format sensor will obtain a greater actual focal length and a greater magnification factor. An equivalent focal length can be calculated by multiplying the lens' actual focal length in mm by the multiplication factor.

Equivalent Focal Length and the Multiplication Factor

In using a camera with an APS-C format, such as a Nikon D300 or a Canon EOS 40D, it is important to know that the behavior of the lens will change in the presence of these smaller-format sensors, because of the effect of the relationship between the diagonal length of the sensor and the focal length of the lens.

The concept of the normality of the lens was discussed in chapter 2. There is always a normal lens for each particular sensor format, and a normal lens for a 15.6 × 23.6-mm APS-C sensor will have a focal length equal to about 28 mm. If an f = 50-mm lens is used on a camera with a sensor of this format, there will be a virtual lengthening of the focal length of the lens.

Because a greater focal length corresponds to a greater magnification factor, this relationship can be expressed by a multiplication factor, which indicates how much the magnification factor will increase. For Nikon DX-format cameras, the multiplication factor will be 1.5×; hence an f = 50-mm lens will have an actual focal length of 75 mm (50 × 1.5 = 75). The actual focal length times the multiplication factor gives the *equivalent focal length*.

Manufacturers indicate the multiplication factor of all cameras equipped with smaller-format sensors among the technical specifications. This is useful for calculating the equivalent focal length of the lenses. To summarize, a lens with a focal length of 50 mm, considered normal for a 24 × 36-mm full-frame sensor, when fitted onto a DX-sensor camera, will have a focal length equivalent to about 75 mm. Thus, it will behave like a telephoto lens, with known consequences on the magnification factor. A Canon APS-C sensor measures 14.8 × 22.2 mm and has a multiplication factor of 1.6×. An f = 300-mm lens, combined with this sensor, will have an equivalent focal length of 480 mm (300 × 1.6 = 480).

Using an f = 100-mm macro lens with a smaller-format sensor, the operator can attain a magnification ratio of about 1.5:1 or 1.6:1 depending on the size of the sensor, far greater than the 1:1 ratio attained with the same lens and a full-frame sensor. With analog single-lens reflex (SLR) cameras designed for dentistry, such as the Yashica Dental Eye, an additional lens is required to attain a greater magnification ratio. With the reduced size of the APS-C format sensor and the higher multiplication factor, the operator has a greater magnification ratio at his or her disposal without resorting to additional lenses; in the field of close-up photography, this undoubtedly is a great advantage.

[
Each lens projects an image circle of a defined size onto the sensor. When the image circle is larger than the size of the sensor, there is a magnification effect because the image itself is cropped. One advantage of this effect is that it uses the central part of the image circle, which for optical reasons is always of a better quality than the periphery.
]

Image Circle and the Vignetting Concept

In addition to the equivalent focal length concept, a second factor influences the magnification ratio: the projection of an image circle onto the sensor. This image circle is the result of the recomposition of the light rays from the framed scene onto the plane of the sensor by the system of lenses. A lens designed for a 24 × 36–mm format projects an image circle precisely related to these dimensions. When the same image circle is projected onto a sensor with smaller dimensions, only the central part of the image circle will be used, resulting in a cropping of the projected area and a magnification of the image itself (Fig 4-6). The main advantage of this effect is that, when using lenses designed for a 24 × 36–mm format on smaller-format sensors, only the central part of the image circle is recorded, avoiding the digital vignetting effect and achieving a better image quality. Because dental photography is a magnification ratio–priority technique, the effects of equivalent focal length and cropping, derived from the use of a smaller sensor, are beneficial.

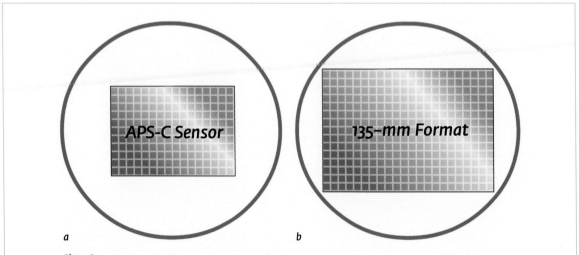

Fig 4-6
The area of an APS-C–format sensor (a) is smaller than the image circle (blue circle) projected by an f = 100–mm macro lens designed for the 24 × 36–mm format sensor (135-mm sensor [b]). The result is a magnification effect and an improvement in the overall quality of the image because the central part of the image circle is used, and the digital vignetting effect is eliminated. The central portion of the image is of a better quality than the periphery because of optical vignetting.

[
The vignetting effect is the loss of brightness in the corners of an image; it can be mechanical, optical, or digital in origin. Using a lens designed for a 24 × 36–mm sensor on a camera with a smaller-format sensor avoids digital and optical vignetting. Using a lens designed for a smaller-format sensor on a camera with a full-frame sensor will result in unacceptable mechanical and optical vignetting.
]

Conversely, it is not advisable to use lenses built for smaller-format sensors on cameras with full-frame sensors because the image circle projected by the lens will not cover the entire area of the sensor, creating vignetting at the corners of the image (Fig 4-7).

Vignetting is a reduction in image brightness at the periphery of an image as compared with the center. In this case, vignetting is caused by the insufficiency of the image circle in covering the entire area of the sensor. *Mechanical vignetting* is caused by external physical objects, such as filters or lens hoods, and optic elements

positioned inside the lens for design purposes. Optical vignetting is the attenuation of the light at the periphery of the image because of an excessive angulation of the peripheral light rays with respect to the optical axis. *Digital vignetting* is connected to the way the photosensitive elements are built; each one can be represented by a photonic well, or a "little bowl," which is completely filled by light rays only when they come from directly above. The more obliquely the light ray strikes the photonic well, the more it is intercepted by the edges of the well itself and thus attenuated.

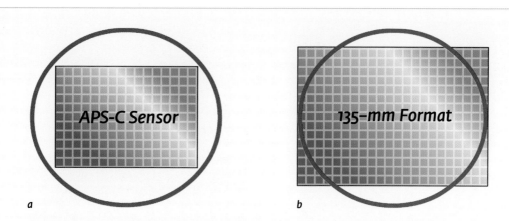

a   b

Fig 4-7
The image circle (red circle) projected by a lens designed for the APS-C format (a) is insufficient to cover the area of a 24 × 36–mm format sensor (b). The resulting mechanical vignetting causes a loss of brightness at the periphery of the image with respect to the center. It is important to remember that lenses designed for 24 × 36–mm format sensors can always be used on cameras with a compatible mount and a smaller-format sensor, bearing in mind the practical consequences of this choice. However, while it is possible to fit a lens designed for the smaller-format sensor onto a full-frame–format camera, the resulting mechanical vignetting and loss of image quality make this option inadvisable.

When used with a smaller-format sensor, a lens with a focal length of 100 mm will have a longer actual focal length and a different actual magnification ratio than indicated on the focusing ring. The specifications inscribed on the focusing ring need to be corrected and interpreted in light of this concept.

Actual and Nominal Magnification Ratio

A traditional f = 100–mm macro lens gives both the selected magnification ratio and the maximum possible magnification factor (the first numeric value, usually 1, of the ratio) on the focusing ring. These figures reflect the 24 × 36–mm sensor format for which it was designed (Figs 4-8 and 4-9a).

Because of the equivalent focal length concept, if an APS-C–format sensor is used with this lens, the specific multiplication factor of the camera must be applied, and thus the actual magnification factor will be 1.5:1 for the Nikon D300 and 1.6:1 for the Canon EOS 40D (Figs 4-9b and 4-9c). The nominal magnification ratio is indicated on the focusing ring, but the actual magnification ratio will differ depending on the format of the sensor used in combination with that lens (Fig 4-10).

It is not possible to provide information, in absolute terms, about the magnification ratio to be used, because it is strictly linked to the specific dimensions of the subject in the frame. For this reason, it is not particularly useful to give strict guidelines regarding either the magnification ratio to be set on the lens or the distance from the object. After a few attempts and a little practice, an operator will have no difficulty deciding which magnification ratio to set preliminarily on the focusing ring (Table 4-1) and will easily understand at what distance from the subject he or she should be positioned to obtain the correct magnification for the desired image.

In conclusion, the use of smaller-format sensors is advantageous in dental photography. However, this advantage is lost when a wide-angle lens with a short focal length is used. The use of smaller-format sensors is contrary to the intrinsic aim of the wide-angle lens, which is to attain a wide angle of view and a lesser magnification ratio.

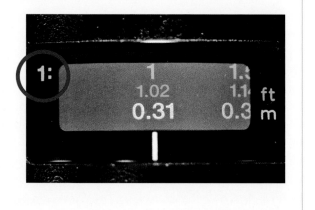

Fig 4-8
The focusing ring shows the magnification ratio for a Canon f = 100–mm macro lens. The first number (red circle), indicates the maximum possible magnification ratio. This lens is designed for a full-frame sensor, which is why the magnification ratio shown varies with different sensor formats.

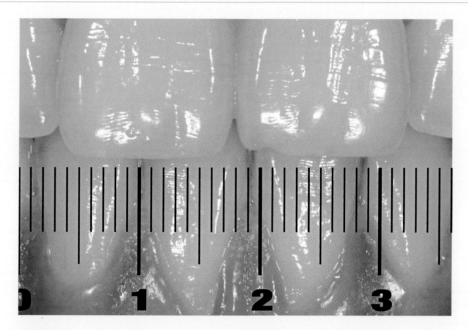

Fig 4-9a
A 1:1 magnification ratio attained with a full-frame sensor; this is the same magnification ratio as shown on the lens' focusing ring.

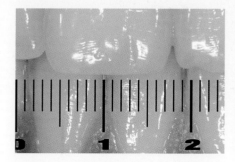

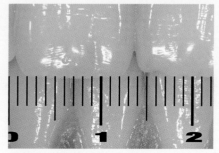

Fig 4-9b
This image has been taken with a Nikon D300 camera and a Nikkor f = 105–mm macro lens, with the focusing ring set on a 1:1 magnification ratio. The camera has a DX-format sensor (15.6 × 23.6 mm), which has a multiplication factor of 1.5× and an actual maximum magnification ratio of 1.5:1. The magnification ratio shown on the lens' focusing ring is clearly nominal and not actual, because it refers to a 24 × 36–mm sensor. Dividing the 36-mm width by the 1.5 magnification ratio, related to the different dimensions of the sensor format, results in a 24 mm–wide image.

Fig 4-9c
The same image has been taken with an f = 100–mm macro lens and 14.8 × 22.2–mm Canon sensor, which has a multiplication factor of 1.6×, and a actual maximum magnification ratio of 1.6:1. The magnification is greater than that shown in Fig 4-9b because the 36-mm image width divided by 1.6 gives an image width of 22.5 mm. The image is 1.6 times greater than the object, the outcome of the lens-sensor interaction.

113

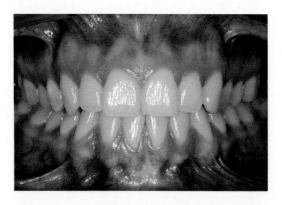

Fig 4-10a
This image has been taken with a Canon EOS 5D camera equipped with a CMOS full-frame sensor and f = 100–mm macro lens. A magnification ratio of 1:1.5 is indicated on the focusing ring.

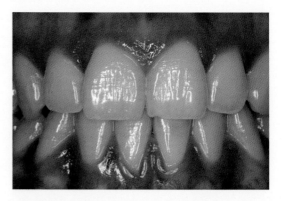

Fig 4-10b
This image has been taken with a Canon EOS 40D camera equipped with a CMOS APS-C–format sensor and an f = 100–mm macro lens. A magnification ratio of 1:1.5 is indicated on the focusing ring, but the actual magnification ratio is greater because of the equivalent focal length concept. The actual magnification ratio is about 1:1 because 1.6:1.5 is close to 1:1.

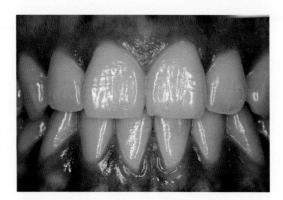

Fig 4-10c
This image has been taken with a Canon EOS 5D camera equipped with a CMOS full-frame sensor and an f = 100–mm macro lens. A magnification ratio of 1:1, life size, is indicated on the focusing ring. Each actual 1 mm of the object corresponds to 1 mm on the sensor. This is the maximum magnification possible with this lens combined with this sensor. This image is very similar to Fig 4-10b.

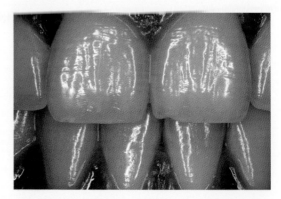

Fig 4-10d
This image has been taken with a Canon EOS 40D camera equipped with a CMOS APS-C–format sensor and an f = 100–mm macro lens. A nominal magnification ratio of 1:1 is indicated on the focusing ring, but the actual magnification is greater, 1.6:1. Each 1 mm measured on the sensor is 1.6× greater than each actual 1 mm of the object. This is the maximum magnification possible with this lens combined with this sensor.

[
The analog-to-digital converter transforms the electric currents generated by the sensor into the numeric values of the binary code. These two numbers supply the information necessary to describe the image.
]

Analog-to-Digital Converter

To obtain digital information, the electric signals provided by the photodetectors of the sensor must be converted into digital, numeric values by a device called an *analog-to-digital converter*. This physically transforms electric currents into numeric data that are stored on the camera's memory card. The combination of sensor and analog-to-digital convertor transforms light into numbers. These numbers represent elementary, binary, digital information, using only two numbers (0 and 1), each of which is called a *bit*. A bit represents the smallest unit of information; typically, eight bits are grouped together to form a *byte*, the basic unit of memory size. A quantity of bytes, and therefore of information, is usually discussed in terms of its multiples: kilo, mega, giga, tera, etc.

The analog-to-digital converter has a certain sampling frequency, which is an indicator of performance and quality; a converter that samples at 12 bits per channel (or per photodetector) can express 4,096 different levels of brightness on the same pixel. The higher the number of bits per channel, the more accurate the return of the tonal shades onto the image. Some cameras, such as the Nikon D300, allow the operator to choose between two analog-to-digital conversion options: 12 or 14 bits per channel. This difference might appear minimal, but instead it is significant; 12 bits per channel can express 4,096 different levels of brightness, while 14 bits per channel can express an amazing 16,384 different levels of brightness.

Table 4-1 Preliminary magnification-ratio settings according to the subject in the frame

Subject	24 × 36–mm sensor	APS-C sensor
Complete arch	1:1.5	1:2.2
Anterior teeth	1:1	1:1.5
Face	1:5	1:8

The pathway from subject to image (Fig 4-11): the light strikes the sensor, which generates extremely weak electric currents via the photoelectric effect, proportional to the intensity of the light. The currents are measured and transformed into binary-code numbers by the analog-to-digital converter. The digital data is processed and stored on the camera's memory card, which is transferred to the computer, the final medium for viewing an image.

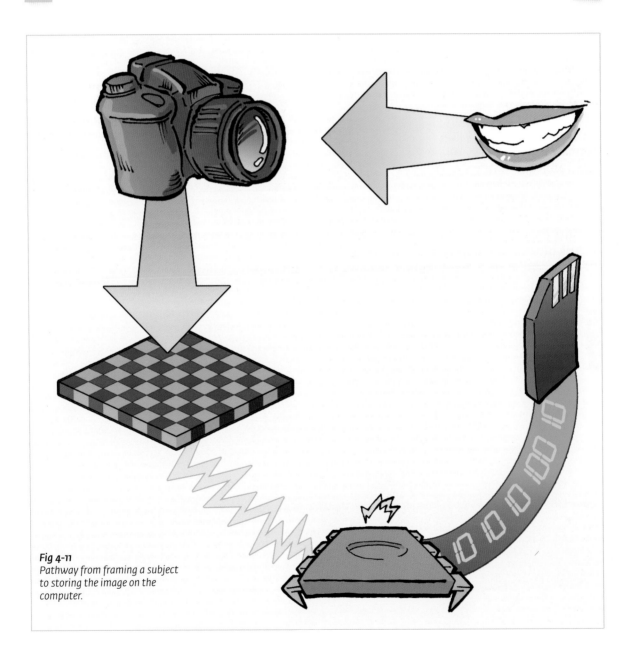

Fig 4-11
Pathway from framing a subject to storing the image on the computer.

Image file formats are the codes that transform data from digital to visual. Various types exist, but the most common are raw, Joint Photographic Experts Group (JPEG), and Tagged Image File Format (TIFF).

Image File Formats

An image is described by an ordered set of bits—simple numbers—so a convention or code is necessary to interpret the correct meaning of the bit sequence. This code is called the *image file format* and is identified by initials or by an extension, which is a dot and a series of letters listed after the name of the file. There are three common formats.

The raw format is a particular method of storing the data needed to describe an image. Its fundamental characteristic is that there is no loss of data or image quality when the file is transferred to a storage medium. JPEG is an acronym for Joint Photographic Experts Group, a committee of experts who defined the first international standards for image compression. Presently, JPEG is the most widely used format for image compression.

The tagged image file format (TIFF) is a noncompressed universal image format, which is quite commonly used because it allows the specification of numerous added indications and information regarding color calibration. TIFF is widely used by the press and professional printers. This format is highly appreciated for its ability to maintain perfect image quality each time the image is saved (Fig 4-12). A drawback to this high quality, however, is the vast storage size of the files, so a practitioner may prefer to abandon TIFF in favor of the raw or JPEG formats.

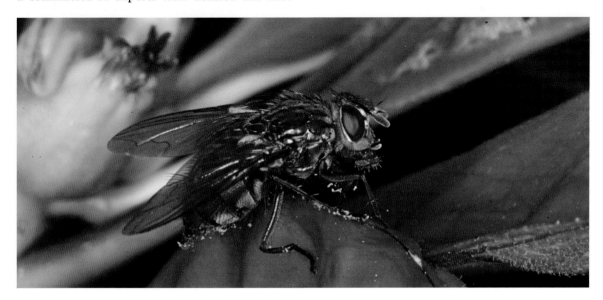

Fig 4-12
A close-up image of the common housefly.

[
JPEG is the most versatile and widely used image file format. It provides an excellent balance between quality and storage size. JPEG accommodates various levels of compression, but the corresponding decline in quality is a drawback to this format.
]

JPEG format

The versatile and widely used JPEG format compresses the image data into smaller files so that a larger number of images can be stored on the memory card. Furthermore, it performs the necessary compression for rapid and efficient transmission of image files via the Internet.

Image compression eliminates repetitive or redundant data or predictable content within a file and cancels visual information that is difficult to perceive with the human eye. JPEG compression thus involves the loss of data and, subsequently, quality. If the degree of compression is minimal, this data loss is insignificant and concerns nonfundamental information. This imperceptible decline in quality is called *lossless compression*. Higher levels of compression correspond to a progressive and significant loss of information and quality called *lossy compression*.

Each time we open a file, it becomes decompressed, and at every closure, it becomes recompressed. If a file is opened in an editing program rather than a normal reading mode, and slight modifications to the file are carried out, the file will be compressed yet again upon saving the changes. This compression, different from the previous one, will result in a progressive decline in the quality of the image and the appearance of artifacts and imperfections. Even a simple rotation of the image causes a different compression upon saving the file. It is therefore advisable to maintain two files, one in a raw format and one in the JPEG format.

Raw format

The data supplied by the analog-to-digital convertor is in a raw format and is like a digital version of a film negative. This format includes the entire amount of information acquired by the sensor.

In raw image files, the actual resolution of the image, or the total number of pixels comprising the image, coincides with that of the sensor. This file is referred to as *raw* because the image, captured by the camera's sensor, is registered in its numeric form after conversion from analog to digital, without further processing or correction by the camera.

Raw files contain many bytes: a 12-megapixel sensor can generate a raw file of 20 MB or more, which uses much storage space on the camera's memory card.

A disadvantage of the raw file format is that these files can only be viewed with specific software provided by the camera manufacturer or with advanced retouching programs. If the operator intends to send a raw file, the recipient must have suitable software to view it. To overcome this difficulty, the software company Adobe Systems has begun providing a free digital negative (DNG) converter utility program, which is able to convert raw data specific to a make (for example, Nikon defines raw files with the extension .nef) into a raw format usable by ordinary image-processing software such as Photoshop (Adobe Systems).

It is important to note that the conversion from the raw format into DNG is a form of image processing that might, from a medicolegal

> *Raw files represent the native format of the analog-to-digital converter and are a true "digital negative." This format preserves the entire amount of information acquired by the sensor and enables the operator to make reversible modifications to the images, without any loss in quality, with special software.*

stance, detract from the value of the data. Because subsequent corrections are possible, the raw format allows the acquisition of less-than-optimal images regarding exposure, white balance, etc. This processing, or so-called lightroom development, allows the operator to make reversible corrections to the settings while maintaining image quality at the highest level (Fig 4-13). Obviously, some parameters of an image are irreversible; depth of field, focus, and perspective must be optimal at the stage of image capture because they cannot be subsequently corrected. The software for viewing raw files provided by the camera manufacturers usually permits the photographer to perform a certain amount of processing and correction of the image without resorting to more complex software.

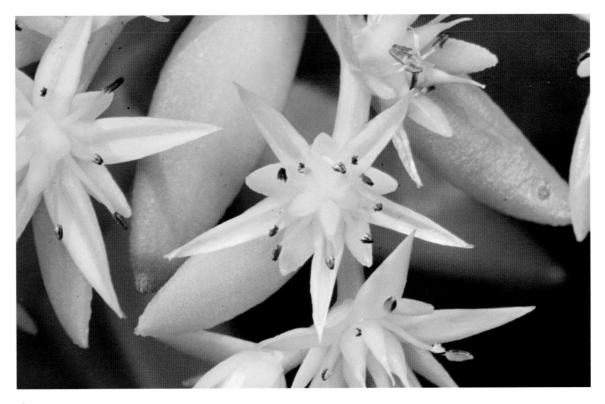

Fig 4-13
Advanced retouching programs can improve a photograph, such as these flowers, long after capture of the image.

> *Unless medicolegal standards change, we can assume that image files in raw format hold the same legal value as traditional film. The camera is fitted with a processor able to transform the native raw-format data into files of other formats that are easier to handle. It is always a good idea to store the images in the raw format and, if the camera permits it, at the same time create a JPEG file of the image.*

Legal value of the raw format

In addition to studying the technical aspects of digital technology, it is also important to reflect on the legal value of digital images in general and, in particular, images in the raw file format. Digital images lend themselves to manipulation with extreme ease using the numerous retouching programs. A photograph can be modified according to one's personal requirements or possibly even for fraudulent purposes. It seems clear that digital images cannot have the legal value of a corresponding analog image recorded on film, although this is not always true, because even traditional analog photographs can be modified or manipulated for illicit purposes.

As a matter of relatively recent technologic innovation, there has yet to be any consolidated legislation in the field of digital photography. It should first be pointed out that there is no law that forbids digital data–recording methods for documentary purposes. As in any other field, suspicions of falsification by modification or alteration can only be supported when there is certain proof that the alteration has indeed occurred, and the burden of proof is on the accuser. In light of this statement, paradoxically, it is the raw file format, rather than the analog image, that offers the greatest guarantee of authenticity. It is an original format, which, by definition and intrinsic characteristics, has not undergone any manipulation following its simple acquisition.

In the raw file format, information relating to the image and the camera that captured it is written into the digital-image file—the date, the time, and many other technical parameters—providing a means to verify the reliability of the file and, in the field of dentistry, its objective reality. It is inconceivable that lawmakers would ignore innovations, would not take into account the advantages offered by technology, and would not keep up with the times; eventually, legislative bodies will have to address this technology, as they have done on other occasions and with other innovations. For now, however, we can assume that the medicolegal value of image files in the raw format cannot be contested, at least not until there is a coordinated effort to the contrary on the part of lawmakers or the law.

[*Shooting menus are used to vary certain characteristics of the images, depending on the taste of the operator; however, because the dentist needs to document reality as faithfully as possible, it is advisable to intervene as little as possible in these parameters.*]

Image Processing

Digital cameras are equipped with a second processor, in addition to the analog-to-digital convertor, that converts raw-format files to the JPEG format to facilitate the viewing of the images.

This conversion procedure involves a compression of the image file, which is useful in reducing file size and storage space usage in the memory and optimizing the number of shots available. In this second phase of processing, corrections to the image also generally take place, either via the manufacturers' default settings, or by the operator to suit his or her personal taste (see "Shooting menus").

The camera's *quality settings* command is used to select the degree of compression and, therefore, the degree of image quality. It is important to remember that each successive manipulation or compression of the JPEG file will result in an irreversible loss of data and image quality. If image corrections or processing are anticipated, it is always a good idea to make a master file. Modern cameras have the option of recording raw and JPEG files at the same time, which automatically creates an original master file and a default JPEG format for processing, which seems to be the most suitable solution for dental purposes. Another advantage of this option is that the JPEG file obtained from the raw file will be of higher quality, after use of retouching program like Photoshop, than one taken directly from the camera itself.

Shooting menus

Traditional analog-photography film has characteristics relating to color and image sharpness that vary from manufacturer to manufacturer. These qualities cannot be modified because they are determined by the manufacturing process. Other factors affecting an individual roll of film include the state of its preservation over time and minute variations in the chemical reagents used for the production of single batches of film.

This variability means that certain films are more suitable than others in particular situations. For example, Ektachrome (Kodak) conveys the azure of the sky extremely well (Fig 4-14); Kodachrome 64 KR (Kodak) guarantees an excellent reproduction of the complexion and of colors, with a very accurate grain and high contrast; Agfachrome (Agfa) captures grays

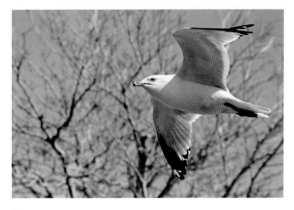

Fig 4-14
This analog photograph of a soaring seagull was taken using Ektachrome film, which captures the azure of the sky extremely well.

> The resolving power of an optical system is the ability of the system itself to perceive as distinct two points extremely close to each other. This parameter can be useful in assessing the efficiency of the eye or, more often, a microscope.

and complexions very well; and Fujichrome (Fujifilm) brings out shades of green.

Characteristics that are not modifiable for traditional film are variable in digital photography. Apart from the degree of compression, the in-camera system processes the images according to parameters set by the operator using the shooting menu.

The parameters that can be controlled via menu options are sharpness, contrast, color saturation, and hue. The photographer can also opt for a monochrome image of black and white on a scale of grays. Moreover, the original raw image format allows these characteristics to be further manipulated at the postproduction stage. Because a dental photographic image should be a document that conforms as closely as possible to reality, it is better to select few alterations among the various options on the menu. However, a slight increase in the sharpness of the image—the degree of definition at the edges of the object—is recommended.

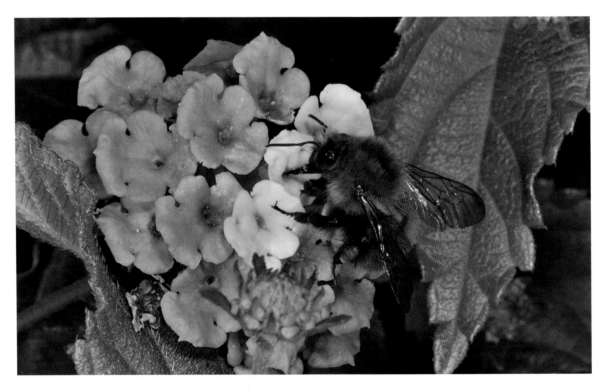

Fig 4-15
On this high-resolution image, individual hairs can be distinguished on the thorax of the bee.

[For a digital image, the term resolution *indicates the quantity of pixels that describe the image. It is an indicator of image quality; a greater number of pixels corresponds to a sharper image that is richer in information. The resolution value can be calculated by multiplying the number of pixels along the horizontal and vertical sides of the image.*]

Resolution and Image Quality

The final quality of an image is related to numerous factors, including the number of pixels provided by the sensor, the quality of the lenses and the camera's processor, the structure and format of the sensor, and the degree of compression of the image. Image resolution is closely related to image quality, so this concept requires clarification.

The term *resolution* can have different meanings depending on the context in which it is used and, because this can cause confusion, it is necessary to clarify the various meanings the term can express. The expression *power of resolution of an optical system* refers to the ability to perceive as distinct two very close points: the greater the resolution power, the shorter the distance between two points that can still be perceived as distinct. When this distance is less than the power of resolution of the instrument or optical system, the points will appear to be joined. The power of a microscope is, therefore, assessed by means of its ability to perceive as distinct two very close points. The word *resolve* has its origins in the word *dissolve*, to separate.

On average, a healthy human eye can distinguish six lines per mm; a calculation of the spaces between the lines gives a resolution of 12 lines or dots per mm, corresponding to about 120 dots per cm or 300 dots per inch; beyond this density, the dots appear as a single uninterrupted line.

In photography, *resolution* refers to the quantity of pixels forming the image; resolution is the parameter by which we communicate the quantity of visual information present on an image (Fig 4-15). The digital sensor contains a defined number of photodetectors, which will generate a certain quantity of pixels. The number of megapixels that a sensor provides is one of its most publicized and important characteristics and has a significant effect on its marketing potential.

Thus, the resolution of a digital image is given by the quantity of pixels, or quantity of information, in its two spatial dimensions. With traditional film, the resolution of an image is calculated by multiplying the dots present on the horizontal and vertical sides. For a digital image, the resolution, or the quantity of megapixels, is calculated by multiplying the pixels present on the horizontal and vertical sides. This calculation is analogous to the dimensions of the film format, in the sense that an image with a higher number of megapixels corresponds to a film with a larger format, which is thus richer in information. A fundamental difference is that the sensitive surface of film is always entirely exposed, while the exposed area of the digital sensor can be reduced or enlarged using the in-camera processor, thus changing the number of pixels. The ability to vary the image format, and thus the resolution of the image, is established at the image-acquisition stage, when the dimensions of the so-called digital

123

> *Digital sensors provide images with differing resolutions or image formats: small, medium, or large. The term* format *also refers to the proportions between the two sides of the image, similar to the format of the sensor.*

negative are selected. Moreover, the image can be captured by the camera in various formats: large, medium, or small (Fig 4-16).

Resolution is important to the way the image is made available for viewing; the higher the resolution, the larger the size of the print that can be made while maintaining excellent image quality. It is not impossible to obtain a large-format print from a small-format negative, but a loss of sharpness of the image will result, which increases the graininess of the photo. By moving the pixels further apart to obtain a larger print, the eye will begin to perceive the space between each pixel, giving the viewer a grainy impression of the image.

An image with a specific resolution or digital format can be printed onto paper of different sizes. The paper size will dictate the space between the pixels, whether closer together or further apart. Thus, another meaning of the term *resolution* applies to the methods and quality of printing. *Print resolution* refers to the density of pixels on a print, measured in dots per linear inch (dpi) or pixels per inch (ppi). The higher the dpi value of a print, the sharper the image will be (Table 4-2). The maximum resolution perceptible to the human eye is about 300 dpi, or approximately 120 dots per cm; it is useless to print at a higher resolution. When progressively lower dpi values are used for printing, a more and more grainy image will result, as the eye perceives the individual dots of the image. The dpi value is also used to express the resolution capacity of a screen. Its quantity of pixels determines the sharpness of its images and, consequently, its quality.

If a print of a specific size and resolution is desired, the required pixel resolution of the digital image can be calculated prior to taking the shot. For example, a 20 × 30–cm photograph with 300-dpi resolution is planned. The following steps should be taken to determine the quantity of pixels needed to obtain the desired result. First, the centimeters are converted into inches (1 inch = 2.54 cm). The print corresponds to a 7.9 × 11.8–in format. These values are multiplied by 300, the density of dots required; 2,400 × 3,600 dots is about 8 million dots. Therefore, a 20 × 30–cm photograph with 300-dpi resolution requires an image of about 8 megapixels.

The same calculation can be done in reverse to determine the size and quality of a print, given the resolution of the image. An 8-megapixel image has a pixel resolution of about 2,400 × 3,600. Three different formats of varying quality can be printed from this file. The pixel resolution is divided by the desired print resolution to arrive at the dimensions of the print. At a print resolution of 100 dpi, the print will 24 × 36 inches (61 × 91 cm). At a 200-dpi print resolution, the print will be 12 × 18 inches (30 × 45 cm), because 2,400 ÷ 200 = 12 and 3,600 ÷ 200 = 18. At a print resolution of 300 dpi, the print will be 8 × 12 inches (20 × 30 cm).

> For a print, the term *resolution indicates the degree of sharpness of the print. Printing on large-format paper requires image files of large dimensions. An image file can be printed at various degrees of resolution. If a print of a specific degree of quality or dpi is planned, the image resolution can be calculated in advance.*

Table 4-2 Relationship between image resolution and print resolution

Image resolution	Dimensions of the print at 100 dpi	Dimensions of the print at 200 dpi	Dimensions of the print at 300 dpi
18 megapixel	90 x 130 cm	45 x 65 cm	30 x 45 cm
8 megapixel	60 x 90 cm	30 x 45 cm	20 x 30 cm
2 megapixel	30 x 40 cm	15 x 22 cm	10 x 15 cm

Fig 4-16
The Canon EOS D40 has many choices for image format. The far left column has options for large, medium, and small formats, with either lossless compression or higher, lossy compression. The next column adds the option of saving in two formats at the same time, raw and JPEG, with decreasing quality for the JPEG format only. The third column is for the small raw format, which has fewer pixels than the full raw format, and also includes a JPEG file. The number of pixels for the image format selected is specified in the horizontal blue box at the top. The brackets on the right contain the shots remaining with the selected degree of resolution.

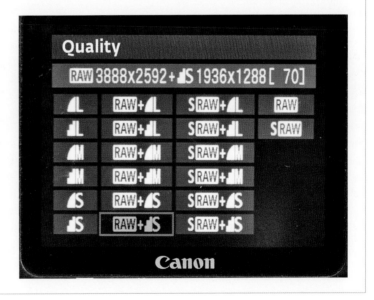

Image depth is a parameter that expresses the intrinsic quality of pixels, or the quantity of digital information they contain. It is measured in bits per pixel (bpp). Image depth is the third dimension of the digital image.

Image Depth and Color Space

The resolution of an image is primarily expressed in two dimensions, the number of pixels on its horizontal and vertical sides. This definition of resolution is insufficient to describe image quality, because it is a purely *quantitative* concept, which, although essential, does not fully indicate the quality of each pixel in terms of the wealth of data and visual information contained in each one.

The brightness and the various hues and nuances of color are information relative to each pixel that can also be expressed. An image can have three dimensions, just as a physical space is identified geometrically in three distinct planes. The third dimension for images, apart from height and width, is the quantity of information present in each pixel concerning brightness and color. These are intrinsic qualities of the pixel. While the other two dimensions of the image, the horizontal and vertical sides, are numeric, the third dimension is virtual.

This parameter, or third dimension, is also referred to as *the color depth of the image*. An image that is said to have great depth is one that contains innumerable variations and gradations of color and brightness.

The image depth is quantified in bits per pixel (bpp). High bpp values indicate better variety and portrayal of the nuances of color in the image.

Chromatic interpolation

The photodetectors in digital sensors can perceive the intensity of the light but are unable to discriminate individual light wavelengths, which are the different hues of color. All photodetectors must be covered by a selective filter, the Bayer filter or color filter array, to differentiate the various nuances of hue. These filters are sometimes referred to as *RBG filters* in reference to the primary colors red, blue, and green.

The function of these filters is to force each photodetector to supply information relative to the brightness of only one primary color. Each pixel must contain at least three primary colors, because all others are obtained by blending. Information about other hues must be calculated by the image processor using a mathematic process called *chromatic interpolation* or *demosaicing*. To recompose the entire range of colors present on a specific pixel, the processor uses the information captured by the adjacent photodetectors, which also have recorded only one of the three color components. The information from each photodetector is normally a variable number ranging from 8 to 16 bits, according to the sampling frequency, which is the parameter that expresses the power of the analog-to-digital converter. The final number of bits needed to describe a pixel is calculated by multiplying the number of bits relative to each channel by three, the number of primary colors. Of this quantity of bits, only one-third have actually been measured and come from the sensor; the other two-thirds

> *Every single sensitive element of the sensor supplies information concerning only one primary color, red, green, or blue. Chromatic interpolation is the mathematic process that calculates the missing hues necessary to complete the color of a pixel. Color space is the mathematic model for representing nuances of color; conceptually, it is equivalent to the color palette of a painter.*

have been estimated and calculated by the image processor.

Unlike traditional digital sensors, the Foveon X3 sensor is configured with three photodiodes on three different levels of a single photosite. Each one is specific for one primary color, resulting in greater accuracy of color, because the measurement value of each wavelength is actual, not calculated.

Color depth is a characteristic related to the structural quality of the sensor and the camera. Average- to high-priced cameras, such as the Nikon D300 and the Canon EOS 40D, have a color depth of 14 bits per channel. There are 14 bits for each of the three RGB primary colors in the raw format, so each pixel has a color depth

of 42 total bits. Some cameras in the high-priced bracket can supply images with a 48-bpp color depth. The compression of data that occurs in the JPEG format reduces the color depth to 24 bpp. This is one reason why the raw file format is more suitable for professional printing.

Color space is a mathematic model for representing color, similar to the color palette of a painter (Fig 4-17). In general, the two color spaces available for cameras are sRGB, developed by Hewlett Packard and Microsoft, and Adobe RGB, developed by Adobe Systems; the former is simpler and more versatile, and the latter is more complete and is better suited for image processing before printing (Fig 4-18).

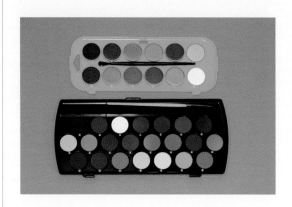

Fig 4-17
A color palette can encompass different numbers of colors with various nuances or variations. A color space is the virtual palette containing a more or less complete range of colors.

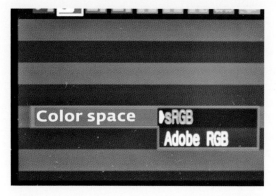

Fig 4-18
The Canon EOS 40D camera has two color space options, sRGB and Adobe RGB.

[
The images from the analog-to-digital converter are stored on a special solid-state electronic device called a memory card. The most common memory-card formats are CompactFlash by SanDisk and Secure Digital by SD Card. They are technically defined as electrically erasable programmable read-only memory devices and are erasable and rewritable ad infinitum.
]

Memory Cards

After the camera processor has acquired and processed an image, its file must be stored. The *memory card* is a removable device inserted into a digital camera for the storage of images.

The main types of removable memory available for SLR cameras have been MicroDrive, made by Hitachi, and CompactFlash, made by SanDisk (Fig 4-19), although the Secure Digital (SD) and Secure Digital High Capacity (SDHC) card formats, licensed by SD Association, are becoming more common. These cards take up less physical space in the camera.

The MicroDrive is a miniature hard disk that works on the principle of magnetization and has moving mechanical parts. The others are memory cards containing semiconducting electronic elements and do not have moving mechanical parts. Semiconductor electronic devices are solid state, whereas traditional electronic devices have valves made of glass and are very fragile. CompactFlash and SD memory cards, which are preferable to MicroDrives because of their durability, versatility, and memory capacity, are categorized as electrically erasable programmable read-only memory (EEPROM).

A CompactFlash card can theoretically be written to, erased, and electronically rewritten ad infinitum. The capacity of memory cards varies; CompactFlash cards are sold at modest prices with 16 GB of memory, but they are also available with a capacity of 32 GB. The evolution of this form of data storage and the progressive increase in its memory capacity appear unstoppable.

A memory card should be chosen according to its capacity (Table 4-3). The image resolution of all intended photographs and the number of photographs to be taken will both determine how much memory capacity is required (Fig 4-20). If the desired image resolution is known in advance, the approximate number of shots that can be stored on the card can be easily calculated by simple division. The dimensions of the image file vary depending on the scene framed, so the capacity of the card is approximate.

Memory cards are further differentiated by the data transfer rate, the speed of writing and reading data. The most efficient cards have a transfer rate of 30 MB/s, but advances in technology may make possible cards with rates of 300 MB/s. While the transfer rate can be very important for those who need to take numerous shots in rapid succession, it is less important for clinical purposes; however, a high transfer rate or speed is useful during transfer of the image to the computer.

Because digital SLR camera users often make use of the high-definition video mode, manufacturers are compelled to design and produce memory cards with an increasingly high transfer-rate capacity. For example, Panasonic has created a new category of cards, Secure Digital Extended Capacity (SDXC), which have shown a capacity of 64 GB and a transfer rate of approximately 100 MB/s in laboratory testing.

Further consideration of the concepts related to the data transfer speed of the cards currently in use, which are more than adequate for clinical purposes, is pointless, because the extraordinarily rapid evolution of technology will render the characteristics of these devices obsolete in an extremely short space of time.

In summary, the use of a card with at least 4 GB is recommended to avoid unexpectedly finding oneself with a full memory card.

Table 4-3 *Available shots as a function of memory-card capacity and image resolution*

Card capacity	Shots available			
	1-MB resolution	**2-MB resolution**	**6-MB resolution**	**12-MB resolution**
128 MB	120	60	20	9
512 MB	500	250	80	40
1 GB	1,000	500	160	80
2 GB	2,000	1,000	320	160
8 GB	8,000	4,000	1,300	650

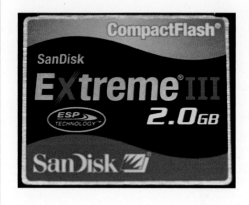

Fig 4-19
This CompactFlash memory card has a 2-GB capacity.

The transfer of image files from a memory card to a personal computer is a fundamental operation in the handling and storing of digital images.

Image Transfer to a Personal Computer

Once images have been stored onto a memory card, they must be transferred to a computer, following the specific procedure of the computer operating system in use. The Windows operating system, for example, has two options for image transfer.

The images can be downloaded without removing the card from the camera. Most cameras are sold with a cord that connects the camera to the universal serial bus (USB) port on the computer (Fig 4-21). After connecting the camera to the computer and clicking the "My computer" icon on the desktop, the contents of the memory card will appear on the screen. The images can be transferred into the desired file using the "copy and paste" command.

Images can also be downloaded by removing the card from the camera and inserting it into a card reader connected to the computer (Fig 4-22); the remaining steps are the same as above. The downloaded images can be catalogued as desired or required. It is strongly suggested that the data be saved in a backup file, because magnetic media can be subject to malfunctioning and might jeopardize the very existence of the data, which would nullify all the precious work carried out.

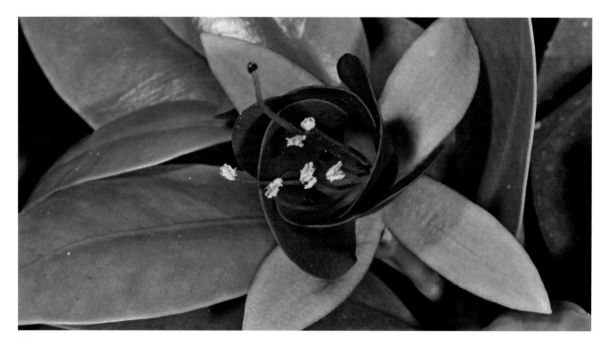

Fig 4-20
A memory card of a certain capacity will hold fewer high-resolution images such as this close-up photograph of a flower.

Fig 4-21a
Images can be transferred to a personal computer with a USB cable.

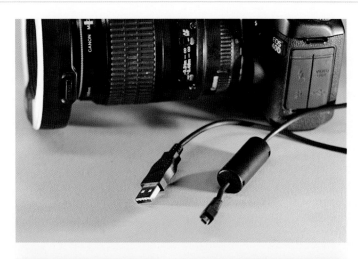

Fig 4-21b
The port on the far right of this Nikon D300 is for the USB cable. Other ports are for high-definition and video signals.

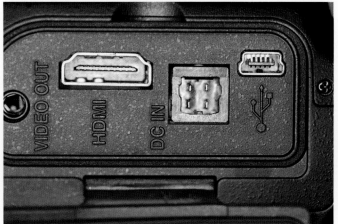

Fig 4-22
The memory card can be inserted into a card reader, which is connected to the computer with a USB cable.

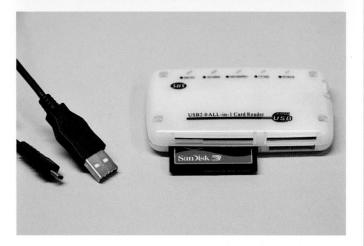

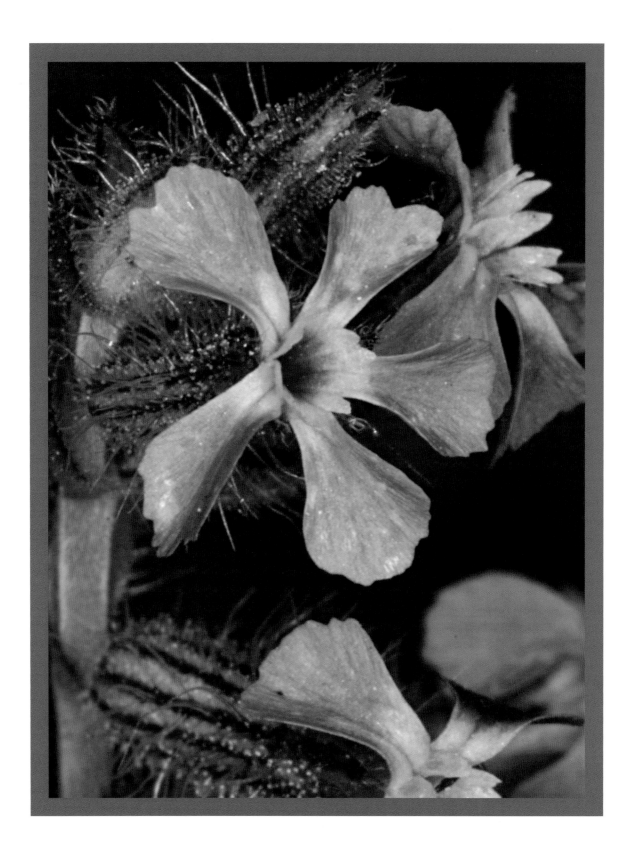

Chapter 5

The Role of Photography in Clinical Practice

[
Photography is a powerful diagnostic instrument because it can suspend time and make space relative. Practitioners can perfect their diagnoses while cultivating their powers of observation and grasp even the most apparently insignificant details. It must be considered a powerful instrument of professional growth.
]

A New Concept: The Photograph As a Diagnostic Instrument

Photography must no longer be considered a privilege for a few practitioners, but a necessity for all those who love their profession and seek to find ever-increasing satisfaction in it. When performed correctly, photography is a great advantage to the modern practitioner in arriving at a diagnosis, which is the most important part of medicine.

Ever more advanced and high-tech diagnostic methods, instruments, and tests, which would have been unimaginable a few decades ago, have burst into our everyday lives. Technology is extremely useful for the practitioner and advantageous for the patient. For example, consider the technology of three-dimensional diagnostic imaging and computer-guided implant surgery. However, practitioners easily develop a tendency to delegate to technology their fundamental role as the careful observer of the patient's condition.

Medicine is the art of scrupulous observation of details and signs—the semiotics of the classical medical tradition—by which the practitioner comprehends the patient's uniqueness and history and formulates an effective therapeutic plan. Photography has often been undervalued as a diagnostic instrument, but in light of the previous statement, it seems appropriate to examine photography more thoroughly and to share knowledge of it as a clinical tool.

Why use photography in diagnosis? It is noninvasive and allows practitioners to continue their examination indefinitely; the photograph is a way of suspending time and making space relative. Time is suspended because a careful examination of the patient's photos can be delayed to a more opportune time, and the patient does not have to be physically present; space becomes relative because an image can be enlarged to show details that might otherwise have been overlooked (Figs 5-1 to 5-3).

Examination of the patient can often be interrupted by negative circumstances beyond the practitioner's control. A difficult surgical procedure with unexpected complications will not predispose the practitioner toward a calm examination of the next patient and can make it more difficult to detect important details.

Moreover, the practitioner's level of experience and sensitivity to details changes over time. A practitioner can look at a photograph at a later date, even years later, and can capture a detail never before perceived. A photograph is an immediate form of communication and transmits a variety of information in a captivating and direct way. Most importantly, however, it is a way of training and improving our insight and powers of observation, because of the constant practice that it requires.

In the practice of dentistry, photography should be given the same dignity as the clinical examination and other instruments. No one technique or instrument is comprehensive in itself; the practitioner must use all of them together to formulate a diagnosis or, more correctly, a diagnostic assessment. In economics, many individual items form a budget. Likewise, a dental diagnosis is the result of a precise and scrupulous patient history, careful listening to the patient, a clinical examination, targeted radiologic examination, a study of models mounted on articulators, and

now, photographic examination. If the role of photography is interpreted in this way, photographic equipment must be considered on a level with other instruments in clinical practice that require the investment of adequate economic resources.

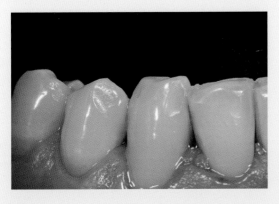

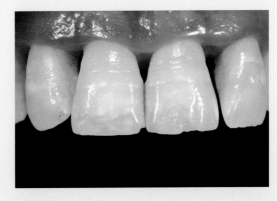

Fig 5-1
Wear facets are clearly visible on the dentition of a man, aged 21 years, with a complaint of bruxism. On this image, the practitioner can fully appreciate details that might have been overlooked during an examination, however accurate. Image taken with a Nikon D300, f = 105–mm macro lens, R1C1 flash system, and two SB-R200 Speedlights.

Fig 5-2
Distinct characteristics of the maxillary incisors are visible in this photograph, taken with a Nikon D300, f = 105 mm– macro lens, and R1C1 flash system.

Fig 5-3
This image of the maxillary central incisors was taken with a Canon EOS 40D at f = 100 mm and an MR-14EX ring flash. When a central incisor must be restored with prosthetics or a conservative restoration, studying the structure and color of the teeth on photographs can be invaluable.

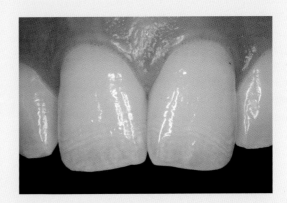

[
Photography allows us to improve communication with patients, because visual language is immediate, comprehensive, and powerful. Better communication between practitioner and patient undoubtedly creates an improvement in the overall quality of oral therapy and in the patient's involvement in the treatment itself.
]

Communication with the Patient

All are aware of the importance and value of images and vision in cognitive, relational, and general communication. The value and communicative power of images have been understood since ancient times. Cave drawings were the original visual expressions of emotional tension. There has always been evidence of this need for images. For example, the Codex Purpureus Rossanensis is an ancient Gospel manuscript illuminated with miniature illustrations, which dates back to the fifth century AD. This codex demonstrates a need to accompany the scripture with images that evoke power and spread the message of faith (Fig 5-4).

The importance of photography in communicating with a patient is rooted in the fact that everyone, whether aware of it or not, communicates more easily by means of images. The immediacy and comprehensibility of visual language, made manifest through images, help the patient to understand their real state of health. How much information would actually reach patients if practitioners were limited to oral communication only? For example, a dentist can say, "After observing your bitewing radiographs, I would like to inform you that you have a Class 2 caries lesion on the mesial aspect of tooth number 2." This is a scientifically complete message, but it is expressed in technical language, and so it is not particularly comprehensible to nonexperts. The patient will understand, generically, that he has a problem but will not be able to appreciate its complexity. However, if the practitioner shows the patient an image of the teeth in question (Fig 5-5) while discussing these details, communication becomes more effective. The patient's compliance, ie, his or her assent to and joint responsibility in the treatment, increases. Survey studies have shown that many patients complain about excessive use of technical terms and jargon. A photograph of a caries lesion can be immediately and easily understood, increasing the patient's acceptance of the treatment plan.

Moreover, patients tend to forget the pain and discomfort once treatment is complete. They may forget their pretreatment condition and thus downplay the value of treatment results. In these cases, a good photograph is worth more than a thousand words and may help to diffuse any tense situations that arise with the patient.

Another circumstance in which a photograph can be very helpful is in the treatment of edentulous patients, in which the practitioner wants to re-create long-lost facial harmony. An old photograph that shows the patient's own facial features, expression, and natural smile will help the practitioner to understand the patient's individual characteristics. This leads to appropriate clinical choices that reproduce or even improve the patient's physical appearance.

Fig 5-4
Table 14 of the Codex Purpureus Rossanensis depicts the parable of the Good Samaritan. (Courtesy of the Diocesan Museum, Rossano Cathedral, Calabria, Italy.)

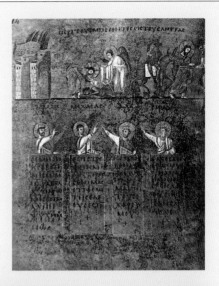

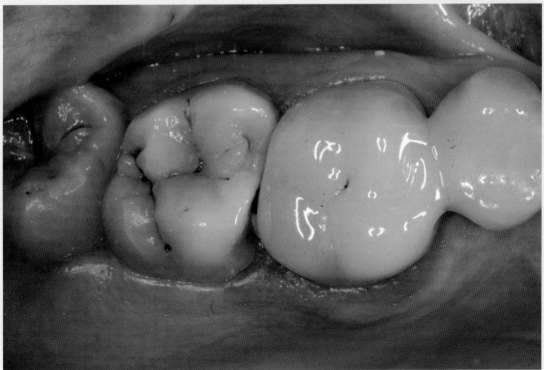

Fig 5-5
This image shows a caries lesion on the mesial surface of the maxillary right second molar. The amalgam tattoo palatal to the first molar is likely secondary to an amalgam buildup in the presence of injured gingiva. The location of this caries lesion on the second molar may be related to poor protection of the adjacent tooth during the buildup procedure on the first molar.

[
A photograph is a useful legal document for demonstrating the correctness of one's work, but it is even more useful in avoiding litigious situations, because it allows the dentist to demonstrate the patient's state of health prior to treatment. Many patients forget pretreatment status and may downplay or unjustly question the dentist's work.
]

Medicolegal Value of Photographic Documentation

The importance of complete medical records in contentious legal situations is well known. Medical records and documentation of the patient's pretreatment condition, supported by photographs of the relevant stages and the conclusion of treatment, demonstrate the quality of the practitioner's work and can serve as proof of appropriate treatment in court. It is certainly reassuring to the dentist to have the medical records in order, together with photographs and necessary data (Fig 5-6). Moreover, photographs can help the dentist to avoid litigation in the first place. As noted previously, all practitioners have experience with patients who, having reached a state of well being, minimize or even forget the experience and negative emotions connected with their earlier condition; they forget the condition of their pretreatment mouth. For this reason, it is an excellent habit to verify the progress of the treatment plan with photographs throughout the course of treatment. These can be shown to the patient while discussing treatment progress in relation to the starting point. This also serves to strengthen both the patient's motivation to complete treatment and his or her faith in the dentist's work.

Photographs may also encourage uncooperative patients to accept responsibility for their dental health. For example, periodontal patients, when asked about their poor oral condition, often reply, "But that's impossible, doctor—I brush my teeth three times a day!" This patient is implying that the ineffectiveness of the treatment must be the dentist's fault. In the author's experience, this can be easily be remedied with a simple photograph. When confronted with photographic evidence, the patient often immediately reevaluates the effectiveness of his daily hygiene regimen (Fig 5-7).

In certain circumstances, a failure to photograph the initial and final oral status of a patient is self-destructive on the dentist's part. In some situations the patient's expectations are naturally elevated, such as tooth whitening, cases with an extremely high esthetic value, and prosthetic implant rehabilitation, and the practitioner must proceed with a proportional amount of caution. At a time when accusations of malpractice are rising exponentially, like a potentially lucrative fad, dentists cannot, and must not, be unprepared to defend their actions and safeguard their peace of mind. Otherwise, dentists run the risk of being held hostage to their patients because they are unable to demonstrate, in a convincing fashion, the patient's preexisting oral status and the quality of their work (see Fig 5-6).

Photographic examinations, whether on film or in a raw digital format (see chapter 4), provide proof, difficult to refute, of the correctness of the dentist's actions and the state of health prior to treatment. The very act of having recorded important and salient diagnostic data demonstrates due diligence on the part of the dentist to the judge.

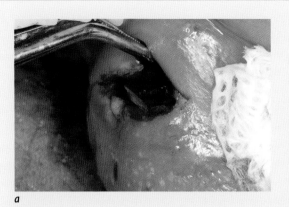
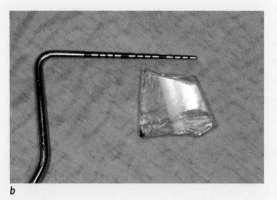

a

b

Fig 5 -6
A fragment of glass remaining after a car accident 4 years earlier is removed from buccal tissue. It was noted at the time of the initial examination. The patient had complained of symptoms, but subsequent treatment of the area by another practitioner did not improve the situation. During the course of a dental examination, the dentist suspected the presence of the fragment, and it was located by palpation. (a) The glass was removed with the aid of a surgical microscope. (b) The actual dimensions of the fragment after removal.

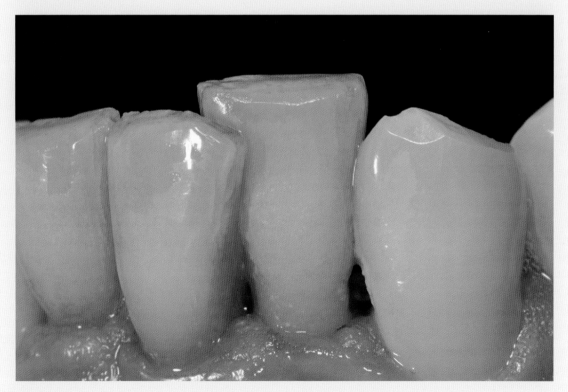

Fig 5-7
This patient's hygiene status at a follow-up appointment after initial treatment is poor. The photograph shows unmistakably poor daily oral hygiene, and, as a periodontal patient, he has a negative prognosis.

[
Photography is a privileged means of communication and a powerful didactic instrument for the entire scientific community because it allows practitioners to judge their own work in a realistic manner, measure themselves against other professionals, and make constant progress.
]

Communication with the Scientific Community

The correct use of photography allows the practitioner to transmit data in a clear and universal language to the entire scientific community, creating opportunities for dialogue and mutual enrichment. Imagine how sterile medical conferences would be if the speakers were limited to mere oral reports or writing complemented by a few images! A photograph allows for the rapid communication of consolidated knowledge and technical innovations. Above all, it allows for the long-term control of the validity of the techniques themselves. For these reasons scientific associations, such as organizations that administer the board certification process for medical specialties, require their own members and aspiring members to document cases according to very precise and standardized operational protocols.

In the following chapters, the specifics of documentation as required by the major scientific organizations will be provided. A reference collection of photographs documenting various clinical stages is useful for many different purposes, including scientific and medicolegal evidence as well as communication with patients, the dental laboratory, and one's clinic staff, whether they be doctors or auxiliary staff (Fig 5-8). Moreover, images can be used to create operational protocols, which can be shared among other professionals in the clinic or in the medical community at large. In fact, the responsibility of educating clinic staff often falls to the practitioner because formal training of staff is often inadequate. Training presentations created with programs such as Power-Point (Microsoft) help the growth and development of the team, which will prove productive and gratifying in the long term.

Photography As an Instrument for Self-Assessment

The operators themselves are the first to benefit from photography when it is used to assess the effectiveness of treatment.

Documentation of surgery and the subsequent recovery allows operators to assess their own work in a detached manner by asking, "Could that incision have been made in a different way?" or "Has that kind of suture helped or slowed down recovery?" (Fig 5-9). Moreover, photographs facilitate interaction with and guidance by more expert colleagues. It is necessary to overcome the natural reluctance to photograph one's work, for fear of having it judged too harshly; however, professional growth happens when one is accustomed to looking for and recognizing one's own mistakes. It is not pleasant, but instead embarrassing, to have to admit to possible mistakes, but only through intellectual humility can a practitioner move forward along the path of science and professionalism. The greatest ally of a person of science is an ability to doubt his or her own certainties.

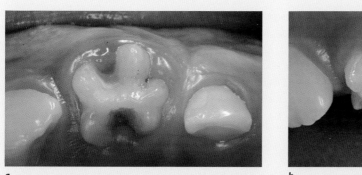
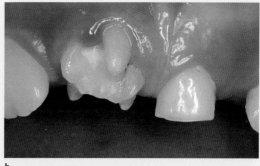

a b

Fig 5-8

Images of a malformed supernumerary maxillary central incisor in a girl, aged 7 years. Because this dental anomaly is rarely seen, it is important to document it. These images are useful for the education of clinic staff and other dental professionals.

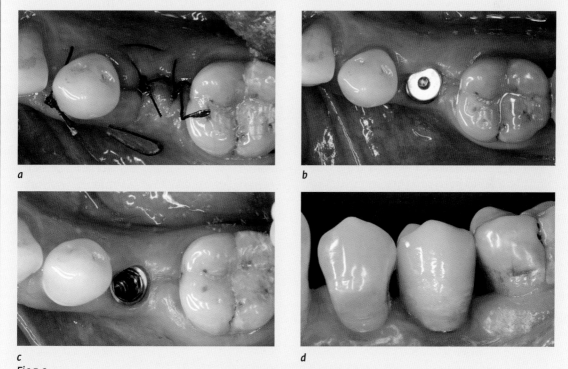

a b

c d

Fig 5-9

(a) An image of an implant site 8 days postoperative. During stage-one surgery, the implant was inserted with vestibular dehiscence. A graft of equal parts autogenous and heterogenous bone, covered by a resorbable collagen membrane, was placed over the site of dehiscence. (b) After 3 months, recession of the soft tissue has exposed the healing cap. The graft lacked sufficient volume to compensate for the physiologic contraction of the soft tissues and the graft itself. (c) Healing is assessed after removal of the healing cap. (d) After insertion of the definitive restoration, the lack of soft tissue volume is apparent in the perception of the gray appearance of the implant site. Because mandibular premolars are typically not in the esthetic zone, the patient decided against a connective tissue graft, which would have eliminated this imperfection. (Courtesy of Barbagallo Dental Laboratory, Lamezia Terme, Calabria, Italy.)

In present times, photography is a precious instrument for dental diagnosis and documentation. The numerous advantages it offers, especially in the perception and communication of information relating to the color and structure of teeth, makes it indispensable in conservative and prosthetic clinical dentistry. The photograph allows us to complete and optimize communication with the dental laboratory.

Photography for Communication with the Dental Laboratory

Success in prosthetic and restorative dentistry can be achieved solely through a harmonious relationship with the dental laboratory. The dentist and the dental technician are not two distinct professional figures, linked merely by a working relationship, but hierarchically and physically separated; they are, rather, professionals with different roles on the same working team, striving together toward professional enrichment and growth.

The dentist is obligated to make it possible for dental laboratory technicians to inspect the patient's hard and soft tissues so that they can contextualize the case and adapt their efforts specifically to that particular patient. This can be achieved simply by sharing photographic images; the patient and the technician do not need to meet, except for the most crucial stages of a complex case. Therefore, for the technician as well as the dentist, photography extends time and space because the patient's photographs are available for as long as necessary for the technician to fully grasp that particular condition (Fig 5-10). This will allow the skilled craftsman to appreciate details that would otherwise be extremely difficult to represent and communicate with a mere description on paper. Imagine how much more gratifying it is for a technician to create a porcelain restoration for a maxillary central incisor while an enlargement of the contralateral tooth is on a screen in front of him.

In esthetic cases, it is the explicit duty of the dentist, and a sign of respect for the work of others, to provide the technician with photographs of the case so that they can best demonstrate their skill.

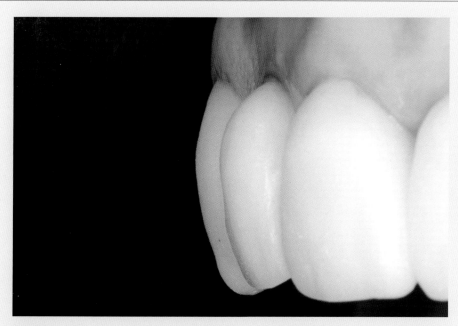

Fig 5-10a
An image of a three-unit full-porcelain fixed partial denture, prior to glazing, highlights the inadequate emergence profile of the pontic that replaces the lateral incisor. This photograph is sent back to the laboratory with the casts for the necessary corrections.

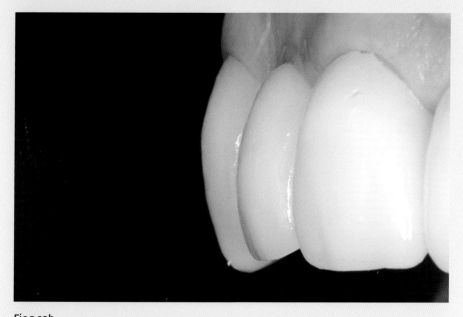

Fig 5-10b
The dental laboratory has corrected the emergence profile. (Courtesy of Aiello-Sirianni Dental Laboratory, Catanzaro, Calabria, Italy.)

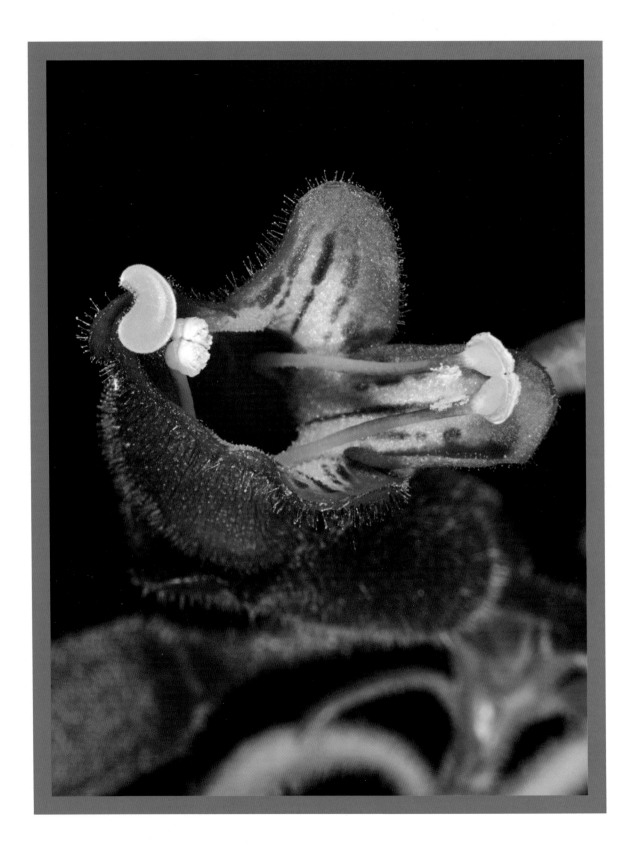

Chapter 6

Camera Settings
for Dentistry

> *Exposure and metering modes are automatic settings controlled by the camera's processor, created for standard situations to facilitate the photographer's work. More often than not, these programs are not suitable for the specific requirements of dental photography.*

Chapters 1 through 4 covered the general principles of photography and its techniques; Chapter 5 highlighted the advantages of and justification for dental photography in the creation of a highly valuable scientific document. This chapter will present the ideal camera settings for clinical purposes. Moreover, the usefulness of the available exposure modes and the effectiveness of the autofocus function will be discussed.

Automatic Exposure Settings

Originally, single-lens reflex (SLR) cameras were fully manual, simple electronic devices. The only sophisticated component was the exposure meter, which provided information about the brightness of the scene but did not directly intervene in the camera's shooting parameters.

When using a fully manual SLR camera, the operator chooses the film sensitivity at the point of purchase and the aperture–shutter speed exposure combination. This simplicity of operation does not mean that a splendid photograph cannot be taken with a manual SLR camera, but it does mean that everything depends on the technique and skill of the photographer.

Modern cameras have evolved considerably because of the continuing miniaturization and perfection of processors and electronic components. All cameras now have automatic settings at various levels of sophistication depending on the manufacturer. Automatic settings mainly control the fundamental shooting parameters of exposure and focusing, which simplify camera use so that the operator can avoid making serious mistakes. However, even with modern cameras, it is always possible to work in a manual exposure mode, which allows the operator to freely choose whatever shooting parameters he or she wishes.

The manual exposure mode is labeled on the camera by the letter *M*. In this mode, the operator selects the timing and aperture and decides whether or not to use the autofocus function. For this reason, the manual mode cannot be considered an automatic setting in the true sense of the words. From a technical point of view, automatic exposure program modes are predefined settings controlled by the camera's processor. They allow the operator to handle the parameters related to the aperture–shutter speed combination independently and rapidly and obtain correct exposure and focusing. It is important to note that, in this sense, correct exposure relates to the logic of the camera, which does not always coincide with the intentions of the photographer.

AUTOMATIC EXPOSURE PROGRAM MODES

- P: Fully programmed mode
- Av or A: Aperture value or aperture priority mode
- Tv or S: Time value or shutter priority mode

The automatic settings have been created to facilitate camera use. The operator chooses the parameter that he or she considers to be a priority, and the camera's processor subsequently sets all other parameters. With all program modes, the operator has the option to deactivate the autofocus function. In P, or *fully programmed mode*, the operator can delegate all decisions to the camera and concentrate on framing and taking the shot (Fig 6-1).

In *Av, aperture priority mode* or *aperture value mode*, the operator sets a specific aperture and allows the camera to set the exposure time. In *Tv, shutter priority mode* or *time value mode*, the operator sets the exposure time and allows the camera to select the aperture value. Cameras have functions that allow the operator to select a particular ISO speed, forcing the exposure and deliberately under- or overexposing the image. In P mode, it is possible to vary the exposure combination by choosing a different aperture–shutter speed combination, which, because of the law of reciprocity, has no effect on exposure (see chapter 1). Changing the exposure combination does influence other characteristics of the photo, such as depth of field or sharpness of an image of a fast-moving subject.

In Fig 6-2, the same composition has been photographed using various program modes, with and without activation of the autofocus function. A critical analysis of the results will justify the camera settings recommended at the end of this chapter. It is the authors' opinion that the best images are those taken with minimum aperture and deactivation of the autofocus function.

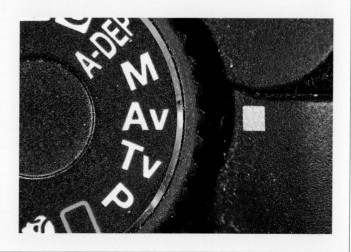

Fig 6-1
The four main automatic exposure program modes are seen on the dial of the Canon EOS 40D. In the image, Av, or aperture priority mode, has been selected. In this mode, the operator selects the aperture according to personal requirements, and the camera's processor subsequently sets the shutter speed (or time) to obtain the best exposure. The operator can vary the aperture–shutter speed combination at any time.

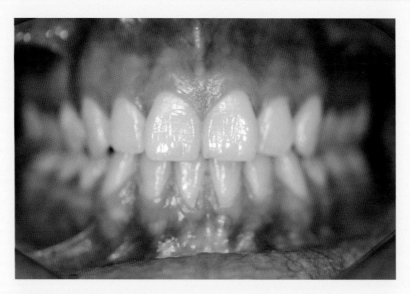

Fig 6-2a
*Photograph taken using the P program mode with the autofocus function activated.
The values automatically set by the camera are t = 1/60 s and f/4. The depth of field is
minimal. The camera has chosen the two maxillary central incisors as the focal point;
the depth of field is so shallow that lateral incisors appear out of focus.*

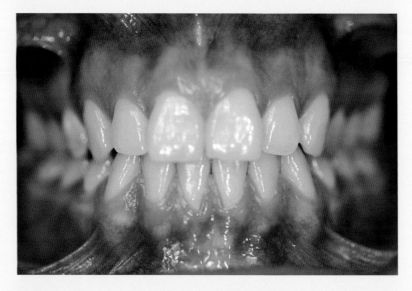

Fig 6-2b
*Photograph taken using the P program mode with the autofocus function deactivated.
The values automatically set by the camera are t = 1/60 s and f/4. The focal point is the
two maxillary canines, and the shallow depth of field is limited to a small area around
them; the teeth distal to the canines and the central incisors appear out of focus.*

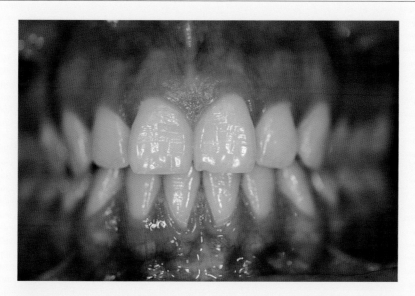

Fig 6-2c
Photograph taken using the Tv program mode at t = 1/200 s, synchronized with default flash, with the autofocus function activated. The camera has automatically set the aperture value at f/3.3. The depth of field is insufficient.

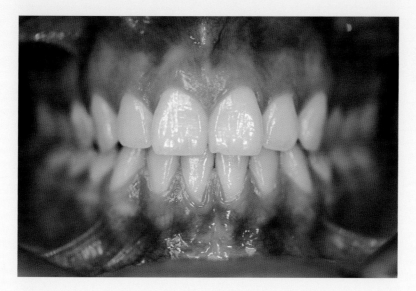

Fig 6-2d
Photograph taken using the Av program mode at maximum aperture (f/3.3) with the autofocus function activated. The camera has set t = 1/60 s. The camera has chosen the two maxillary central incisors as the focal point. The depth of field is insufficient.

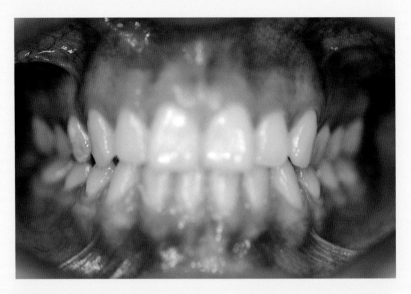

Fig 6-2e
Photograph taken using the Av program mode at maximum aperture (f/3.3) with the autofocus function deactivated. The operator has positioned the focal point on the maxillary canines. A lack of sharpness is apparent because of the shallow depth of field.

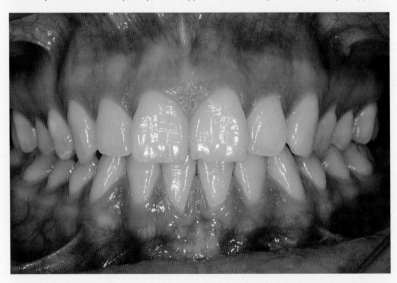

Fig 6-2f
Photograph taken using the Av program mode at minimum aperture (f/45) with the autofocus function activated. The excellent depth of field is attributable to the quality of the lenses. Although the focal point has been automatically positioned by the camera on the maxillary central incisors, only a slight loss of sharpness on the most posterior teeth is observed. Image taken with a Nikon D300, R1C1 flash system, and four SB-R200 Speedlights.

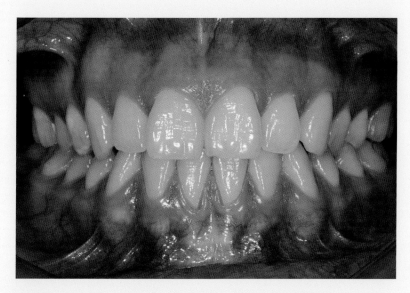

Fig 6-2g
Photograph taken using the M mode with the autofocus function deactivated. The operator has set the parameters at t = 1/200 s synchronized with default flash and minimum aperture (f/45). Image taken with a Nikon D300, R1C1 flash system, and four SB-R200 Speedlights. The focus has been set on the marginal gingiva of the mandibular canines.

> *The autofocus function is invaluable for general use, but in dental photography it must be avoided in favor of manual focusing. The autofocus function prevents the practitioner from selecting the most suitable focal point for the desired composition.*

Automatic Focus Settings

People who take photographs only occasionally or without any particular pretensions are rarely concerned about the problem of the focal point, and they delegate this task to the camera.

The professional or skilled amateur photographer, on the other hand, will tend to use focusing, or the lack thereof, as a powerful means of expression; for example, an effective image frequently requires blurring of the background to eliminate visual tension or to emphasize the framed figure (Fig 6-3).

In the field of documentation, correct focusing is not optional. The practitioner does not have to take artistic photos but is obliged to document reality as faithfully as possible. In light of this premise, the practitioner should gain an understanding of the working logic of the autofocus functions available on cameras and assess them critically in the context of dental requirements.

There are three manners of operation for the focusing function (Fig 6-4). In the *fully automatic focusing mode*, the camera's processor selects the point or points on which to focus, on the basis of its own calculations; then, the lens' motors focus the optics accordingly. In the second mode, the operator selects the points on which to focus, and the camera executes task of focusing by motorization of the lens. In the third mode, *fully manual focusing mode*, the operator selects the focal point using the viewfinder and sets the focus manually with the focusing ring.

Although the fully automatic mode is an easy, logical choice for most operators, it contradicts the obligation of the practitioner to document reality, as already emphasized. The truthful representation of reality does not require the use of artistic effects such as blurring or the use of tools such as filters or illumination. In dentistry, photographs must be focused correctly in all areas and, to achieve this result, the dentist must be able to exercise total control over focusing. In comparing images taken with the same exposure program mode, with and without the autofocus function (see Fig 6-2), it seems clear that, for clinical purposes, the best photographs are those taken with the autofocus function deactivated, or in fully manual mode.

Another fundamental reason to deactivate the autofocus function is the strict relationship between the magnification ratio and the focal distance (Fig 6-5). The act of focusing the lens involves a variation in the focal length and thus in the magnification ratio. If focal point selection is delegated to the in-camera processor, the camera will invariably alter the chosen magnification ratio. In practice, when the autofocus is activated, the adjustment in focus and the change in magnification ratio are so rapid that there is no possibility of control on the part of the operator. The operator is not able to choose the most important parameter for the purpose of documentation, the magnification ratio. The best images are achieved by working in fully manual mode, wherein the practitioner selects the focal point and consequently performs the focusing maneuver as well, using the lens' focusing ring. Focusing is a complex maneuver and requires a specific technique, which involves moving the camera toward and away from the subject. This is, in the author's experience, one of the greatest difficulties faced by those attempting dental photography for the first time. However, with a clear idea of the principles and technique, correct focusing will soon become automatic.

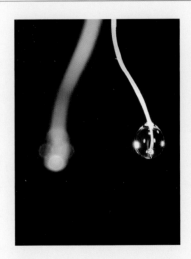

Fig 6-3
The magic of a single drop of water; in the background, another blurred drop. Image taken with a Nikon D300 at f = 105 mm, f/45, t = 1/250 s, R1C1 flash system, manual exposure.

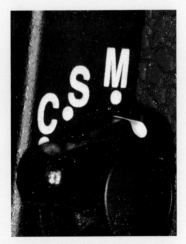

Fig 6-4
The autofocus can be deactivated directly on some cameras, such as the Nikon D300, with a button on the camera itself; however, all lenses have a means of disabling the internal motor that executes the autofocus function.

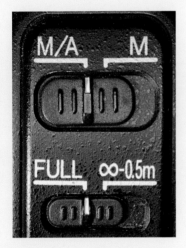

Fig 6-5
The upper switch on this lens turns the lens-integrated motor on and off. The lower switch increases the minimum focusing distance. Increasing the minimum focusing distance reduces the magnification ratio, so this option is not recommended. The minimum focusing distance should always be set at "full."

The depth of field refers to the space in front of and behind the focal plane. Objects within this space are sharply defined on the photographic image. The extent of the depth of field is regulated by the aperture, and the operator can vary this parameter to achieve maximum sharpness in the photograph.

Depth of Field

The ability to control the depth of field is the fundamental reason why the operator, not the camera, must choose the focal point. The focal point and focal plane have been described previously.

The latter term refers to the plane of space where the light rays, after passing through the lens, converge to recompose the framed image onto the sensor plane. The area where objects are perceived as sharp includes the object on which the photographer focuses deliberately and a variable area in front of and behind the focal point. This extent, the depth of field, is delimited in space (Fig 6-6).

This concept is of fundamental importance, because a photograph for documentary purposes must not contain blurred areas because of incorrect use of depth of field; therefore, the practitioner must be in complete control of the depth of field and must know how to handle it effectively.

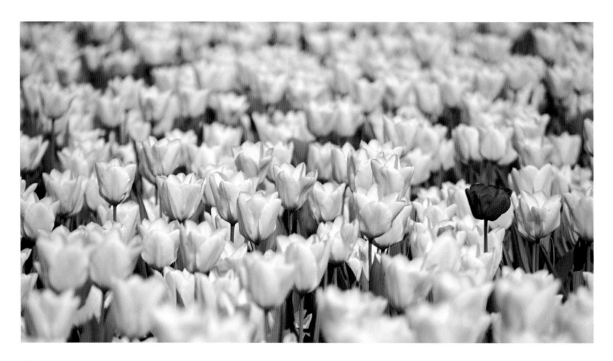

Fig 6-6
In this example of depth of field, the area in front of and behind the plane of the main subject, a red tulip, appears out of focus. Image taken with a Canon EOS 20D, f/6.3, ISO 100, t = 1/800 s.

Close-up dental photography has two priorities: magnification ratio and depth of field

Factors That Influence Depth of Field

Very precise parameters influence the depth of field; the most noteworthy of these is the degree of aperture.

The diaphragm or aperture is the device that allows the gradual and variable passage of light; it is a mechanism that regulates the amount of light. It is also a means of controlling the depth of field. From this point forward, the practitioner should consider the main function of the aperture to be regulation of the depth of field. In particular, when the degree of the aperture decreases, the depth of field increases. Increasing the degree of aperture has the opposite effect, making the area of sharpness more shallow (Fig 6-7). Moreover, the depth of field is asymmetric in relation to the focal plane; the area in which objects are perceived as sharp extends two-thirds behind the focal plane and one-third in front of it. This asymmetry affects the choice of the most appropriate focal point that will fully exploit the depth of field. This concept is so important that the practitioner must learn to consider the aperture solely for this function.

If the first fundamental rule for clinical photography is control of the magnification ratio, the dental photographer's second fundamental rule is priority of depth of field. Mastery of these two factors must become second nature for the dentist. In summary, dental photography is close-up shooting dependent on the magnification ratio and depth of field.

APERTURE AND DEPTH OF FIELD
APERTURE IS THE FUNDAMENTAL DEVICE THAT GOVERNS DEPTH OF FIELD; INCREASING THE DEGREE OF APERTURE DECREASES THE DEPTH OF FIELD, AND VICE VERSA

Low f-stop values = high aperture values = shallow depth of field	High f-stop values = low aperture values = deep depth of field

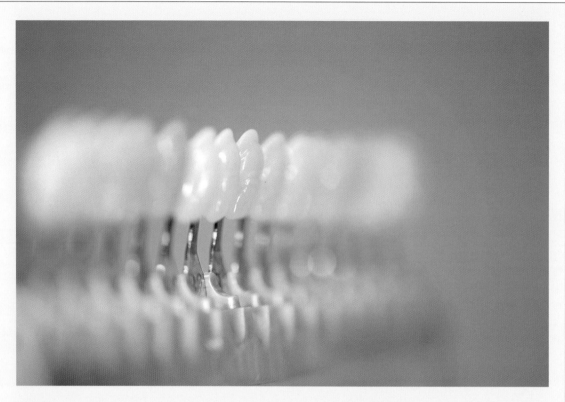

Fig 6-7a
An image of a shade guide taken from a lateral perspective with maximum aperture (f/3.3); the focus is positioned midway along the shade guide, and these elements appear sharp, while all other elements are out of focus. By definition, the depth of field is the area of space in which objects are perceived as sharp. In this image, the depth of field contains only the two elements.

Fig 6-7b
This illustration highlights the approximate depth of field of a dental arch photographed at maximum aperture. The depth of field is asymmetric with respect to the focal plane (dashed line), with two-thirds of its extent behind and one-third in front of the plane.

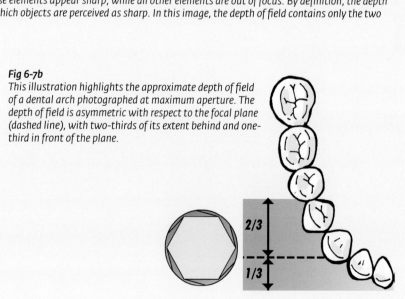

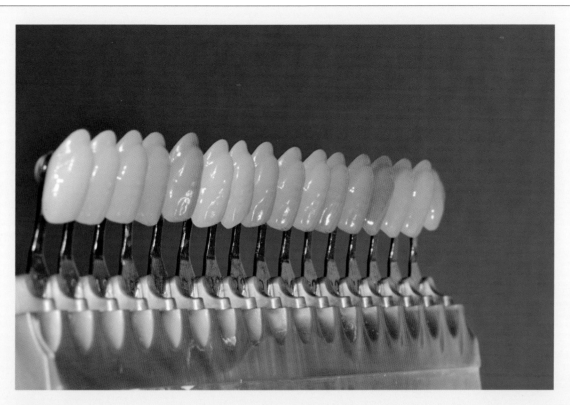

Fig 6-7c
When the shade guide is photographed with minimum aperture (f/32), the depth of field increases. Moreover, the background appears darker, because the aperture is more closed, and therefore the total amount of light striking the sensor is less. The focal point is on the darker central elements of the shade guide. The asymmetry of the depth of field is apparent, and the elements closer to the camera appear slightly less sharp than the ones further away.

Fig 6-7d
This illustration highlights
the approximate depth of field of a dental arch
photographed at minimum aperture.

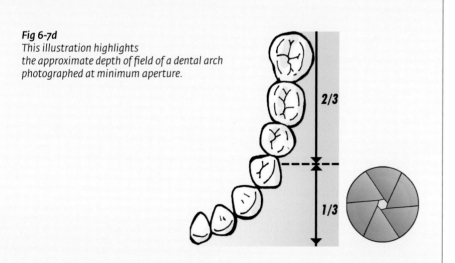

[
Wide-open apertures cause loss of sharpness and reduce the depth of field because they allow for the perception of blurred image circles called circles of confusion. Diffraction mottling is the result of alteration in the path of light rays as they interact with the edges of the aperture diaphragm.
]

Circles of confusion

Circles of confusion are the reason why higher degrees of aperture correspond to shallower depths of field.

The light that strikes the sensor travels from the subject through a system of round lenses, and thus it is conical in shape. This cone of light, which reproduces the image on the sensor, always maintains its depth. It is present on the various planes of space as a circular image, or circle of confusion, parallel to the plane of the sensor and extending in front of and behind it. When the degree of aperture is wide, the circular images immediately in front of and behind the plane of the sensor are very large and can therefore be perceived by the human eye as disks instead of points, and the image will no longer appear sharp. When the degree of aperture is small, the eye will perceive the corresponding images as points, and the image on the sensor will appear sharp.

The size of the aperture affects the dimensions and the visibility of the circles of confusion. Compact cameras, which have minimum apertures as compared to SLR cameras, have a greater depth of field than the latter.

Diffraction mottling

Reduction of the aperture to increase the depth of field is limited by diffraction mottling. This optical phenomenon occurs when light passing through a very small aperture interacts with the edges of the diaphragm. The light rays scatter and change direction, which results in a loss of detail and sharpness of the image. For this reason, f-stop values of f/9 or f/11 allow for maximum image definition by minimizing diffraction mottling while offering good depth of field. Manufacturers, who are well aware of these issues, design macro lenses to maintain the maximum f-stop value (or minimum aperture) compatible with limited diffraction mottling; however, these factors depend on manufacturing decisions and vary from make to make.

Often, the photographer must make a compromise between flawed focusing of the image due to shallow depth of field and a slight loss of detail due to diffraction mottling. It is the author's opinion that it is preferable to accept the latter as the lesser of two evils; loss of sharpness caused by insufficient depth of field is much more perceptible by the observer than that caused by diffraction mottling.

[
An increase in focal length results in a greater magnification ratio and a shallower depth of field. With very high magnification ratios, the depth of field tends to become more symmetric with respect to the focal plane.
]

Relationship Between Focal Length and Depth of Field

Focal length is a second factor, in addition to aperture, that influences the depth of field. As focal length increases, there is a corresponding decrease in the depth of field. The depth of field also decreases as the magnification ratio increases because of the direct correlation between the magnification ratio and the focal length. This relationship is especially noticeable when using a surgical microscope, where very high magnification such as ×25 corresponds to a depth of field only a few mm deep. Moreover, as the magnification ratio increases, the depth of field becomes more symmetric with respect to the focal plane.

A third factor that influences depth of field is the distance between the framed subject and the lens. Because of the inversely proportional relationship between the magnification ratio and the lens-object distance; if the object is brought closer to the lens, the magnification ratio will increase, and consequently the depth of field will decrease.

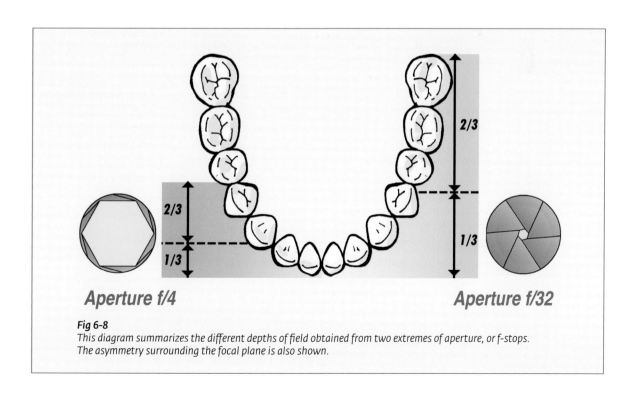

Aperture f/4

Aperture f/32

Fig 6-8
This diagram summarizes the different depths of field obtained from two extremes of aperture, or f-stops. The asymmetry surrounding the focal plane is also shown.

[

The various automatic exposure and focusing settings are not useful for the special requirements of dental photography; their use should be excluded from routine work. The concept of depth of field has extraordinary value, so to maximize it, the dentist is obliged to use the manual program, the maximum f-stop value, and a flash to compensate for the exposure.

]

Camera Settings Related to Clinical Requirements

In summary, maximizing the depth of field and the extent of the area of sharpness requires working with minimum aperture for all intraoral photographs; however, for extraoral photographs, a wider aperture can be used. Depth of field is inversely proportional to the magnification ratio, and the lower magnification ratio and shallower depth of field required for extraoral photographs allow the use of lower f-stop values, or wider aperture.

As a general rule, a high f-stop value or smaller aperture implies a decrease, in absolute terms, in the amount of light that strikes the sensor. According to the law of reciprocity, the reduction in light can be offset by increasing the exposure time considerably. If the amount of light is reduced, the exposure time must be increased; however, significant increases in exposure time inevitably result in blurred photographs.

Therefore, an additional source of light, the flash, becomes indispensible in optimizing exposure in the presence of a small aperture while maintaining acceptable exposure time. The subject of the flash is very important and is examined thoroughly and exhaustively in chapter 8.

The above considerations have been integrated into the recommendations for ideal camera settings listed in the box on the next page.

Automatic exposure program modes: It is advisable to forgo these modes and to work in fully manual mode because this allows the operator to choose the time and aperture according to clinical needs. Alternatively, the Av mode can be used if the value suitable for the desired image is set.

Aperture: Minimum aperture is recommended for all intraoral photographs. When the magnification ratio is low, as in extraoral photographs, values of f/11 or even f/9 should be used to optimize the power of the flash. For photos of the smile or lips, an intermediate aperture such as f/22 is sufficient.

Exposure time: Exposure should be synchronized with the flash; this occurs automatically with dedicated flash units. Otherwise, a suitable setting is t = 1/125 s.

Autofocus: This option should be deactivated in favor of working in fully manual mode. Motorization of the lens should be turned off.

Sensor sensitivity: Standard ISO speeds of 100 or 200 are recommended, depending on the characteristics of the camera. In the presence of additional light sources such as a flash, it is necessary to minimize background electronic noise, which can be generated at high ISO speeds.

White balance: Generally, the auto white balance function fully satisfies dental photography needs. Alternatively, the flash mode can be selected, if the result of using the automatic mode is unsatisfactory.

Measurement of exposure: It is recommended to select a mode that calculates the exposure based on the whole scene in the frame, weighted toward the center. Other modes of measurement may be preferable in the presence of strongly contrasting levels of brightness, or when the camera's design characteristics require it.

Correction of exposure: For intraoral photographs, the camera should be set for a slight overexposure of ⅔ or 1 exposure value (EV) to compensate for the camera's tendency to underexpose in the presence of white objects (see chapter 3).

SUMMARY OF RECOMMENDED CAMERA SETTINGS

Exposure program:	Manual exposure mode or Av mode	**ISO speed:**	100 /200
Autofocus:	Deactivated	**White balance:**	Auto white balance or flash mode
Lens motorization:	Deactivated	**Shutter speed:**	Synchronized with flash
Aperture:	Minimum aperture (f/32) in intraoral images, relatively open (f/11) in extraoral images	**Measurement of exposure:**	Calculated on entire scene, weighted toward the center
		Shooting menu:	Standard or neutral

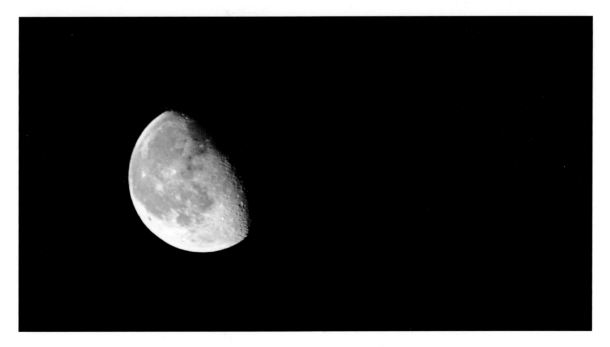

Fig 6-9
This image of a waning moon was taken with a very low magnification ratio, 1:∞, which allows the depth of field to extend for hundreds of kilometers even with a fairly wide aperture. Image taken with a Canon EOS 20D, f = 70-300-mm lens (Sigma), f/9, t = 1/30 s; the M mode and a tripod were used.

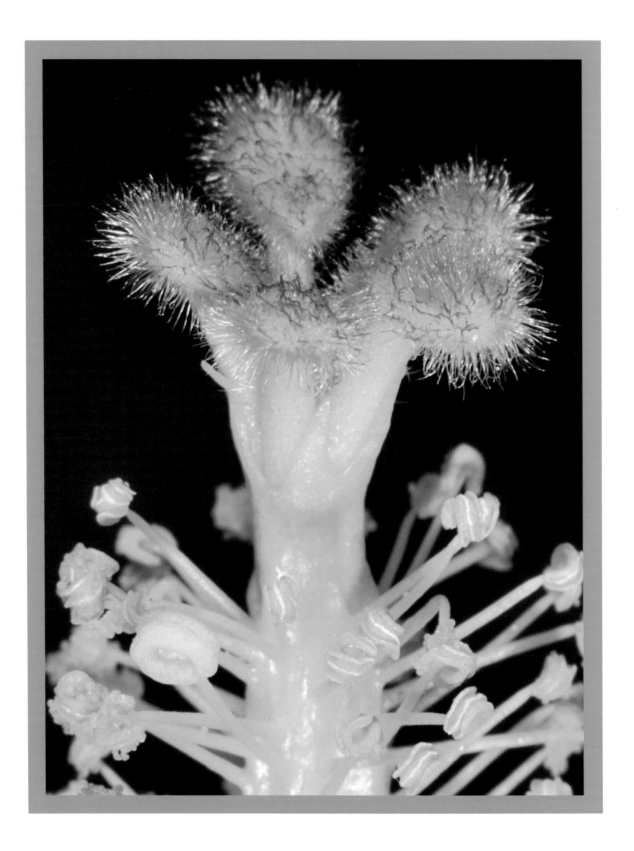

Chapter 7

The Orthography of Images

[*The term* frame *is used to mean the area of space included and visualized in the photographic image. What makes up the frame is the choice of the magnification ratio, which is the mere expression of the photographer's will.*]

Concept of Framing

The frame is the area of space included and visible in the photographic image. As previously discussed, the magnification ratio is the means used to distinguish elements that are important to include in the image from those that must be excluded.

To repeat the one essential rule that underlies the reasoning and methods of close-up dental photography, the two priorities are magnification ratio and depth of field.

A corollary of this general rule is that the choice of the magnification ratio determines the frame. Related to this rule are two problems particular to dentistry. First, the practitioner needs to use soft tissue retractors and specially shaped mirrors for many types of images, especially for posterior and occlusal views. Second, the center of the frame often does not coincide with the desired focal point. There is often a difference between the point at which the camera is aimed and the point to be put into focus. The tasks of framing and shooting are facilitated when these two points coincide. When these points differ, additional effort and thought are required to obtain an excellent documentary photograph.

Accessories for Intraoral Photography: Retractors and Mirrors

All intraoral images require the use of accessories to retract the soft tissues and allow correct framing with respect to the desired magnification ratio. Moreover, they remove unwanted peripheral elements or elements of visual tension. Cheek retractors are made of plastic or metal, in various shapes and sizes, and are chosen according to the image to be taken (Figs 7-1a and 7-1b). Some photographs require the aid of mirrors, which are also available in a variety of shapes to reflect the targeted area (Figs 7-1c and 7-1d). Without the aid of these devices, it is impossible to directly photograph the complete arch from the occlusal aspect, because to do so would exceed the anatomical limitations of the patient's mouth opening (Fig 7-2a). Similarly, it is not possible to take a lateral view without a mirror, because the cheek requires complete retraction (Fig 7-2b).

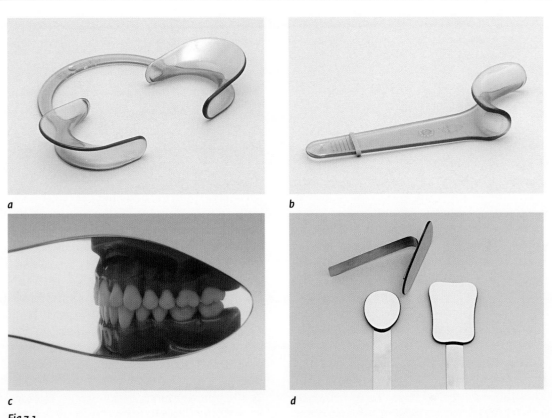

Fig 7-1
Cheek retractors (a and b) and mirrors (c and d) are available in various shapes and sizes for different kinds of images and patients.

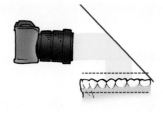

Fig 7-2a
An occlusal photograph of the entire arch requires the use of appropriate mirrors. This image cannot be framed directly because of the anatomical limitations of the patient's mouth opening.

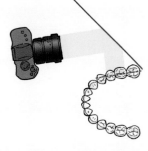

Fig 7-2b
The presence of perioral tissues prevents the practitioner from taking certain shots directly. In this lateral photograph of arches in occlusion, the use of appropriately shaped mirrors is necessary to photograph a reflected, rather than direct, image. The image will not be real, but instead will be reflected and inverted; with appropriate programs for handling the image, it is easy to invert the image again and render it true to life.

[
Special retractors for the perioral soft tissues are required to frame an intraoral shot correctly. In addition to retractors, some photographs also require the aid of specially shaped mirrors, whose reflecting metal layer is deposited directly onto the surface to avoid the formation of secondary images.
]

Characteristics of Mirrors for Dental Photography

Mirrors for clinical photography have special characteristics that differentiate them from those for everyday use. The reflecting layer of ordinary mirrors is deposited by vacuum electrolysis on the surface opposite the reflecting side. This layer, generally aluminum, is covered by the glass itself, which both supports and protects it.

Two problems result from this position of the reflecting layer. First, the mirror's reflecting power is reduced. Second, a double image is reflected by the shiny surface of the glass, called a *ghost image* (Fig 7-3a).

To avoid these two problems, mirrors for scientific and medical use are constructed differently. The reflecting metal layer is deposited directly onto the surface of the glass support (Fig 7-3b). Because the glass does not cover and protect the reflecting layer, these mirrors are incredibly delicate and must therefore be cleaned with extreme care and nonabrasive materials to avoid scratching the surface.

To increase its reflecting power and to avoid corrosion problems, the metallic layer is often treated with rhodium vapors. This metallic element has an extremely high power of reflection and also protects the mirror from corrosion.

Aiming and Focal Points

The aiming point is the center of the frame chosen by the operator using the magnification ratio. The focal point is the area of the frame to be perceived most sharply. This point is important because it divides the depth of field into two generally asymmetric parts. The operator must select the correct extent of the depth of field and position of the focal point.

In a frontal view, the aiming point must be chosen so that the framed subject is perfectly symmetric. Specifically, when the practitioner photographs the arches in occlusion from a frontal view, the aiming point is the intersection of the line between the two arches and the median line between the central incisors. This position divides the vertical and horizontal space into equal parts and frames the four quadrants symmetrically (Fig 7-4). The practitioner will be naturally inclined to focus on the chosen aiming point, but the result will be unsatisfactory because of the depth of field. Focusing on the central incisors results in a blurred image of the molar area, because the depth of field extends behind and in front of the focal plane. Focusing on the central incisor wastes the extent of image sharpness that is in front of the central incisors themselves.

> *To obtain an ideal image, it is essential to distinguish the aiming point, which represents the center of the correct frame, from the focal point, which is the area of the arch where the practitioner should focus to obtain optimal depth of field. In some frames, the two points may coincide, but most often, they are different.*

Because the depth of field extends one-third in front of and two-thirds behind the focal plane, the correct focal point will be the mesial aspect of the canines in a short arch and the distal aspect of the canines in a particularly long arch. This will divide the areas perceived as sharp according to the extent of the depth of field (see Fig 7-4).

Moreover, the practitioner must play an active role in focusing because it is not possible to delegate the task of focal point selection to the autofocus device. For these reasons, the practitioner must use the fully manual focusing mode.

In summary, the practitioner must first correctly compose the frame according to the magnification ratio and spatial symmetry. To do so, the camera is aimed at the center of the image as seen on the viewfinder. Then, the practitioner focuses on a suitable point that will exploit the maximum depth of field. Although in certain circumstances the aiming and focal points may coincide, conceptually, they must be kept distinct (Figs 7-5 and 7-6).

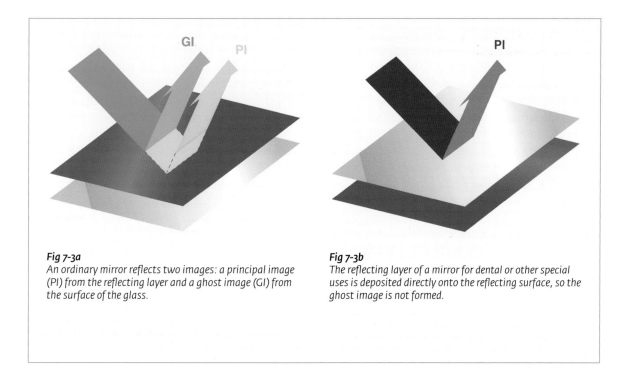

Fig 7-3a
An ordinary mirror reflects two images: a principal image (PI) from the reflecting layer and a ghost image (GI) from the surface of the glass.

Fig 7-3b
The reflecting layer of a mirror for dental or other special uses is deposited directly onto the reflecting surface, so the ghost image is not formed.

167

[
The correct focusing technique is synchronized adjustment of the lens' focusing ring and the operator-subject distance. After setting the desired magnification ratio with the focusing ring, the practitioner focuses the image with small backward and forward movements and simultaneous minimal adjustments of the focusing ring.
]

Focusing Technique

Mastering the correct focusing technique is often problematic for the aspiring clinical photographer. The importance of the magnification ratio in the composition of the frame has already been emphasized. Other essential elements of a good photograph are exploitation of the depth of field and selection of a correct focal point.

It is important to bring these two parameters, magnification ratio and focusing, in harmony with each other, but practical considerations make this task difficult. The author considers the 105-mm macro lens to be the gold standard for lenses for dental photography. Its focusing ring, which adjusts the magnification ratio, also sets the focus. This is not a design flaw on the part of the manufacturers, but a necessity that originates from optical principles. As the practitioner moves closer to the subject to increase the magnification ratio, the light rays reflected from the subject are recomposed as an image on a focal plane positioned behind the sensor; the opposite happens upon moving away from the subject. The act of focusing involves moving the lens away from or nearer to the sensor, until the focal plane coincides with the sensor. This maneuver is essentially a small variation of the focal length, which is the distance between the optical center of the lenses and the sensor plane. However, the focal length is strictly linked to the magnification ratio; as the focal length increases, the angle of view decreases, and the magnification ratio

increases. In summary, the act of focusing with the macro lens' focusing ring alters the focal length and the magnification ratio because these two parameters are inseparable.

The focal length inscribed on a lens is the focal length with the focus set at infinity for reasons of standardization. When the focus is adjusted, the distance between the center of the lens and the focal plane is altered. This distance, by definition, represents the focal length.

In clinical practice, the following steps should be taken to focus the image. First, because the magnification ratio is the priority for composition of the frame, this parameter must be set with the focusing ring, according to average reference values that will be given in part two of this book. However, a single magnification ratio that is strictly valid for every standard type of image does not exist, because each mouth has its own dimensions, so the practitioner must make slight adjustments to the magnification ratio using the lens' focusing ring.

Second, once the correct magnification ratio has been set, it is almost always necessary to adjust the focus; however, it is important to remember that by varying the focus, the magnification ratio, which was previously chosen and set, is altered.

Third, after the magnification ratio has been finalized, the practitioner no longer focuses using the lens focusing ring, but by moving closer or further away from the subject with slight backward and forward movements. Obviously, the practitioner must still make minimal adjustments to the magnification ratio with the focusing ring. He or she will learn that the magnification ratio and focus are set by two synchronized adjustments: the focusing ring and the distance from the subject (Fig 7-7).

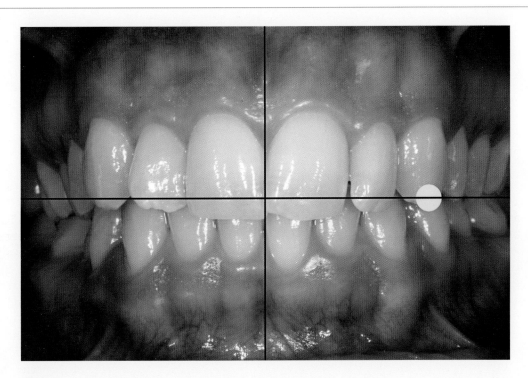

Fig 7-4
In this frontal view of both arches in occlusion, the aiming point is the center of the frame, represented by the intersection of the two lines. This does not coincide with the focal point (yellow dot), which is the mesial or distal aspect of the canine, depending on the anteroposterior dimensions of the arch.

Fig 7-5
In this occlusal view of the maxillary arch, the aiming point is the center of the frame, and the focal point is the gingival margin of the second premolar.

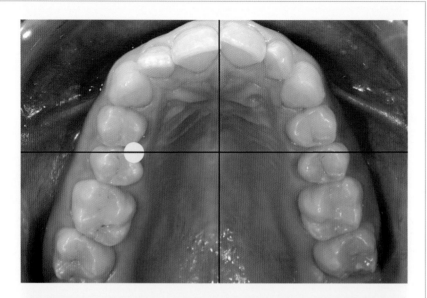

Fig 7-6
In a lateral view taken with a mirror, the aiming point and focal point may coincide.

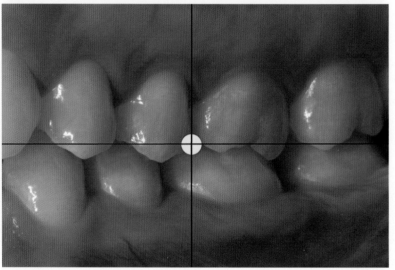

> The spatiality of the frame is the photographer's perspective or viewpoint of the subject framed in the image. It is the pure and simple expression of the photographer's will and an irreversible element of the shot because it cannot be corrected by an image-retouching program.

Spatiality of the Frame and Orthography of Images

The analysis of the focal and aiming points is a good transition to the concept of the *spatiality of the frame*. This term means the way in which the photographed object is positioned in space with respect to the observer's point of view. The spatiality of the frame is decided by the photographer at the moment that he or she selects a particular perspective; it is the pure and simple expression of the photographer's choice or skill. Unlike other parameters, such as exposure or magnification ratio, which can, to some extent, be subsequently corrected at the final stage of image processing, the perspective of the frame is irreversible (Fig 7-8).

At the moment of choosing the perspective and taking the shot, the perspective and the focal point can no longer be corrected. The fundamental concept that underlies the philosophy of dental photography, ie, that it is a field of scientific photography for documentary purposes, makes the perspective or the spatiality of the frame an essential element for the reproducibility of that frame and the effectiveness of communication. The orthography of a language is a set of codified rules that enables people to correctly communicate in writing with others who use that same language. Because photography is, at its essence, a medium for writing with light or a writing system of visual language, it is the author's opinion that an "orthography of images" must exist. The correct spatiality of the frame can, and must, represent the orthography of images, or the correct formal writing of a particular image. Only by writing an image correctly can the practitioner create a visual message that is immediately comprehensible and universally legible without effort on the part of the observer.

The practitioner's efforts must be directed toward excellent documentation because the aim is to achieve what the ancient Greeks called *kalligraphia* (beautiful writing) with light and images (Fig 7-9). The correct method and rules will obtain excellent results in a systematic manner, not in a fortuitous or random way. To quote John Ruskin, "Quality is never an accident; it is always the result of intelligent effort."

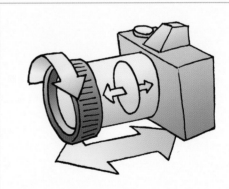

Fig 7-7
The act of focusing is performed by simultaneously maneuvering the lens' focusing ring and moving the camera away from and closer to the subject. Both actions contribute to the determination of the final magnification ratio.

> *A dentist who photographs writes documents with light; as in all other forms of writing or communication, there must be rules, or orthography, for its correct form. The spatiality of the frame represents the orthography of the image or the correctness of visual writing. With these rules of spatial orthography, the practitioner is able to assess the correctness of an image from the point of view of its documentary value.*

Fig 7-8a
This image has been taken from a lateral and superior perspective. Most of the two left quadrants and part of the two right quadrants are not visible in the image, and it will be difficult to reproduce because there are no clear planes of reference. This parameter of an image cannot be corrected by any retouching program.

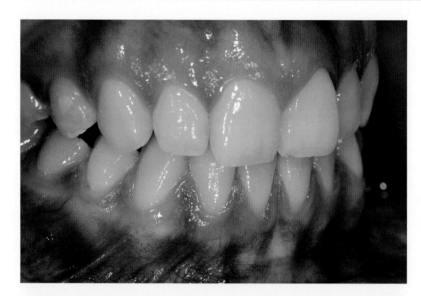

Fig 7-8b
This image has been taken from an inferior perspective and is not acceptable as a scientific document because it appears to have been taken at random without precise rules of spatiality. This photograph is not correctable.

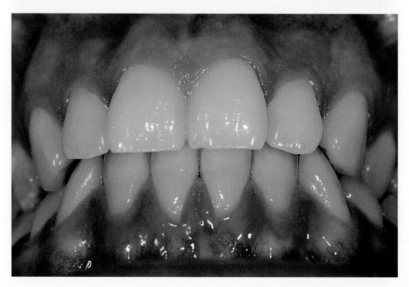

[
The zero-coordinate rule is the fundamental principle for the orthography of an image because it allows the practitioner to create images that are reproducible with respect to the two reference planes of space.
]

The Fundamental Rule for the Orthography of Images: Zero Coordinate

The first two rules for the orthography of images have been discussed: magnification ratio priority and depth of field priority. The third rule, and a natural complement to the others, is the zero-coordinate rule.

These three concepts, in the author's opinion, represent the essence of a rational, scientific approach toward clinical photography. The third rule has been introduced because, with its simplicity and immediacy, it can greatly benefit all those who are taking their first steps in dental photography.

The formulation of this concept was inspired by general anatomy, a discipline in which the position of organs and tissues in space are described using virtual spatial planes of reference. By analogy, dental photography requires planes of reference for the correct orientation of an image in space. In fact, all aspects of professional dental practice involve planes of reference. For example, the prosthodontist visualizes the three spatial planes of the tooth to achieve perfect parallelism of the tooth preparation. In the same way, the implantologist must always take into account specific planes of reference when inserting a prosthetically guided implant.

There are two planes of space that concern dental photography:

- The sagittal plane, which coincides with the median line of the face and teeth; this is the classic plane of general anatomy.
- The axial plane; in the anteroposterior dimension, it represents the occlusal plane; from a frontal view, it coincides with the smile line.

The practitioner must learn to mentally visualize these planes because an image must be framed with respect to and in relationship with them. The zero-coordinate rule originates and takes its meaning from these planes of reference. This rule establishes that the observer must not perceive any angulation of the two planes of reference, but only a visual angle of 0 degrees (Figs 7-10a and 7-10b).

If the arch is observed by standing exactly in front of it, the observer's eyes are at an angle of 0 degrees with respect to the sagittal plane; in other words, the observer does not perceive a plane, but an absolutely vertical line. As the observer moves laterally (Fig 7-10c), the angle between the eyes and the plane increases, so that the plane becomes more and more visible and is fully visible when the observer is perpendicular to it, at an angle of 90 degrees to the plane (Fig 7-10d).

The zero-coordinate rule establishes that any change in perspective with respect to the sagittal plane creates an unwanted asymmetry, which prevents the observer from perceiving the photographed subject correctly (Fig 7-10e).

APPLICATION OF ZERO-COORDINATE RULE FOR SAGITTAL AND AXIAL PLANES
FRONTAL IMAGES: THE OBSERVER MUST NOT PERCEIVE ANY ANGULATIONS OF THE TWO ORTHOGONAL PLANES OF REFERENCE, SAGITTAL AND AXIAL, WHICH MUST BOTH APPEAR AT 0 DEGREES. THE AXIAL PLANE, CORRESPONDING TO THE SMILE LINE, MUST NOT SHOW ANY INCLINATION.
LATERAL IMAGES: THE OBSERVER MUST NOT PERCEIVE AN ANGULATION OF THE AXIAL REFERENCE PLANE. WITH THE USE OF MIRRORS, IT IS ACCEPTABLE TO HAVE A MINIMUM ANGULATION OF THE SAGITTAL PLANE, WHICH IS NORMALLY PERPENDICULAR TO THE OBSERVER'S EYES.

Similarly, when the perspective of the axial plane changes, the observer will perceive a change in angulation, not laterally, but from above or below (Fig 7-10f). In observing the smile line, which is the axial plane from a frontal view, the zero-coordinate rule is in effect when the smile line appears perfectly horizontal, without any inclination with respect to the frame (see Fig 7-10a).

Any changes in perspective from 0 degrees are extremely difficult to measure and to reproduce, making any attempt to precisely replicate the image problematic; in scientific photography, the only easily reproducible angles of perspective that can be manually set are 0, 90, and 180 degrees.

A mask for the fixation of the skull and its connection to the camera could make any image reproducible, even one taken at an arbitrary angle, but its use would be a lengthy and unrealistic task, especially if this mechanism existed only for photographic purposes.

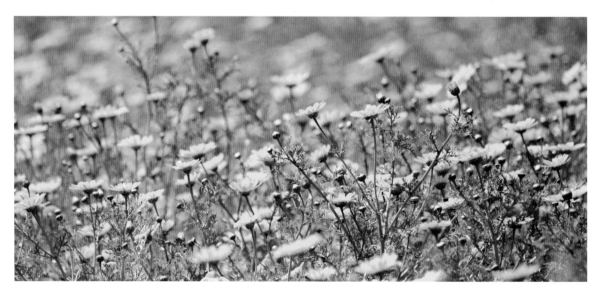

Fig 7-9
This image is an excellent example of kalligraphia. The photographer has used the subject matter and light to convey emotion.

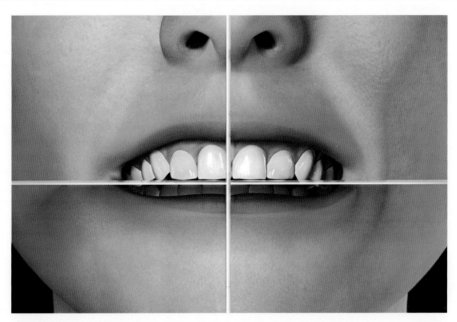

Fig 7-10a
The two planes of reference at right angles to each other. The planes appear as lines and can be considered virtual from this perspective.

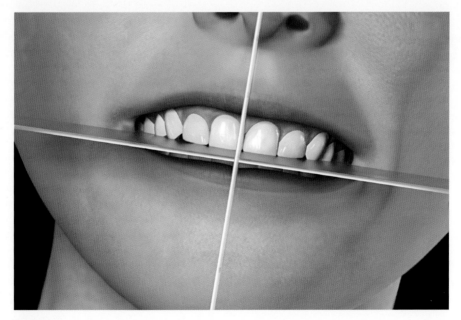

Fig 7-10b
The smile line is seen at an angle; this is totally unacceptable in a clinical photograph.

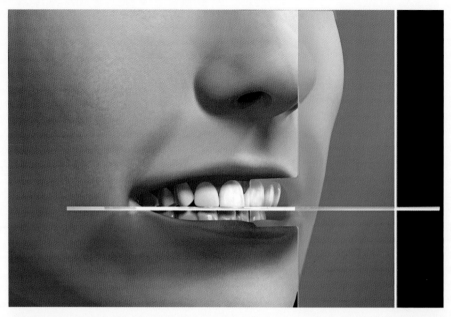

Fig 7-10c
As the perspective becomes more lateral, the sagittal plane can be perceived. Because the observer's perspective is at an angle, this is not a zero-coordinate view.

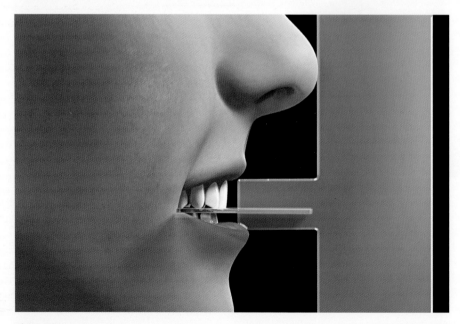

Fig 7-10d
From a fully lateral perspective, the sagittal plane is perpendicular to the observer. The perspective of the axial plane has not changed; it is still seen as a line.

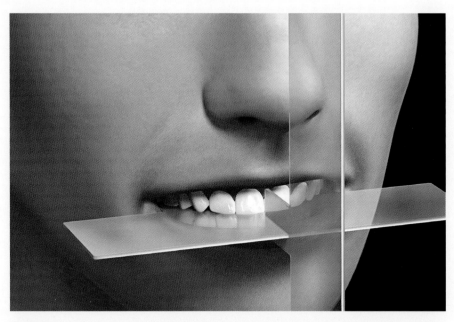

Fig 7-10e
From this perspective, both planes are perceived as planes rather than as lines. This condition is difficult to reproduce photographically, because the precise angle of vision in degrees is unknown.

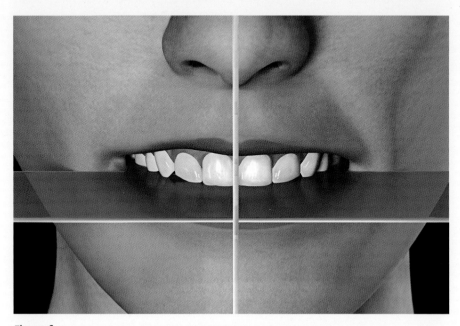

Fig 7-10f
As the observer's perspective becomes more superior, the axial plane can be perceived. This is not a zero-coordinate view.

> [*The zero-coordinate rule provides a precise reference point for frontal images; in lateral or occlusal images taken with the aid of mirrors, it is not possible to position oneself perfectly, but the zero-coordinate rule provides a valid criterion for a frame that is reproducible.*]

Zero-Coordinate Rule Applied to Various Images

It is clear that the zero-coordinate rule is subject to variation according to the type of image framed. This rule remains valid for all intraoral frontal views, such as views of the arches in occlusion, the anterior teeth, or the incisors, because both planes, axial and sagittal, are perceived as lines rather than as planes.

In theory, the concept of zero coordinate is different for lateral views because the sagittal plane is not at 90 degrees, or perpendicular to the observer's eyes. In practice, the concept changes very little: the plane of reference of lateral views is the axial plane, which must be perceived at an angle of 0 degrees by the observer. The universality of this rule can be demonstrated as follows. In lateral views, the frame and, therefore, also the observer's eyes must be perpendicular to the sagittal plane. Because the sagittal plane is always perpendicular to the axial plane, this statement simply reiterates the fact that the axial plane must be perceived at 0 degrees, as a line rather than a plane.

The use of mirrors complicates this rule because the spatiality of the frame then refers to the planes of space represented in the mirror. It will not always be possible to frame a photograph in a mirror and adhere to the zero-coordinate rule, but the rule serves as a valuable reference point for achieving the best possible image (Fig 7-11).

In summary, for intraoral images practitioners should position themselves correctly with respect to the two planes of space, which provide clear reference points for image perspective and spatiality. Doing so will make the image reproducible and, therefore, comparable over time. The concept of the orthography of images is a valid instrument for obtaining excellent images, from both a documentary as well as an esthetic point of view.

For extraoral images, the zero-coordinate rule should be followed in frontal and lateral views as necessary for basic documentation of a case; however, it is correct and sometimes desirable to search for unusual perspectives that will bring out particular expressions of the patient or other details considered important and worthy of being documented. Moreover, some situations require the use of unusual perspectives that deviate from the zero-coordinate rule in intraoral shots.

General rules governing the orthography of images are necessary, but they do not always allow for exhaustive documentation of details or unusual aspects that the practitioner would like to communicate. Because the photographic medium is noninvasive, it permits the practitioner to explore and to search for distinct views for effective communication, especially in the field of esthetic dentistry. These images can be defined as creative photographs.

Creative Photographs

In general, operational protocols exist out of necessity, to avoid errors and to simplify matters, but this does not mean that they are appropriate or effective in all situations. It has been said that "as a rule, there must be an exception to every rule," which can be interpreted to say that the operator must always have a minimum of discretionary power.

No rule should prevent the practitioner from playing with light and searching for particular perspectives if they help to document or describe facts and situations that do not fully emerge in the usual views (Fig 7-12). A particular perspective can be effective in revealing aspects such as the texture of surfaces, the three-dimensionality of teeth, or other subtleties that the operator intends to bring to the attention of the observer.

Because photography is a noninvasive technique, the search for a novel or particular detail using this medium can be an incentive for practitioners to enrich their daily activity by continually refining their sense of observation and curiosity. Thus, new frames and new perspectives can be explored, particularly in areas with high esthetic value such as the anterior teeth.

In cases where esthetics is of maximum importance, the practitioner's task is facilitated because the use of mirrors is unnecessary; cheek retractors and a black background are all that is needed to heighten contrast (Figs 7-13a and 7-13b). In this type of image, accessory lighting plays an important role. Extra flash units provide the light needed to reveal the three-dimensionality of the teeth or their surface texture (Fig 7-13c). In fact, light from unusual angles allows the photographer to create particularly effective and impressive images, which will have a unique documentary value and will, above all, fully convey the esthetic power of a natural tooth or a perfect restoration.

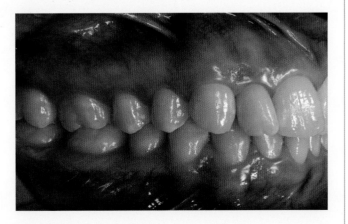

Fig 7-11
In this lateral view of the patient in occlusion, the zero-coordinate rule has been followed with respect to the axial plane only; however, the image is correct and legible.

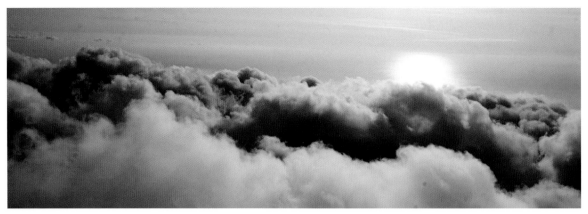

Fig 7-12
The photographer has chosen a perspective that beautifully reveals light and shadows.

Fig 13a
In this example of excellent photographic kalligraphia, the microtexture and macrotexture, which are the extrinsic optical characteristics of the teeth, are clearly documented.

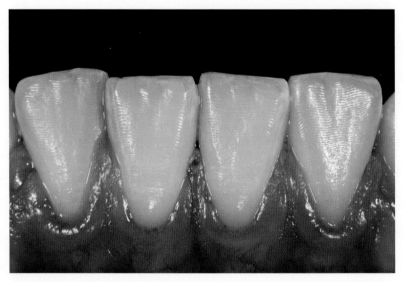

Fig 7-13b
A contrastor has been used to create an image of unusual translucency. This accessory facilitates the study and precise diagnosis of the intrinsic optical characteristics of teeth. In this image, it is clear that the lateral incisor is the aiming point; it is the center of attention of the photograph. For this reason, the zero-coordinate rule has not been precisely followed.

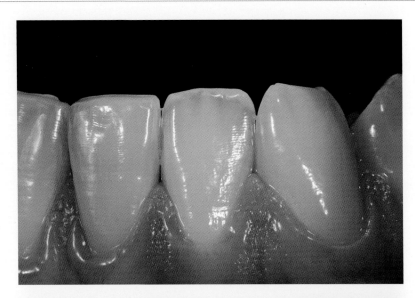

Fig 7-13c
The beauty and delicate spatiality of these incisors can be admired in this image. The unusual perspective highlights the developmental lobes and grooves, which represent the macrotexture or vertical texture of the tooth surface. This image does not respect the zero coordinate rule; it has been taken from an arbitrary perspective and would be difficult to reproduce, but it has esthetic and documentary value.

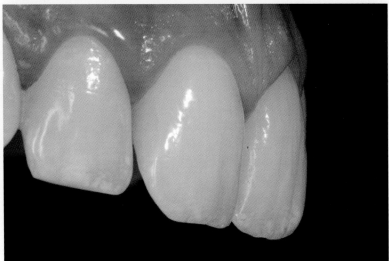

[
In photography, the term contrast *indicates the gradual transition between light and dark areas in the same photograph. Contrastors are accessories that darken the background and thus increase the contrast in an image. They subtly improve the observer's understanding of the intrinsic characteristics of dental tissues, such as translucency and brightness.*
]

Contrast in Photography

In photography the term *contrast* refers to the gradualness of the transition from light to dark hues throughout the various areas of a photograph. A photograph with little contrast will have a smoother transition between the various areas of differing brightness. On the other hand, a photograph with more contrast will have transitions that are sharper and harder and that bring out the differences in brightness among the various components of the picture. Essentially, because visual perception is facilitated by the sharpness of the edges of small elements, high contrast allows the observer to better grasp the details comprising the image.

Contrastors

Contrastors are sterilizable black backgrounds, either metallic or disposable cardboard, which are positioned behind the teeth at the moment of taking the shot (Fig 7-14). Because teeth are light in color, when the natural background of the tongue and oral cavity is replaced with a black background, the contrast between the background and the teeth increases. Consequently, definition of the teeth, including the details that are most difficult to perceive, also increases. Another advantage of the greater contrast provided by the black background is better visualization of the translucent areas of the tooth, such as the incisal edge. The translucency revealed by greater contrast allows the practitioner to appreciate the intimate structure of the tooth; the overall degree of translucency and brightness of that tooth can be perceived (Fig 7-15).

A tooth's degrees of brightness and translucency are inversely proportional to one another. As brightness increases, translucency decreases, and vice versa. This allows the practitioner to assess the enamel's intrinsic characteristics of quality as well as quantity in a particular patient. A color analysis of a tooth shows that it is the dentin, with its natural opacity, that determines the degree of brightness or value of the tooth. On the other hand, increased translucency of enamel tends to lower the brightness of teeth.

Knowledge and consideration of the intrinsic characteristics of dental tissues allows the practitioner to subtly assess and understand the optic properties of teeth; the practitioner can then make an in-depth diagnosis, which is crucial in cases of conservative or prosthetic restorations. When practitioners photograph and document a case before restoration, study of the photographs will prove very advantageous, confirming the basic concept expressed in chapter 5: photography is a powerful diagnostic technique.

The intrinsic optical properties of a body are opacity, transparency, and translucency. An opaque body reflects or absorbs light completely, while a transparent body allows light to pass through it totally. A translucent body allows light to partially pass through it; it is partly reflected by the body and partly diffused within it. The intrinsic optical properties of teeth play a fundamental role in the perception of color.

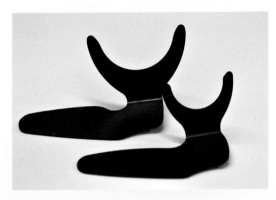

Fig 7-14a
This type of contrastor is used for lateral and occlusal photographs.

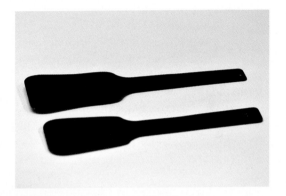

Fig 7-14b
This type of contrastor is used for frontal views.

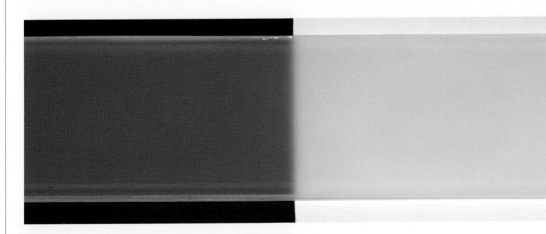

Fig 7-15
A translucent sheet of glass is placed onto black and white backgrounds. The dark background lowers the brightness of the object, allowing the degree of translucency to be fully appreciated.

The degrees of translucency vary from almost total opacity to almost total transparency. In general, the degree of translucency of teeth is linked to the quality and quantity of the enamel, which varies according to age subsequent to the processes of maturation and aging of the teeth. The chromaticity of the tooth, or the overall hue-chroma, relates to the quality and quantity of dentin present.

Intrinsic Optical Properties of Teeth: Translucency

All objects interact with light in a way that depends on the particular characteristics of their composition. The manner of this interaction distinguishes opaque and transparent objects from a purely optical point of view. White objects appear so because they reflect light totally, while black objects absorb it totally; see chapter 3 for a thorough examination of the concept of reflectance.

White and black objects have a characteristic in common: neither allows the transmission of light waves; this property is defined as opacity (Fig 7-16). The opposite property is called transparency, in which light waves are totally transmitted through an object such as a sheet of glass (Fig 7-17).

A property intermediate to these two is *translucency*, in which light waves are partially transmitted and partially reflected or absorbed (Fig 7-18). Inside translucent bodies, there is an extremely irregular diffusion of light waves, which takes on great importance in the perception of the color of the body itself. In opaque objects, there is total or no reflectance, depending on whether the object is white or black; in transparent objects, there is no reflectance; in translucent objects, the degree of

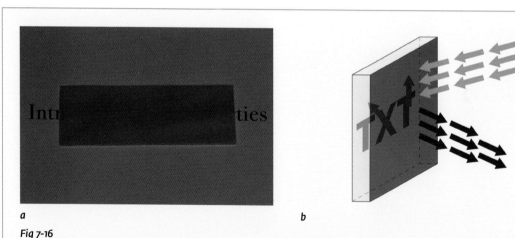

a   b

Fig 7-16
(a) An opaque object does not allow the transmission of light and prevents the observer from perceiving the writing underneath it. Note that the paper with the writing, which is white, appears gray because of the functioning of the exposure meter; this photograph has been taken without any corrections to exposure. (b) The reflectance, the percentage of reflected light, is correlated with the color of the opaque body: a white object exhibits total reflectance of light, and a black object, total absorption. In this case, the reflectance is partial, because the glass is not completely white.

The handling of opacity and translucency in various areas of an esthetic restoration, by correct stratification of the restorative materials, is the key to success. The correct use of contrastors is useful for learning to recognize and diagnose the intrinsic optical properties of teeth and in predicting the effectiveness of whitening procedures.

reflectance is partial and inversely proportional to the degree of translucency.

In summary, the most translucent object has less opacity and reflectance, and thus a greater degree of transparency; the least translucent object has greater opacity and reflectance, and thus a lesser degree of transparency (Fig 7-19). Translucency has great significance for the practitioner because, together with chromaticity, it substantially contributes to the perception of the brightness or value of teeth.

Very translucent natural teeth or restorations lack brightness and tend to lack luminosity. The degree of translucency of teeth is linked to the quality and quantity of the enamel;

these attributes vary with age because of the maturation and aging processes of the teeth. With the passing of time, the enamel becomes more and more translucent because of mineralization processes and intrinsic maturing, but also because of the reduction and loss of surface irregularities, such as texture, lobes, and developmental grooves. A further consequence of the loss of texture and surface characteristics is a reduction in the degree and quality of the diffusion of the light rays inside the tooth itself; this results in the perception of the aging of the tooth. Greater translucency is typical of certain areas of the tooth, such as the proximal areas of the anterior teeth, which

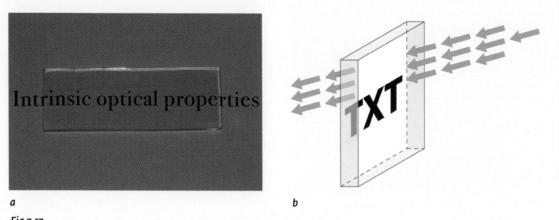

a

b

Fig 7-17
(a and b) *Glass is an example of a transparent object: the sheet of glass allows us to immediately visualize what is written underneath it, which proves the complete transmission of light.*

> The most translucent bodies have less opacity and reflectance and thus a greater degree of transparency; less translucent objects have greater opacity and reflectance and thus a lesser degree of transparency. The degree of translucency of enamel increases progressively with age because of both loss of surface texture and reduced thickness due to wear.

sometimes appear to have a translucent frame (Fig 7-20).

The chromaticity or the hue-chroma combination of teeth is a reflection of the quality and quantity of dentin present; it also varies progressively with time, resulting in the loss of brightness of the teeth that is characteristic of the elderly. Therefore, the translucency, chromaticity, and brightness of a tooth vary from patient to patient in relation to the quality and quantity and reciprocal integration of dentin and enamel. This relationship between translucency and chromaticity is responsible for the overall brightness of teeth. It is important to emphasize that the degree of translucency of a tooth can be a decisive prognostic factor in

whitening techniques (Figs 7-21 and 7-22). It is well known that oxidizing agents, which are responsible for the degradation of colored pigments in the whitening process, mainly affect the dentin, where the majority of the agents responsible for the discoloration are deposited. By carefully studying photographs prior to treatment, the practitioner can better assess the degree of translucency and the quantity of dentin and enamel and thus better predict the effectiveness of the whitening procedures. Teeth are anatomically composed of various complex structures—enamel, dentin, and neurovascular pulp—perfectly integrated in a functional and esthetic harmonious whole, according to a process called *natural stratification*. This anato-

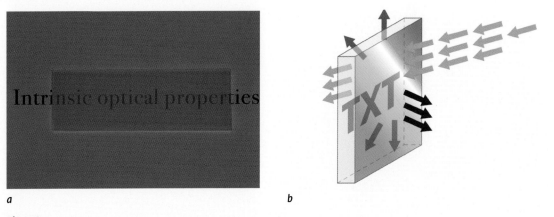

a   *b*

Fig 7-18
A small glass sheet demonstrates the concept of translucency. As the degree of translucency diminishes, the writing underneath becomes less clear, which is a sign of reduced transmission of light waves through the glass and an increased diffusion within the object itself. Because translucency is a property intermediate to opacity and transparency, it can also be considered as a gradation of either property.

> *The overall brightness and the degree of translucency of a tooth are the end result of the qualitative and quantitative integration of enamel and dentin. A high degree of translucency in a natural tooth or restoration equals a reduction in the value or brightness of the tooth itself.*

mical complexity corresponds to a certain optical complexity; the individual anatomical components behave differently in the presence of light. It is a challenge for the practitioner to create a restoration that achieves perfect blending and stratification of materials so as to perfectly simulate the behavior of the natural tooth in the oral environment. This can only be achieved by an accurate knowledge and proper handling of the parameters of opacity and translucency in partnership with the dental laboratory technician.

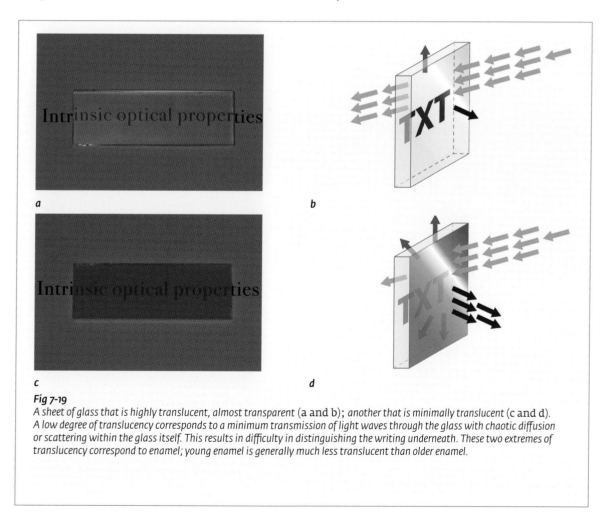

a   b

c   d

Fig 7-19
A sheet of glass that is highly translucent, almost transparent (a and b); another that is minimally translucent (c and d). A low degree of translucency corresponds to a minimum transmission of light waves through the glass with chaotic diffusion or scattering within the glass itself. This results in difficulty in distinguishing the writing underneath. These two extremes of translucency correspond to enamel; young enamel is generally much less translucent than older enamel.

> *The overall surface texture of a tooth increases the overall quantity and quality of the reflected light, amplifying the diffused light and making the tooth appear more luminous. Surface texture also increases the percentage of diffused refraction within the tooth itself, to the detriment of specular refraction; this scattering of light contributes to the perception of the naturalness and depth of the tooth.*

Extrinsic Optical Properties of Teeth: Surface Characteristics

The surface of a tooth consists of horizontal microtexture elements called the *striae of Retzius* and vertical macrotexture elements, including developmental lobes, grooves, and microscopic concavities and convexities. The overall texture of the surface produces a diffuse reflection of light, which greatly contributes to a perception of the tooth's naturalness and depth (Fig 7-23a); furthermore, the diffuse reflection increases the degree of reflectance and, consequently, the tooth's brightness (Fig 7-23b).

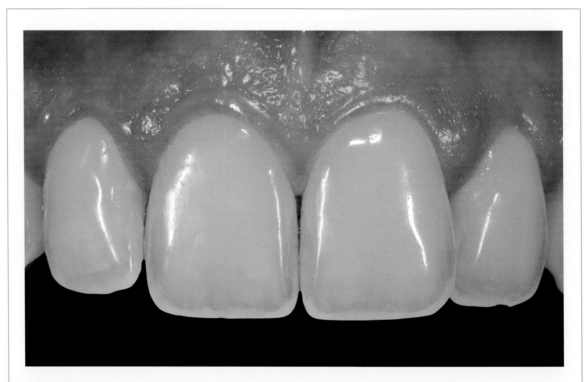

Fig 7-20
The teeth in this image exhibit significant translucency of their incisal edges and proximal line angles, which tends to lower their brightness; the thickness and quality of the enamel and loss of surface texture diminishes the total reflectance and the percentage of diffuse reflection of the light striking the teeth.

Fig 7-21
An image taken with (a) and without
(b) a contrastor. The increase in contrast
obtained with a dark background improves
the perception of the dental structures,
particularly the translucency of the various
areas of the tooth. The image taken with
the contrastor in place presents less visual
tension and is thus more legible. These
teeth have an extremely high degree of
translucency, especially at the proximal
line angles, presumably because of the
thickness of enamel. The prognosis for the
effectiveness of whitening procedures in this
situation is generally negative, because the
images imply a reduced thickness of dentin
available to be whitened.

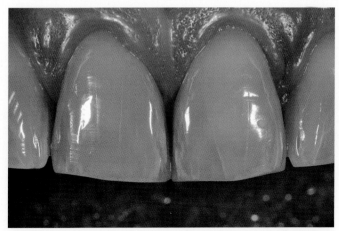

a

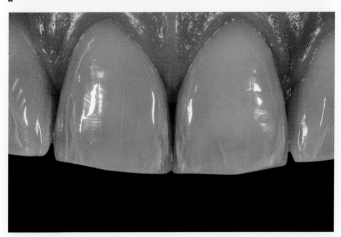

b

Fig 7-22
These incisors exhibit less translucency and
thus more brightness than those depicted
in Fig 7-21. These factors depend on both the
dentin structure and quality and quantity of
the enamel.

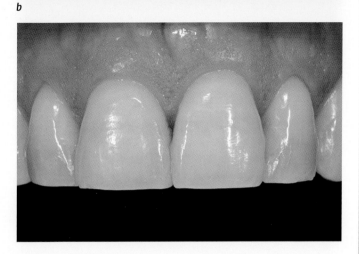

The progressive loss of surface texture because of function and wear increases the percentage of specular reflection, which, along with progressive changes in chromaticity related to age, makes the teeth appear older and more opaque. Perception of the tooth's brightness and overall appearance is, therefore, strictly influenced by the smoothness or irregularity of its surface.

The characteristics of the tooth's surface partially determine the behavior of the light waves that strike it. Three parameters describe this behavior. The first parameter is the quality of light reflection, which can be more specular or more diffuse. The second parameter is the reflectance, or quantity of reflection; more surface irregularity corresponds to a greater reflection of light waves. It is easier for the light waves to penetrate the tooth if the surface is smooth. The third parameter is scattering, or the quality of the internal diffusion of light waves (Figs 7-23c and 7-23d). When the light waves strike the tooth surface, they are partly reflected and partly transmitted, but a variable amount are absorbed and diffused by the body of the tooth. An irregular surface increases the variability of the angle of penetration of the light rays within the tooth and, consequently, the degree of internal diffusion. When the quality of the internal diffusion is more chaotic and irregular, the perception of the depth of the tooth is amplified (Fig 7-24).

A corresponding phenomenon occurs for reflection; the light that irradiates and refracts within the tooth can be either specular or diffuse. Specular reflection is more regular, and diffuse reflection is more disorganized. A given surface will cause both types of reflection at the same time, but increased surface irregularities cause an increase in the quantity of scattering and in the diffuse and random refraction within the tooth (see Fig 7-23c). This also occurs as a result of intrinsic factors, such as the enamel-dentin interface (see Fig 7-23d). It is, therefore, primarily the presence of enamel, with its properties of intrinsic and surface translucency, that causes these optical phenomena, giving teeth their characteristic depth and rendering them so harmonious (Figs 7-25 and 7-26).

Fig 7-23a
When an equal quantity of light waves are introduced, the irregular surface will have a greater percentage of diffuse reflection than specular reflection. Surface texture influences the quality of the reflection. An irregular surface is formed by superficial microtexture and vertical macrotexture components, including developmental grooves, lobes, microconcavities, and microconvexities.

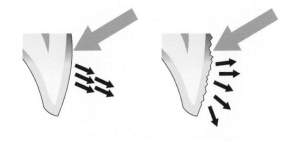

Fig 7-23b
An irregular surface also results in an increase in the reflectance, the total quantity of reflected waves. Light waves are better reflected from the tooth surface if its surface is irregular, making such teeth less translucent and more luminous.

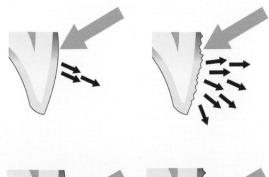

Fig 7-23c
A significant number of light waves do not pass through the object but are diffused within it. This diffusion can be either regular or chaotic, and surface irregularities increase the scattering or the strength and disorder of the waves.

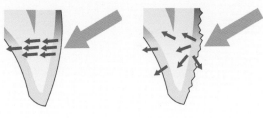

Fig 7-23d
Intrinsic factors also affect the scattering of light waves within the tooth. For example, the enamel-dentin interface modifies the angle of refraction of light. The concept of the correct stratification of restorative materials is based on the diffusion of light within the tooth.

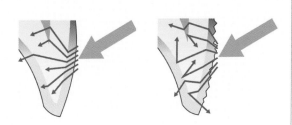

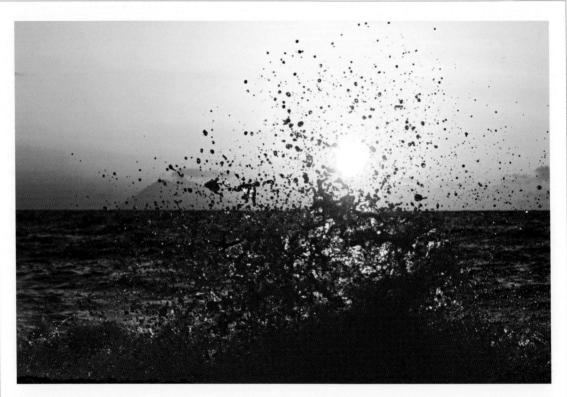

Fig 7-24

The behavior of the light waves that interact with a tooth is similar to that of waves breaking against the beach. The morphologic characteristics of the shore line and the intensity and direction of the waves breaking onto it create myriad droplets of water, which spread out into space in a chaotic fashion but, for this very reason, are still harmonious and evocative. This "dance of the waves" is a metaphor for the dynamism of the color-light interaction in teeth. This image of the active volcano of Stromboli at sunset was taken with a Canon EOS 20D, Tv shutter priority mode, t = 1/800 s.

Fig 7-25
In this image of the central incisors of a young girl, the black background allows better appreciation of the milky opalescence present in certain areas of the enamel, and the greater quantity of enamel itself on the incisal edges. The high value of these teeth is the result of the youthfulness of the enamel and the perfect conservation of the surface texture.

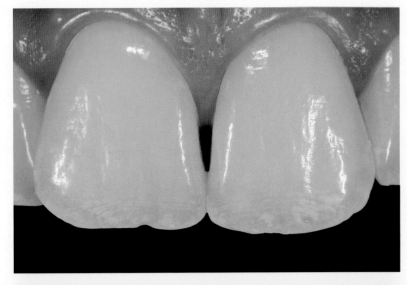

Fig 7-26
The photograph allows for a careful study and assessment of the dental structure. The translucency at the proximal line angles and the enamel defect on the right central incisor are both clearly visible.

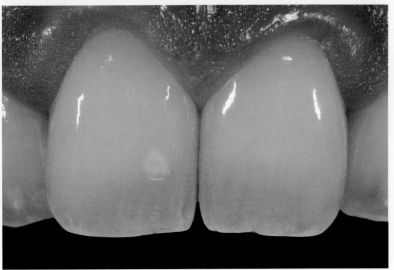

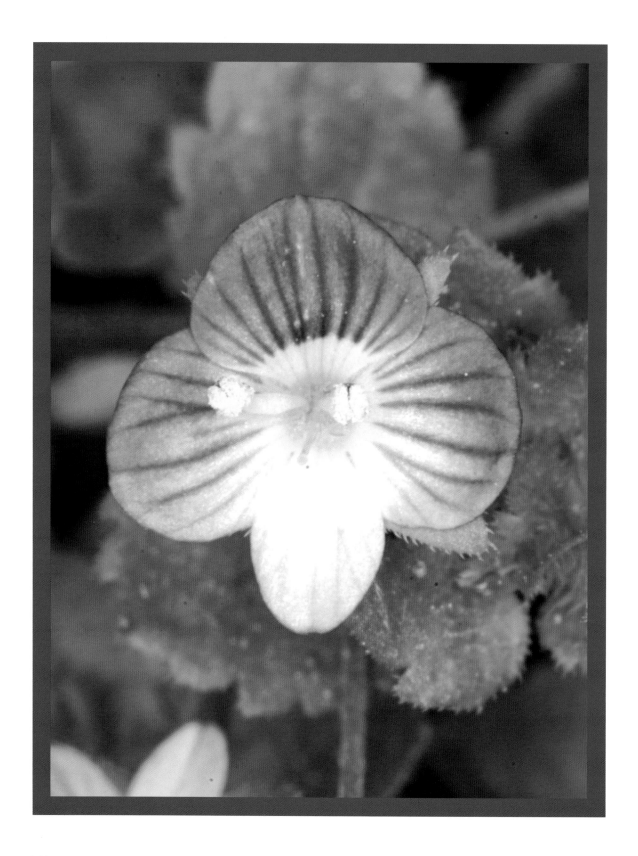

Chapter 8

Flash Units

In dental photography, the use of a flash unit is needed to compensate for exposure, which would otherwise be diminished because of the very high f-numbers required to obtain adequate depth of field. Traditional single-flash units can be built into the camera or positioned on an external flash connection called a hot shoe. *They are not suitable for dental purposes because, in close-up photography, their use will result in a parallax error.*

Traditional Flash Units

In chapter 6, the use of very high f-numbers, or f-stops, for intraoral images was validated because small apertures exploit the maximum depth of field. This means that it is absolutely essential to use additional light sources, such as flash units, to optimize exposure.

Selection of the additional light source is an important issue. The easiest solution might seem to be the use of a flash unit built into the upper part of the camera body. Unfortunately, this option is not feasible for one fundamental reason. This source of light is positioned on a different plane than, and at an angle to, the optical axis of the lens, which corresponds to the central ray that passes through the lens. This causes a parallax error of the light source,

creating unwanted shadows (Figs 8-1 and 8-2). The use of a more powerful flash unit, mounted onto an external flash connection called a *hot shoe*, aggravates the problem without solving it because it is positioned at an even greater angle to the optical axis. This position of the light source, together with the need to get very close to the subject, increases the parallax error and the extent of undesirable shadows, making this solution unfeasible as well (Figs 8-3 and 8-4). Although a flash unit positioned on the upper part of the camera is an excellent and valuable aid for general photography, providing the powerful source of light needed to obtain good exposure (Fig 8-5), it is not suitable for dental requirements. These types of flashes create shadowy areas or uneven illumination in close-up photographs.

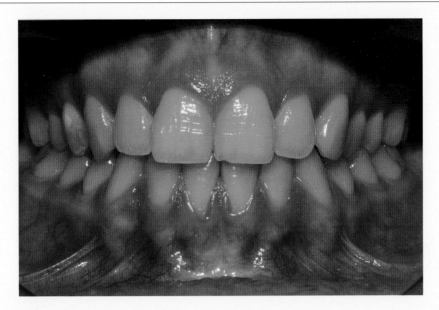

Fig 8-1
This photograph taken with a built-in flash unit appears slightly underexposed, and the upper parts of the posterior areas are in shadow because of parallax error.

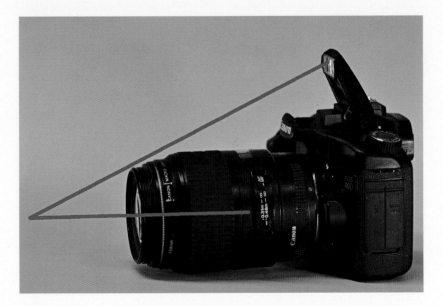

Fig 8-2
The built-in flash unit is positioned above and at an angle to the optical axis, causing parallax error.

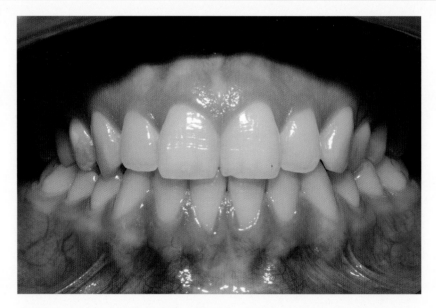

Fig 8-3
This photograph, taken with an external flash unit, has better exposure because of the increased power of the flash unit; however, the flash unit is positioned at a greater angle to the optical axis, which increases the formation of shadows.

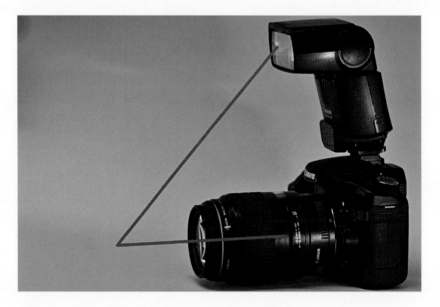

Fig 8-4
An external flash unit mounted on a hot shoe has been added to the camera shown in Fig 8-2. The source of light is further away and at an even greater angle to the optical axis, thus increasing the parallax error.

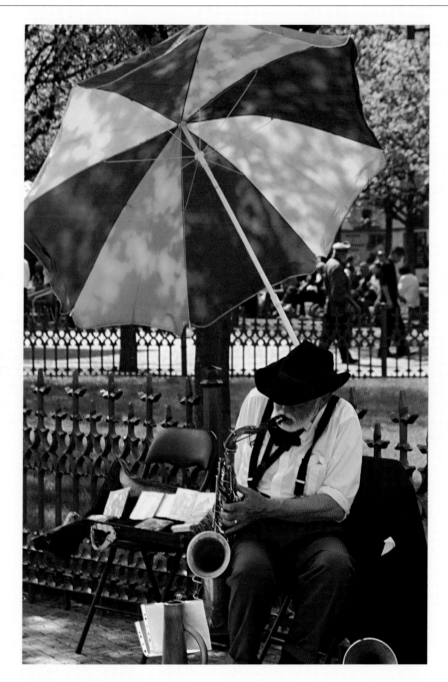

Fig 8-5
For general photography, a flash unit positioned on the upper part of the camera, whether built-in or mounted on an external flash connection, provides the powerful source of light needed to obtain good exposure.

A ring flash is a device with at least two sources of light positioned around the lens on a special ring support. Because the light sources are positioned directly to the side of the optical axis, no parallax errors are created. This type of flash is, therefore, specific to and indispensible for close-up photographs.

Ring Flashes

The limitations of traditional flash units can be overcome by positioning the light source directly at the side of the lens, level with and lateral to its optical axis. These flash devices are located on a special ring mounted onto the front part of the lens, and they are called *ring flashes* (Fig 8-6). The ring flash allows the practitioner to get very close to the subject without creating shadowy areas from parallax error (Fig 8-7). A drawback of this closeness of the flash to the lens is a relative loss of depth and three-dimensionality and a flattening of the image. Practitioners do not have to concern themselves with this issue unless photographic documentation of the highest caliber is required. In summary, the ring flash is considered a necessary, even indispensible, accessory for the dentist-photographer.

The practitioner who intends to benefit even more from clinical photography will have to use additional devices such as twin or supplementary flashes.

One factor that is generally underestimated in dental photography is interference from ambient sources of light such as the overhead dental unit light. Additional light sources may be responsible for errors of exposure because the exposure meter can be deceived in reading the brightness of the scene in the frame by the presence of other very strong light sources. Therefore, photographs should be taken only in the presence of ambient light; however, the consequent lack of light can interfere with correct focusing, so ring flashes are generally fitted with small light sources, called *focus-assist illuminators*, to aid focusing (see Fig 8-6).

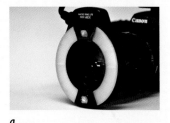
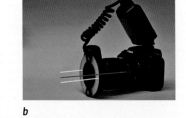

a　　　　　　　　　　　　　　　　　　　　*b*

Fig 8-6
(a and b) *On the Canon MR-14 EX ring flash, the light sources* (yellow lines) *are positioned directly to the side of the optical axis* (red line) *at the 3- and 9-o'clock positions. They can rotate around the ring mount to the 6- and 12-o'clock positions or other positions as required. The small focus-assist illuminators are positioned at the top and bottom, between the two flash light sources; they aid focusing in the presence of minimal light in the framed scene.*

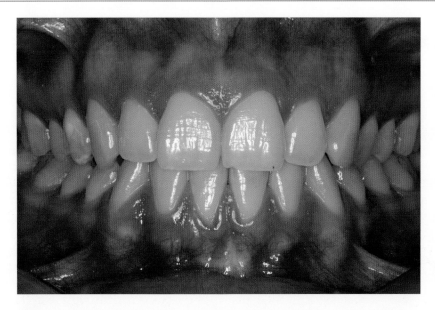

Fig 8-7a
In this photograph taken with a Canon EOS 40D camera, MR-14 EX ring flash, and
f = 100–mm macro lens, the image appears correctly and uniformly exposed, even in the
posterior areas.

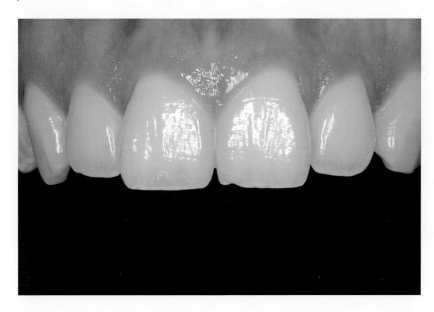

Fig 8-7b
This image of the maxillary anterior teeth was taken with the same equipment.

[
Twin flashes differ from ring flashes in the position of the light sources, which are placed more laterally and further away from the optical axis of the lens. This position brings out the three-dimensionality of the image.
]

Twin Flashes

To avoid the loss of image depth caused by ring flashes, *twin flashes* can be used. These types of light sources are fitted onto a ring mounted around the lens but are positioned more laterally and further away than the ring flash. Their inclination is adjustable, which helps to accentuate the three-dimensionality of the object. The light source used by the authors is the Nikon R1C1 flash system (Fig 8-8), which is a wireless system consisting of one or more SB-R200 Speedlight flash units fitted onto an adjustable ring and mounted onto the front of the lens. A Nikon SU-800 commander unit is positioned on top of the camera. The commander can activate up to eight light sources subdivided into three groups: A, B, and C. The operator assigns each flash unit to a group for a specific exposure setting. A characteristic of this system is that the flash units can be positioned in two ways. First, they can slide along the ring mount to be positioned at different angles to each other, from 45 to 180 degrees apart (Fig 8-9). Second, each light source can be independently tilted on its own axis, altering the angle between the light source and the optical axis of the lens (Fig 8-10). Moreover, additional SB-R200 units can be added to achieve particularly harmonious and impressive lighting effects (Figs 8-11 and 8-12).

This system is particularly versatile and allows the operator to take traditional shots as well as to explore new ways of lighting. One drawback to high magnification is that the practitioner must get very close to the subject, and the patient's perioral tissues may block the illumination of the oral cavity. This is particularly true for images of the posterior teeth. This problem can be solved by moving the SB-R200 units around the ring mount and positioning them close together, 45 degrees apart, rather than 180 degrees apart (see Fig 8-9d).

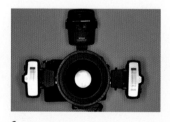
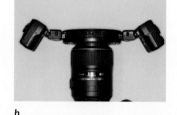

a   *b*

Fig 8-8
(a) *The Nikon R1C1 flash system is comprised of an SU-800 commander unit, mounted on the hot shoe above the camera, and two SB-R200 flash units, mounted on a ring on the front of the lens. As seen here, the flash units are positioned at the 3- and 9-o'clock positions. (b) These flash units are located at a distance from the lens's optical axis, forming an angle that results in better spatial presentation of the image.*

> *Rotating the flash units away from the 3- and 9-o'clock positions, or 180 degrees apart, allows the practitioner to explore new image spatialities and to create photographs of great documentary value. Moreover, added flash units introduce light from unusual angles; the intensity and the direction of the light sources can be varied at will to discover special and impressive effects.*

Creative Use of Flashes

Artificial light can be used in unusual ways to great effect. First, because the light sources are mounted on a ring, they can be rotated around the lens. The standard placement for two light sources is 180 degrees apart at the 3- and 9-o'clock positions (see Figs 8-8a and 8-11a), but they can be moved to the vertical 6- and 12-o'clock positions, maintaining their 180-degree relationship (see Figs 8-9a and 8-12b). This variation in the angle of origin results in a different light reflection on the oral surfaces, bringing out spatial characteristics or surface textures not generally visible with normal lateral lighting.

Second, one or more additional flash units can be placed on opposite sides of the lens, depending on the operator's taste; these so-called servo flash units enrich the overall lighting and improve the perception of the tooth's spatiality.

A third option is to increase or decrease the intensity of the light sources to obtain particular effects. All modern macrophotography flash units, whether ring or twin, can be adjusted in this way. This modification can be done in both through-the-lens (TTL) or manual exposure modes. Experimenting with various light sources is gratifying, especially when photographing areas with extremely high esthetic value, where the perfection of a well-executed restoration can only be improved by an unusual perspective. There are many richly captivating possibilities offered by such lighting systems for whomever wishes to play with light and create exceptional photos.

Fig 8-9a
The twin SB-R200 flash units of an R1C1 system are seen in the 3- and 9-o'clock positions, 180 degrees apart.

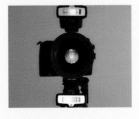

Fig 8-9b
Additional flash units can be added to the mounting ring.

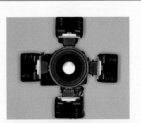

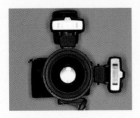

Figs 8-9c and 8-9d
The flash units can slide along the mounting ring to other positions, forming smaller angles such as 90 degrees or 45 degrees.

c

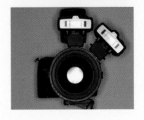

d

[*The emission of light from the flash unit must take place within a definite interval, called* flash sync speed. *In modern cameras with dedicated flash units, this occurs automatically; otherwise, a shutter speed of 1/125 s should be set.*]

Flash Synchronization

The presence of a flash affects how exposure must be handled; the amount of artificial light emitted, together with environmental lighting, must be adequate for the requirements of the shot.

The total amount of light emitted by the flash unit must be regulated according to the required exposure. To obtain this result, the duration of the flash, but not its intensity, can be controlled with exposure settings. This has two consequences: first, the camera must be able to intervene in the setting of the flash; second, the flash pulse must take place within a specific lapse of time. In fact, if the shutter speed is too rapid, the emission of light by the flash may occur after the shutter has closed or before it has opened. Therefore, it is essential for the flash to be synchronized with the shutter speed, which is set at a specific value called *flash sync*

speed. Because intraoral shots are always taken with a small aperture, the exposure setting is controlled, not by the shutter speed, but by the length of the flash's light emission, called the *flash pulse.* This synchronization occurs automatically with a *dedicated flash unit* that is produced by the same manufacturer as the camera and is thus able to communicate with it. Otherwise, the shutter speed must be set at 1/125 s to ensure that the shutter stays open long enough to allow the light of the flash to reach the sensor. Because the subject in the frame is generally stationary, the photograph will not be blurred, even with a somewhat slow speed of 1/125 s.

Exposure and Flash: TTL Mode

In practice, the practitioner has two choices for exposure: relying on the flash's TTL readings or using manual mode. In TTL exposure mode, the

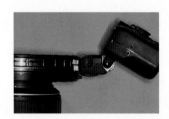

Figs 8-10a and 8-10b
An individual flash unit can be tilted on its own axis.

a

b

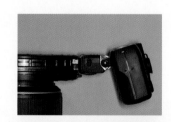

Fig 8-10c
Detail of the mounting mechanism of an SB-R200 unit and the pivot point around which the unit rotates.

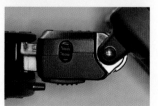

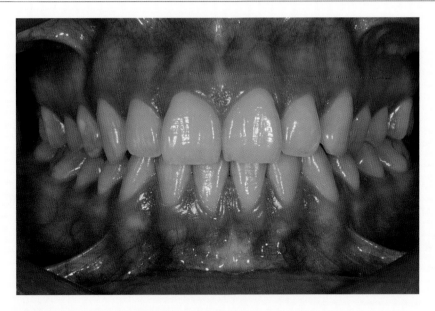

Fig 8-11a
This image was taken with the Nikon R1C1 twin flash system, with two SB-R200 units placed 180 degrees apart at the 3- and 9-o'clock positions.

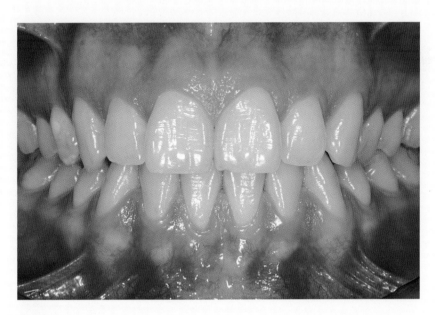

Fig 8-11b
Four SB-R200 units, placed 90 degrees apart at the 12-, 3-, 6-, and 9-o'clock positions, create powerful and impressive lighting effects.

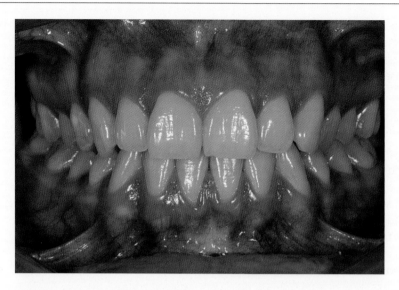

Fig 8-12a
Each SB-R200 flash unit can comfortably rotate on its own axis to illuminate the scene in the frame in a more or less direct way, while maintaining its position on the ring support. In this image, the configuration of the light sources brings out the texture of the incisors, to the detriment of the posterior areas. The photograph is slightly underexposed; any variation in the angle of origin of the light can have both advantages and disadvantages, which is why the practitioner must decide which aspect of the image to favor.

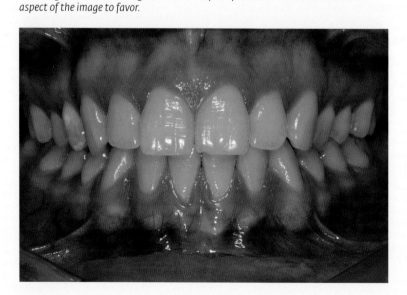

Fig 8-12b
In this photograph, two flash units have been positioned vertically at the 6- and 12-o'clock positions. Notice how the reflections bring out different aspects of the surface texture.

[
When the flash unit is controlled by TTL light readings, exposure is measured through the camera's lens system itself for maximum precision. In manual mode, on the other hand, the operator selects, according to his or her own personal requirements, the exact duration of the flash pulse.
]

camera and the flash are designed to communicate rapidly with each other. Depending on the amount of light that passes through the lens and strikes the sensor, the camera decides on the exposure and very rapidly informs the flash processor when to interrupt the flash pulse (Fig 8-13a). This automatic mode is extremely useful in most situations, but certain circumstances can affect its accuracy.

For example, the presence of metallic objects in the frame, such as dental dam clamps, shade guide supports, or even implant components, can cause reflections that can falsify the camera readings and create undesirable underexposure. In practice, the light of the reflection deceives the exposure meter, which overestimates the amount of light and interrupts the flash pulse before correct exposure has been achieved (Figs 8-14a and 8-15a).

Manual Mode

To avoid the possibility of underexposure, all flash units have a completely manual mode, which allows the operator to determine the duration of the flash pulse (Fig 8-13b).

It is important to recognize that the TTL light-reading system can fail for a number of reasons, so the practitioner must know how to assess correct exposure and, in the presence of incorrect readings by the camera, overcome the problem by choosing to work in manual mode. In such situations, it will be the practitioner who, by trial and error, will establish the correct amount of light; in general, it will only take two or three attempts to achieve the desired result, avoiding the overly brief flash pulse set according to the TTL reading (Figs 8-14b and 8-15b). Photography is a creative medium that is noninvasive for the patient, so the practitioner can always search for new possibilities in documentation.

Fig 8-13a
The flash unit display, starting at the top left-hand corner: the arrow indicates a connection with wireless commander units; the flower indicates the macro function; the initials TTL indicate the exposure mode; the letters A and B indicate the main light-source groups; the 1:1 ratio indicates that the two groups are set at the same power; the symbol CH indicates the radio frequency on which the unit commands the light sources; the symbol C indicates the third group of flash units, which operate exclusively in manual mode.

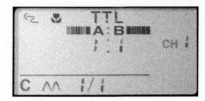

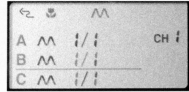

Fig 8-13b
The letter M at the top of the screen indicates that manual mode has been set. The power for each light-source group can be set with consecutive halving: ½, ¼, ⅛, etc.

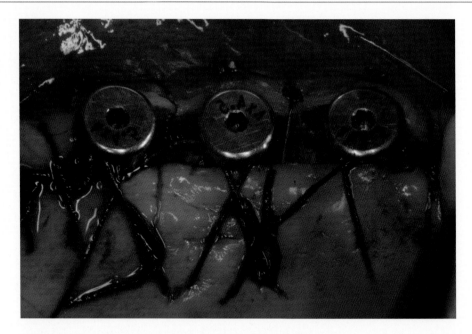

Fig 8-14a
In this photograph taken in TTL mode of stage-two surgery with vestibular connective tissue grafting, metallic reflections from the healing abutments have caused the image to be underexposed.

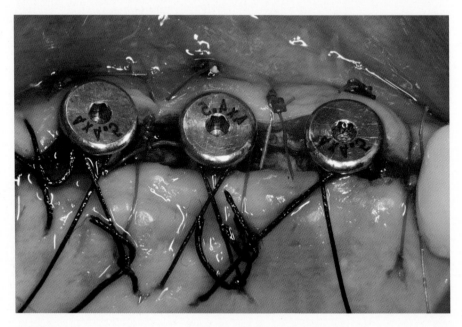

Fig 8-14b
The same image, taken with the flash in manual mode, is correctly exposed.

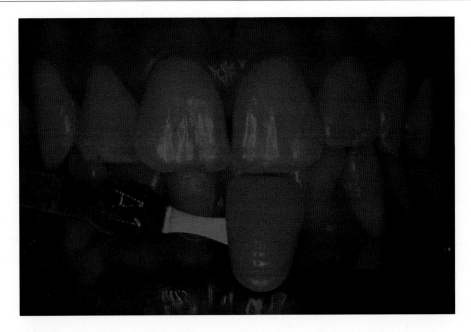

Fig 8-15a
The metallic reflection of the shade guide support has caused this photograph taken in TTL flash mode to be underexposed. The reflection has falsified the exposure-meter measurement.

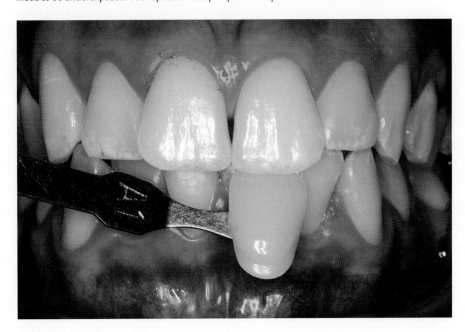

Fig 8-15b
The same image, taken with the flash in manual mode, appears correctly exposed.

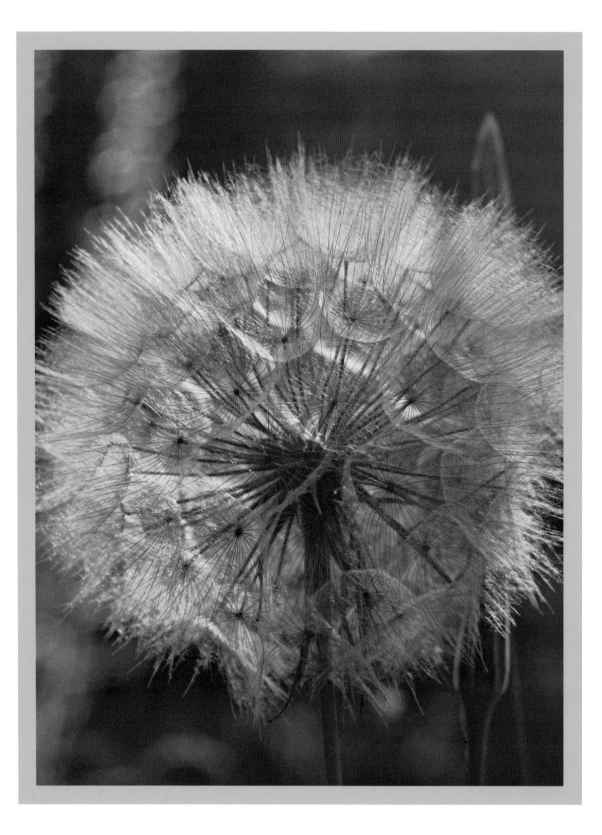

Chapter 9

Photographing
Radiographs

Radiographic images can be directly acquired in digital format and then managed with this modern technology, which also allows for easy transmission of the images via the Internet. The photography of radiographs is a simple, economic way of transferring these images from a traditional format to a digital file, which is an easier way to store, transmit, and utilize diagnostic data.

Normally, radiographs are converted to a digital format using a backlit scanner, which, unlike an ordinary scanner, detects both reflected and transmitted light. Ordinary scanners use only reflected light; the light source is positioned from the same observation point as the image sensor, which perceives the light reflected from the scanned object.

Backlit scanners have a second light source on the part of the scanner behind the object, so light is transmitted through the radiograph in addition to being reflected. Obviously, the object to be scanned must be translucent for light to pass partially through it. The light transmitted through the object to the sensor, together with normally reflected light, allows an optimal reading of the details of the radiographic image.

One of the interesting applications of digital photography is the transfer of a radiographic image to a digital format without using a dedicated scanner. This step is not necessary if the radiographs have been acquired directly in a digital format and subsequently printed. However, it may be useful to photograph a printed digital radiograph when a particular detail has been highlighted, so that it can be emailed to a colleague for consultation or advice.

Recent studies have shown that the conversion of a radiographic image to a digital file does not cause a loss of detail or information; these studies reported a resolution of 1,280 × 960 pixels, which is more than adequate to correctly digitalize the images.

Radiographic Masks

When a radiograph is placed on a lighted viewbox to be photographed, the light around the edges of the radiograph is relatively brighter than the transmitted light, which leads to the image being underexposed. A very simple, economic method of preventing underexposure is to make a mask with black cardboard. A window that corresponds to the dimensions of the radiograph is cut in the cardboard (Fig 9-1).

Film mounts for periodontal images are generally dark in color and are also easy to use as a mask for a single intraoral radiograph. If multiple radiographs must be photographed, the black cardboard can be easily cut and adapted to meet the needs of the practitioner.

[

Light around the periphery of a radiograph on a viewbox interferes with the exposure-meter reading, which leads to an underexposed image that is difficult to read. Radiographic masks are simply contrast mediums made of black cardboard, useful for eliminating peripheral light around a radiograph; their use promotes optimal exposure of the image.

]

Camera Settings

If a backlit scanner is not available, the simplest and most economic method of transferring and storing a radiographic image in a digital format is to photograph it. The best way to obtain a good image of a radiograph is to photograph it when illuminated by transmitted light. This requires that the radiograph be placed onto a lighted viewbox.

Setting the camera to obtain the best results is problematic. Technically, there are advan-tages and disadvantages of photographing ra-diographs, as compared to photographing pa-tients. One advantage is that there is no need to use mirrors or cheek retractors. Most impor-tantly, the subject is immobile; furthermore, it is a two-dimensional object with no depth.

A disadvantage is that a flash cannot be used because it creates reflections that would make the image unreadable. Therefore, an ordinary lighted viewbox for reading radiographs, available in all dental offices, must be used. However, the absence of a flash unit leads to

Fig 9-1a
The large window in this radiographic mask, seen in position on a lighted viewbox, is for photographing panoramic radiographs.

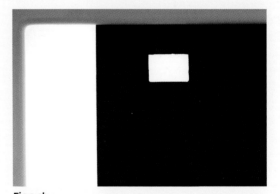

Fig 9-1b
This radiographic mask has a smaller window, suitable for photographing an intraoral radiograph. The cardboard does not fully cover the viewbox surface, and light can be seen at its lateral edge. The masks are made from sheets of black A4 cardboard, which is inexpensive and easily cut to the contour of any radiographic format.

[*The camera settings used in clinical practice are not suitable for photographing radiographs. For this special kind of photography, the fully programmed mode is recommended, with the autofocus function activated and the ISO speed increased to a setting between 800 and 1600. To avoid the presence of chromatic dominants and to standardize the images taken, the monochrome image mode should be selected.*]

problems with the exposure setting. If the settings for clinical situations are used, the light transmitted from the viewbox through the radiograph will be insufficient for correct exposure, so the practitioner must search for other solutions.

Because there is no need for a significant depth of field, a wide-open aperture can be used to allow a greater amount of light to reach the sensor. Furthermore, because the subject is immobile, a longer exposure time can be used; however, there is still a risk of the photo being blurred because lengthier exposure times may allow hand vibrations to become perceptible upon pressing the shutter button. Blurring can be avoided by increasing the sensitivity of the sensor to an ISO speed of 800 or more; this high value is still compatible with an acceptable amount of background noise. The fully programmed exposure mode (P) is recommended to let the camera decide the best aperture–shutter speed combination.

If the effect of micromotion is still perceptible on the photograph with these shooting parameters, there are three options: use a more powerful lighted viewbox, increase the ISO speed to 1600, or use a tripod and the self-timer function to avoid further vibrations when pressing the shutter-release button. If these changes are made, the practitioner will certainly obtain the desired results.

It is important to be aware that undesirable color dominants may appear on the image. They can be avoided by selecting the black-and-white or monochrome mode on the camera's shooting menu. The image will then vary only in the intensity of brightness on a scale of grays, without any variations of hue or unnatural chromatic dominants (Fig 9-2). In theory, the white balance function can be set on a fluorescent-lighting mode, but the monochrome mode makes this setting superfluous. White balance functions are devoted to the correct calculation of the color temperature, which is related to the quality of light; the color temperature varies according to the wavelength, and therefore the hue, of the light waves emitted. The monochrome mode instead favors the amount of brightness, or the intensity of gray on various areas of a radiograph, which allows the observer to perceive details in the image.

SUMMARY OF SETTINGS					
Exposure program	Image mode	Autofocus function	Flash	White balance	ISO speed
Fully programmed mode (P)	Monochrome or black-and-white	Activated	Off	Auto white balance	800 to 1600

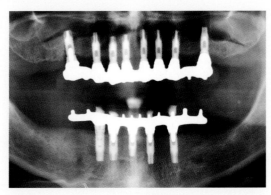

a

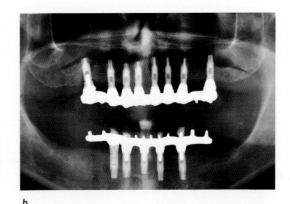

b

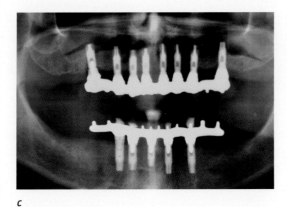

c

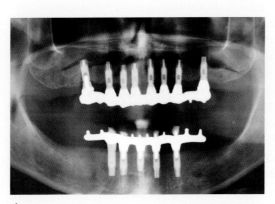

d

Fig 9-2

This panoramic radiograph has been photographed using various camera settings. (a) The recommended settings have been used: P exposure mode with the self-timer function turned on, ISO 800, monochrome mode, and auto white balance. In this gray-scale image, the observer can distinguish anatomical details perfectly, which results in a pleasurable reading. (b) The white balance function has been set on the fluorescent-lighting mode. No other settings have been changed. The image is almost identical to Fig 9-2a. (c) The standard image mode has been set instead of monochrome mode, and the white balance function has been set on fluorescent lighting. As a result, the image is characterized by an unpleasant blue dominant, which is not completely uniform throughout the image. (d) The standard image and auto white balance modes have been selected. The green dominant in this image is less noticeable than the blue dominant of Fig 9-2c, but it is still distracting and undesirable.

[*General concepts relating to spatiality have already been illustrated for intraoral and extraoral images. The zero-coordinate rule for the two planes of reference also must be followed when photographing radiographs.*]

Correct Framing

The correct spatiality when framing an intraoral or extraoral image has been defined with the zero-coordinate rule. Similarly, the practitioner must also choose the correct perspective when photographing a radiograph.

The zero-coordinate rule is also relevant to photography of radiographs. Practitioners must position themselves so that they correctly perceive the horizontal and vertical planes of the radiograph. These two planes are perpendicular to each other, and, most importantly, both are perpendicular to a third plane, the surface of the lighted viewbox. This rule requires that practitioners position themselves directly in front of the illuminated surface, so that the optical axis of the camera lens or eyes is 90 degrees to the surface of the viewbox, and both the horizontal and vertical planes are perceived as lines (Fig 9-3a). When the optical axis is not perpendicular to the plane of the viewbox or the radiograph, undesirable distortions of the image may result (Fig 9-3b).

By analogy, Rinn radiograph-positioning instruments are used to ensure that the x-ray beam is aimed correctly. These tools have been specially designed to precisely position the radiograph or digital sensor parallel to the mesiodistal plane of the tooth. The radiograph holder together with the extraoral aiming ring are used to perfectly position the x-ray tube perpendicular to the radiograph or sensor, avoiding undesirable distortions upon image acquisition.

The concept of image distortion can be understood by thinking about what happens at sunset; as the sun gradually sinks behind the horizon, its angle with the zenith point directly overhead increases, and the light creates longer and longer shadows. Similarly, greater inclination of the radiograph or digital sensor to the axis of the x-ray beam causes greater lengthening and distortion of the radiographic image. If the camera is inclined with respect to the surface of the viewbox, the same distortion can occur. Both errors will falsify the image.

In summary, inclination of the camera's optical axis can be varied with respect to the plane of the radiograph, which leads to distortions in both the vertical and horizontal dimensions (Figs 9-4 and 9-5). To achieve excellent results practitioners must consistently visualize and use suitable reference planes in all aspects of professional practice.

It is the author's belief that one of the greatest initial difficulties in photography, as in most clinical procedures, is adopting the habit of mentally visualizing the appropriate reference planes; it requires constant practice and a desire for self-improvement, which will prove rewarding for the practitioner in the long run.

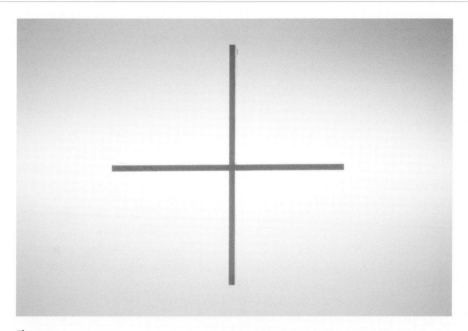

Fig 9-3a
When the observer is positioned at 90 degrees to the surface of the viewbox, the vertical and horizontal planes are perceived as lines. These planes are used for reference.

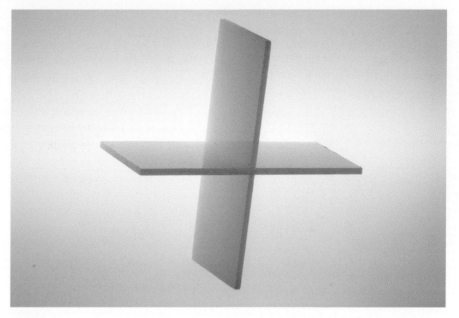

Fig 9-3b
When the observer is positioned at a lateral and superior perspective, the two reference planes are perceived.

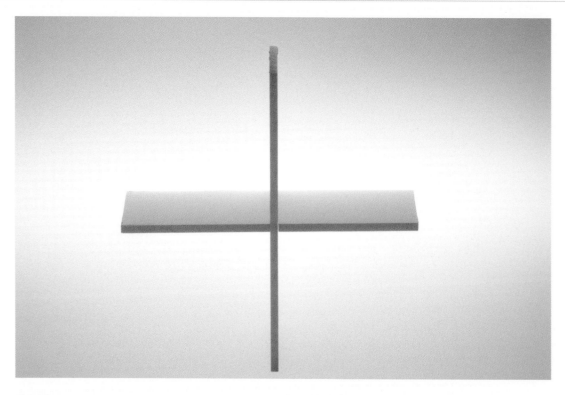

Fig 9-4a
When the position of the observer changes only with respect to the horizontal plane, that plane is perceived; if a similar inclination of perspective occurs at the moment of taking the shot, a distorted image will result. In this example, the vertical plane remains at an angle of 0 degrees to the observer's eyes.

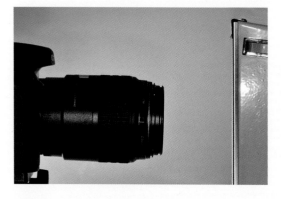

Fig 9-4b
When the optical axis is observed from a lateral perspective, it should appear perpendicular to the surface of the viewbox; the optical axis is positioned correctly with respect to the horizontal plane of reference.

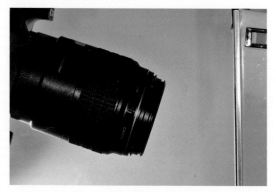

Fig 9-4c
When the camera is incorrectly positioned with respect to the horizontal plane, the perspective changes, and image distortion will result.

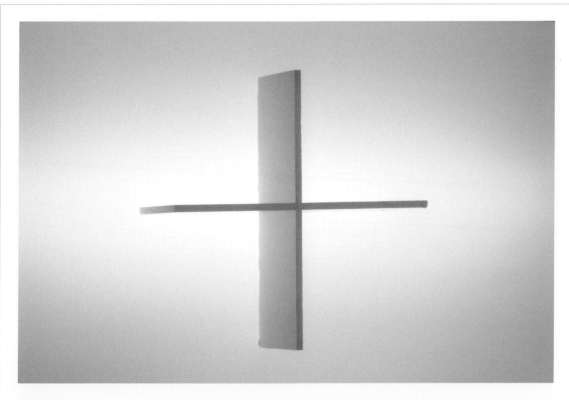

Fig 9-5a
When the position of the observer changes only with respect to the vertical plane, that plane is perceived; if a similar inclination of perspective occurs at the moment of taking the shot, a distorted image will result. In this example, the horizontal plane remains at an angle of 0 degrees to the observer's eyes.

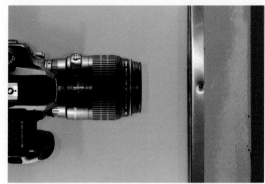

Fig 9-5b
When the camera and viewbox are observed from directly above, the camera's optical axis should be exactly perpendicular to the plane of the viewbox.

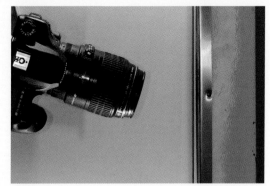

Fig 9-5c
When the camera is incorrectly positioned with respect to the vertical plane, an undesirable perspective is introduced, and distortion of the image will result.

Luca Pascoletti

Part Two

Techniques

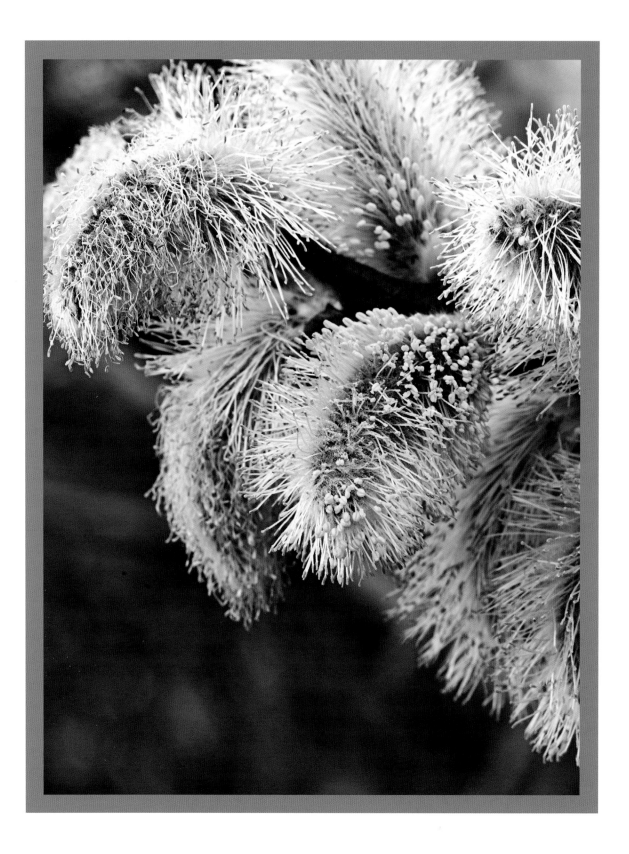

Chapter 10

Equipment and Accessories

The first part of this book presented the theory of photography in dentistry, the many advantages of photographic documentation, and the importance of excellent quality; furthermore, the general principles of photography and specialized techniques were described.

This part of the book focuses on technique; procedures for creating visual documents in an effective and, most importantly, efficient way will be demonstrated. To achieve excellence, priority must be given to ergonomics and to the correct management of technical equipment and auxiliary devices.

With the advent of digital technology, it is possible to document and store a huge quantity of photographic material after a modest outlay of funds. Maintaining a collection of patient photographs is extremely useful for a number of reasons.

In clinical practice, photography is not always easy, especially with patients who are not very cooperative, or who have a small mouth opening. Objectively, some anatomical situations are unfavorable and may be impossible to overcome, such as particular dimensions of the arch or lips. Furthermore, some patients do not immediately understand the need for a photographic examination and, therefore, do not appreciate the maneuvers with mirrors or cheek retractors necessary to obtain good results.

Without a clear and efficient protocol, all photographic procedures will waste time in the long run, which can be discouraging for the practitioner. As already noted, a critical assessment of the results of one's work can prove frustrating, but it is a necessity for those who wish to make professional progress. All operative procedures must be effective and efficient, producing the desired results within a reasonable time and with relative ease.

The aim of photography is to create documents for various purposes:

- Diagnosis
- Communication
- Medicolegal documentation
- Creation of operative protocols
- Education
- Assessment and verification of the quality of one's work
- Creation of photographic archives

Following this line of reasoning, three distinct topics will be developed:

- Choice of suitable instruments
- Criteria for the quality of the visual document
- Synergy between operator and assistant

Cameras and Accessories

In clinical practice, the author uses Nikon equipment: a D200 digital single-lens reflex (SLR) camera, equipped with a Micro-Nikkor f/2.8G VR (vibration reduction) 105-mm macro lens, an SU-800 commander unit, and two SB-R200 Speedlight twin flash units (Fig 10-1). The magnification ratio inscribed on the focusing ring of the 105-mm macro lens always refers to a full-frame 24 × 36–mm sensor. It is important to remember that the actual magnification ratio will be greater when using the same lens on a camera with a classic Advanced Photo System (APS-C) sensor format, such as the D200 (see chapter 4).

Therefore, the recommended magnification ratio values for each photograph listed in chapters 11 and 12 are nominal rather than actual, because they are specific to the camera listed above, which has a smaller-format sensor. The magnification ratios inscribed on the lens'

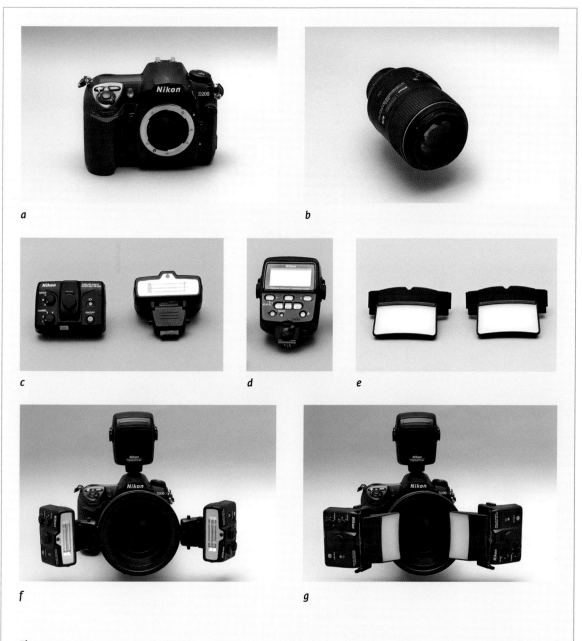

Fig 10-1
*The following Nikon camera components and accessories can be used in clinical photography. (a) D200 camera body.
(b) Micro-Nikkor f/2.8G VR 105-mm macro lens. (c) Wireless remote SB-R200 Speedlight twin flash units. (d) SU-800
commander unit for wireless Speedlights. (e) SW-11 extreme close-up positioning adapters. (f) The lens and the SU-800
commander unit are attached to the camera body. The twin flash units are anchored to an SX-1 attachment ring that is
mounted on the lens. (g) In this image, two SW-11 adapters have been added to the attachment ring; these are excellent for
intraoral close-up shots of the posterior teeth.*

focusing ring only correspond to reality when used with a camera with a full-frame sensor.

Dental photography requires the use of accessory devices, some of which are more crucial than others. There are two pieces of equipment that are indispensible; these are available in various shapes and sizes to suit a variety of situations:

- Intraoral mirrors
- Cheek retractors

The practitioner will find other accessories particularly useful:

- Heat source, such as a Bunsen burner
- Air-water spray
- Saliva ejector
- Contrastor, either cardboard or metal

A detailed analysis of the characteristics of each of these devices and instructions for their use follow.

Intraoral mirrors

The need to respect the spatiality of the image, as dictated by the zero-coordinate rule, makes the use of intraoral mirrors indispensible in certain shots. For example, without the use of a mirror, it would be impossible to correctly frame full-arch occlusal photographs because of the anatomical limitations to mouth opening.

Intraoral mirrors for dental photography are available in three basic shapes (Fig 10-2):

- Large figure eight–shaped
- Small figure eight–shaped
- Bean shaped

The figure eight–shaped mirrors are indicated for the following images:

- Occlusal full-arch views
- Incisal views of the anterior sextants
- Palatal and lingual views of the anterior sextants

The figure eight–shaped mirrors come in two sizes. Both sizes have ends of different widths and a narrower middle part. For photographs of the complete arch, the width of the mouth opening at the level of the labial commissures determines the end to be used. The wider end is preferable whenever possible for two reasons: a larger area of the molar region will be included, and it will be less likely that the edges of the mirror, a source of visual tension, are visible in the image (Fig 10-3).

The bean-shaped mirror is indicated for the following images:

- Occlusal views of the posterior sextants
- Lingual and palatal views of the posterior sextants

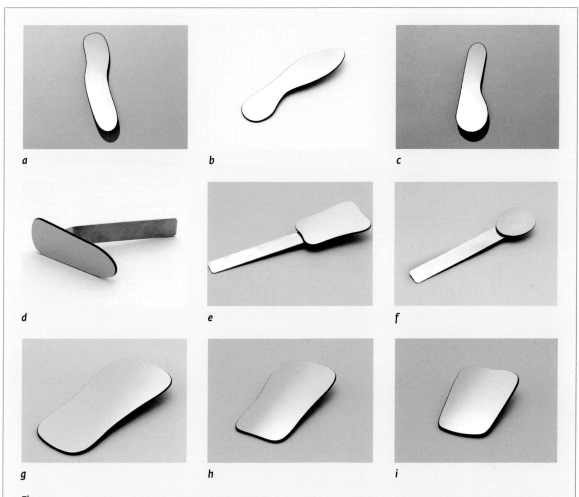

Fig 10-2

(a to i) A variety of intraoral mirrors are available on the market and are appropriate for most images. In choosing which mirror to use, both the area to be framed and the area to be illuminated should be considered. The mirror should be as wide as possible to enable the light to be reflected in the best possible way. For this reason, large mirrors are recommended.

To simplify matters, the two ends of the mirror, the drop-shaped end and the tapered end, are considered separately. Furthermore, each end has two edges: for the drop-shaped end, a convex and a flat edge; for the tapered end, a convex and a concave-convex edge (Fig 10-4).

Cheek retractors

These accessories remove the cheeks and lips from the framed image. Various shapes and sizes are available to satisfy the practitioner's requirements: self-retracting or handheld, large or small (Fig 10-5). The self-retracting version has two wings connected by an arch; the handheld retractor has one or two wings on a support handle. For some images, it is necessary to modify these accessories to

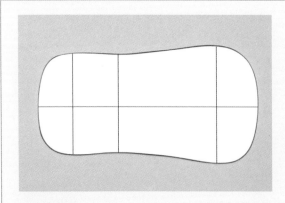

Fig 10-3a
Dimensions of a large figure eight–shaped mirror (Fotoscientifica): maximum length, 156 mm; maximum width, 81 mm; minimum width, 67 mm.

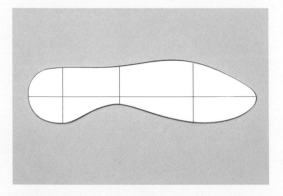

Fig 10-3b
Dimensions of a bean-shaped mirror (Fotoscientifica): maximum length, 175 mm; width at the tapered end, 147 mm; width at the drop-shaped end, 43 mm; minimum width at the level of the isthmus, 30 mm.

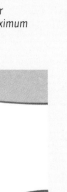

Fig 10-4a
On the drop-shaped end, the upper edge is flat and the lower edge is convex.

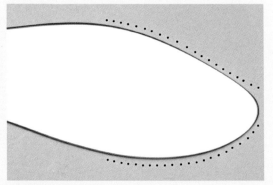

Fig 10-4b
On the tapered end, the upper edge is concave-convex and the lower edge is convex.

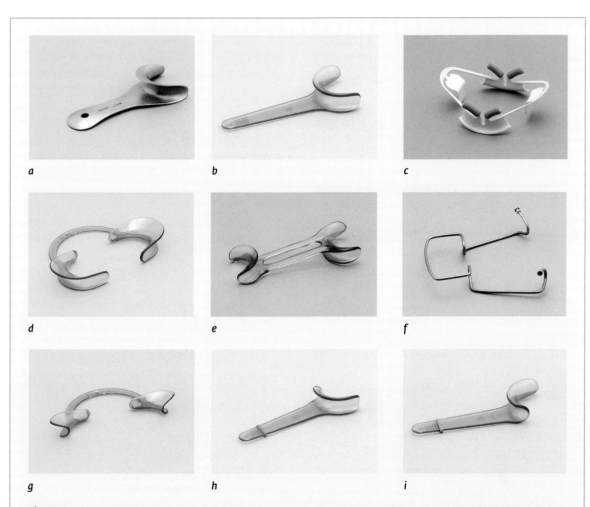

Fig 10-5

Cheek retractors are available in many shapes and sizes. (a) The Maxil retractor (Omnia) is ideal for photographing posterior teeth from a lateral view for orthodontic documentation. This retractor allows the practitioner to photograph as far back as the permanent first molar without using a mirror. (b) The Spandex retractor (Hager & Werken) is used to photograph lateral views with a mirror and frontal views in occlusion. (c) The Optiview retractor (Kerr) retracts the lips and cheeks at the same time. (d) The Spandex self-retracting cheek retractor is used as an alternative to two handheld retractors for frontal views of the arches in occlusion. (e) A double-ended handheld retractor. (f) With a self-retracting wire retractor, the practitioner can take photographs even without being supported in the posterior regions. (g) The Spandex self-retracting cheek retractor with modified wings is ideal for full-arch occlusal photographs; it makes the use of large mirrors possible by not interfering with their placement. (h) This Spandex retractor with modified wing is appropriate for occlusal, lingual, and palatal views of the maxillary right and mandibular left posterior sextants. (i) This Spandex retractor with modified wing is appropriate for occlusal, lingual, and palatal views of the maxillary left and mandibular right posterior sextants.

obtain optimum tissue retraction; these modifications are simple operations and can be carried out in the clinic. For example, a self-retracting cheek retractor is used for the photograph of the occlusal surfaces of a complete arch; however, the retracting wings may interfere with placement of the mirror or framing of the image. If the retractor is modified by removing half of each wing, it can be used to retract the cheeks adequately, position the mirror, and capture the image. The handheld retractor can be modified in the same way. However, it is important to bear in mind that this will produce two retractors that are mirror images of each other: one for the maxillary right and mandibular left sextants, and the other for the maxillary left and mandibular right sextants. It is important to be able to differentiate between the modified retractors, for ease and rapidity of use. A tungsten carbide disk mounted onto a straight handpiece or a small saw should be used to cut the retractor. The edges must be carefully polished with rubber wheels and brushes so that irregularities do not cause the patient any discomfort.

To modify a retractor for images of the maxillary right and mandibular left sextants, the following steps should be taken: first, the retractor is positioned with the handle facing down and the U-shaped wing facing up; second, half of the right wing is cut off. To modify a retractor for images of the maxillary left and mandibular right sextants, the left half is removed. For short arches, such as in children or in distal edentulous areas, a special retractor with very concave wings can be used, which allows the practitioner to forgo the use of mirrors in lateral photographs in occlusion. This technique provides better visualization of the teeth and direct framing of the image.

Additional accessories

In addition to the instruments described above, other accessories are also very useful (Fig 10-6). The saliva ejector and the air-water spray keep the mirrors dry and the teeth and mucosa free from saliva. Contrastors are needed to create a background that brings out the shape and, especially, the various degrees of translucency of the tooth, which is a fundamentally important aspect of esthetic restorations. A source of heat, such as hot water or a flame generated by an alcohol lamp or a Bunsen burner, is necessary to prevent the mirrors from fogging.

The ergonomics of dental practice necessitates rational storage of these accessories to facilitate ease of use; therefore, they should be labeled and stored in ready-to-use containers (Fig 10-7). As a general rule, it is a good idea to use the same instruments as much as possible because changing instruments makes for loss of precious time. For example, after taking occlusal and palatal photographs of the maxillary right posterior sextant, it is logical to proceed to the occlusal and lingual views of the mandibular left posterior sextant because they require the same instruments. It is recommended to maintain at least three containers of photography supplies to avoid delays caused by sterilization.

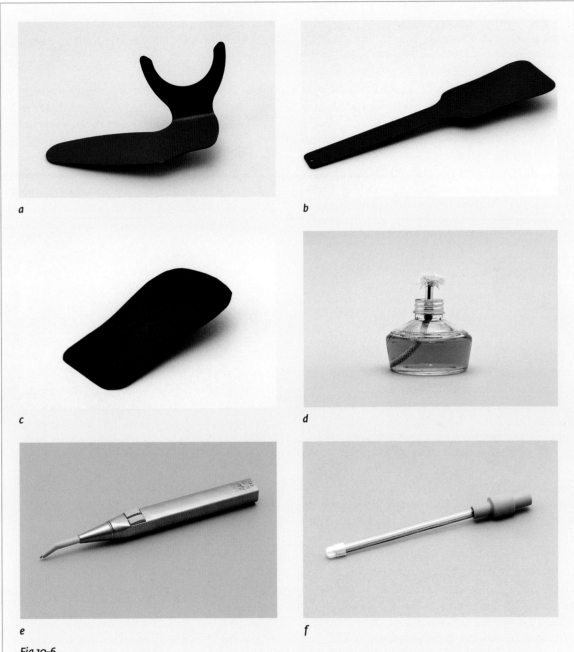

Fig 10-6
(a and b) *Metal contrastors (Nike) are useful for creating a black background whenever the practitioner wishes to emphasize the shape and color of teeth. (c) Disposable black cardboard contrastors are also available. (d) A heat source is used to warm the mirrors to prevent fogging. (e) The air-water spray is indispensible for eliminating the bubbles of saliva that inevitably form between the teeth. (f) A saliva ejector is useful for eliminating saliva and preventing the mirrors from fogging.*

Image Quality

Because the concepts of spatiality and the orthography of the image presented in the first part of this book are fundamental prerequisites to obtaining excellent images, it should be emphasized that all efforts by the practitioner must be directed toward these concepts. To better aim the camera with respect to the planes of reference (see chapter 7), it is extremely useful to display the viewfinder grid, if the camera has this option (Fig 10-8). The quality of the images obtained depends on respecting the rules already set out in the theoretical part of this book, which prioritize magnification ratio and depth of field. These rules can be summarized in the fundamental questions:

- Have I framed everything I need to show?
- Can I see anything in the frame that creates visual tension?

The photographs must not include anything distracting, such as fingers, mirror edges, parts of retractors, saliva ejectors, teeth of the opposing arch, tongue, saliva, lips, or

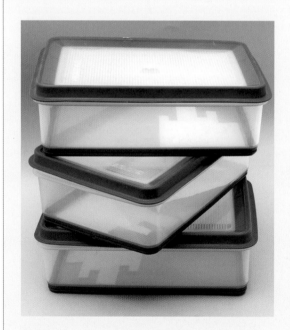

Fig 10-7a
Containers are indispensible for organizing all the necessary accessories. It is a good idea to have several identical containers with all items needed for the various image series.

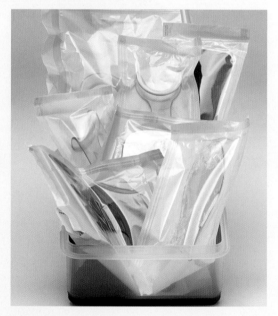

Fig 10-7b
An open container shows the packed and sterilized accessories.

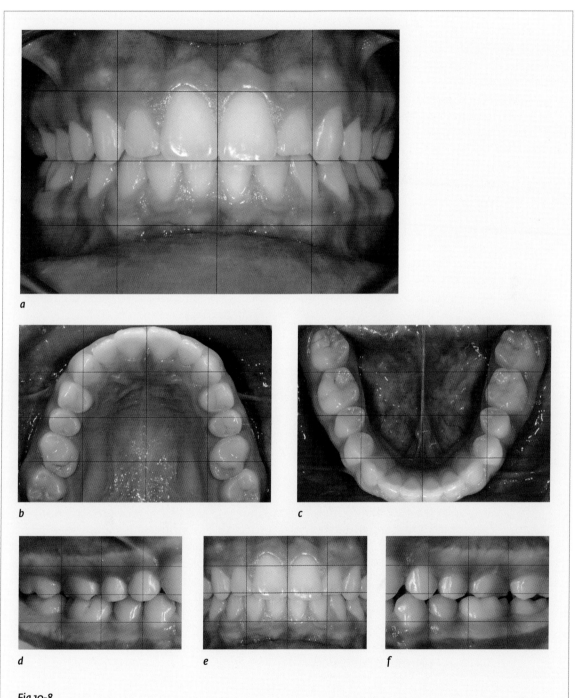

Fig 10-8
(a to f) *Intraoral images illustrate the correct use of the grids on the viewfinder in framing an image according to the zero-coordinate rule.*

nostrils. The photograph must be correctly exposed, and, above all, there must be no areas out of focus; the image must respect the second fundamental rule, depth of field priority. Apart from these parameters, which are fundamental to framing the image, there are other, less important details, which can, nonetheless, prevent the correct reading of the image.

These factors, which can cause visual tension, mainly involve the management of the photographic field or the mirrors: halos, saliva, or scratches on the surface of the mirror spoil the image and frustrate the efforts of the practitioner. Likewise, excessive saliva, residual plaque, or food on the tooth surfaces are disturbing elements, unless the photographs are to serve as pretreatment documentation. To avoid reducing the value of the image, the mirrors must be kept clean with a soft cloth and heated before using to prevent fogging from the patient's breath. The consistent use of a saliva ejector, positioned where saliva is most likely to collect, is extremely useful in avoiding a buildup of saliva. Use of an air-water spray is also recommended to keep the surface of the teeth dry and, if necessary, to clean the mirror. Although image-retouching programs can be used to correct unwanted details, the act of retouching or cropping may alter the quality or the proportions of the image. If the practitioner must retouch a photograph, he or she needs to be careful to always keep the original, preferably in the raw image file format.

Synergy Between Practitioner and Assistant

Previous discussion has established that a visual document should be acquired in a standardized manner, as rapidly as possible for the sake of efficiency and to avoid stress for both the patient and the practitioner. The collaboration of the dental assistant is fundamental in effectively and efficiently photographing the patient.

The assistant is responsible for the following tasks:

- Position the backrest of the dental treatment chair correctly for each view
- Instruct the patient as to the position of the head and tongue
- Choose and correctly handle the retractors and mirrors during the shot

The assistant should be well positioned, preferably seated, for maximum stability and to be able to grasp the mirror as firmly as possible. Mirrors should be held by their edges, as far away as possible from the area to be framed, so as to not obstruct the light from the flash units (Fig 10-9). This maneuver is not easy and requires a great deal of strength, so it can be extremely tiring for the assistant. For this reason, constant practice is absolutely essential, and it is a good idea to photograph on a daily basis. The assistant must be familiar with the photography procedures to anticipate the practitioner's needs, getting into position quickly and correctly and with the appropriate accessories readily available. The assistant's role is fundamental to achieving the desired results, and, like other dental procedures, photography must be considered a four-handed job. In summary, fast and efficient photography requires perfect knowledge of the camera settings, and also of every position of the patient, assistant, and practitioner.

Contrary to other authors' beliefs, the patient should not actively participate in the taking of the photograph, but should passively follow the instructions given by the assistant. This will save the time it inevitably takes to instruct the patient, and, most importantly, it will avoid possible interference by the patient during positioning of the accessories. As a general rule, the practitioner, in addition to being oriented for correct framing of the image, must ensure the stability of the position of the patient and accessories. Ideally, photography should be done from a seated position, but should this not be possible, the practitioner should rest on a stable support, preferably the structure of the dental treatment chair.

In the series of photographs that follow in chapters 11 and 12, the descriptions of the positioning of the patient and the image are often repetitive; however, it is very useful to have all the information required for each shot listed in one place.

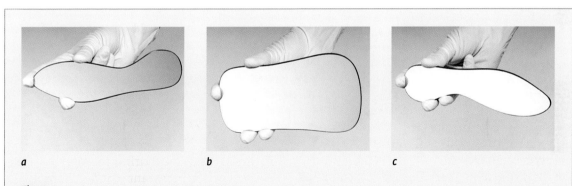

a   b   c

Fig 10-9
(a to c) *The correct grasp of the intraoral mirror in various positions is shown. It is essential for the assistant to have a firm grip on the edge, leaving the maximum surface area free for reflection of light from the flash units. This grasp can be difficult because of the strength needed; however, with constant practice, excellent results can be obtained.*

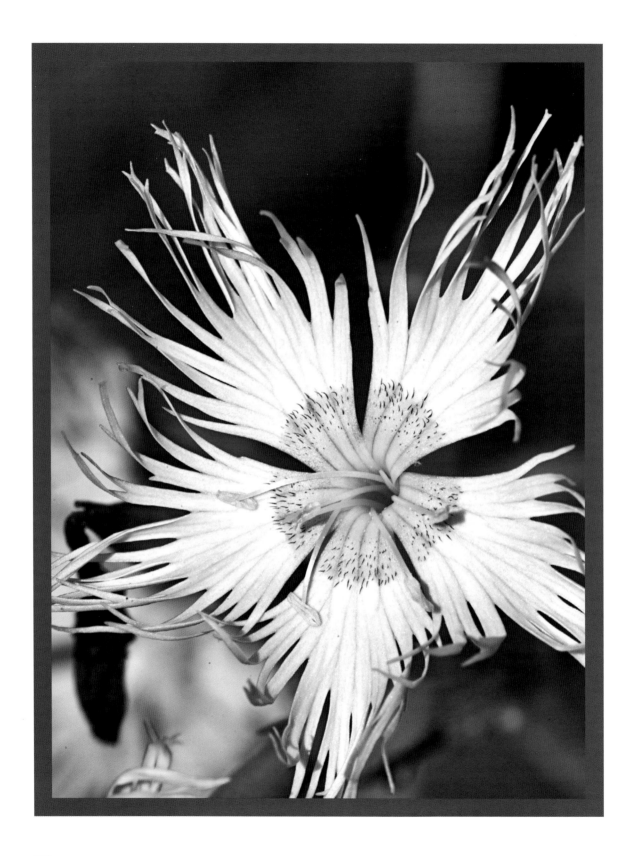

Chapter 11

Extraoral
Series

Neither accessories nor the aid of an assistant are needed for extraoral views. Wheeled swivel are used to allow easy adjustment of position (Fig 11-1). To ensure that the image is repeatable, it is important to always use the same background. Moreover, the same operator-subject distance should be used to preserve the magnification ratio. It may be helpful to make note of this distance in the patient chart. The photographs in chapters 11 and 12 were taken using a camera with a classic Advanced Photo System (APS-C) format, so the magnification ratio inscribed on the lens' focusing ring is nominal rather than actual. The magnification ratio changes when a smaller-format sensor is used because of the concept of equivalent focal length (see chapter 4).

Documenting the patient's profile is a useful technique in dentistry. To highlight the profile of a fair-skinned patient, a dark background can be used, although a lighter background will bring out the radiance of the face. Gray-colored backgrounds are a good compromise for all extraoral photos (Fig 11-2). Photographs can be standardized even further by using a tripod that is always placed in the same position.

The use of the through-the-lens (TTL) exposure mode and at least two flash sources is recommended. The flash units should be inclined so that a beam of light converges toward the focal point. Moreover, the use of auxiliary lateral flash units is advised, to minimize the inevitable shadows that form on the background. Alternatively, the distance between the subject and the background can be increased, which avoids the use of additional flash units if the room is well lit; however, this procedure is not recommended because the quality of the lighting will be too variable and the repeatability of the image will be lost. For the protocols that follow, the degree of difficulty of each shot is rated on a scale from 1 to 5 according to the experience of the author.

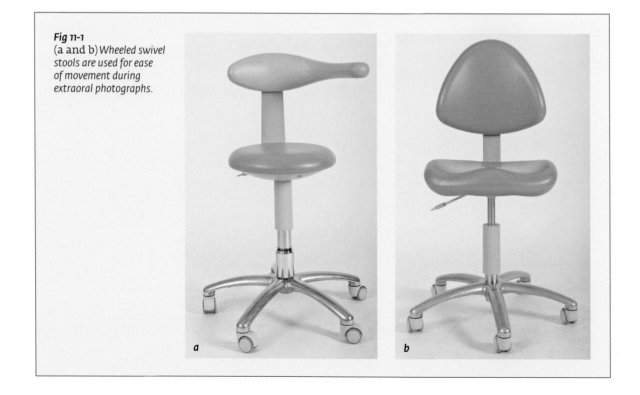

Fig 11-1
(a and b) Wheeled swivel stools are used for ease of movement during extraoral photographs.

a

b

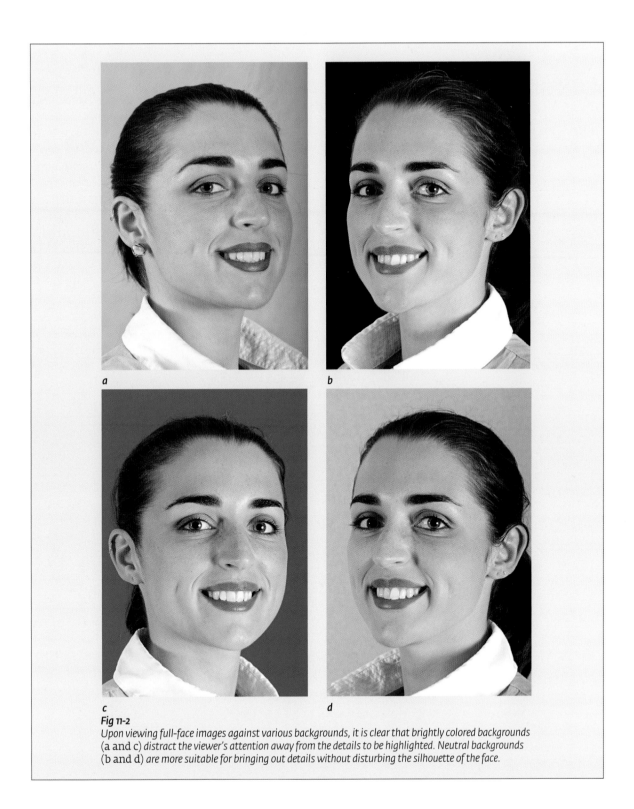

a

b

c

d

Fig 11-2
Upon viewing full-face images against various backgrounds, it is clear that brightly colored backgrounds (a and c) distract the viewer's attention away from the details to be highlighted. Neutral backgrounds (b and d) are more suitable for bringing out details without disturbing the silhouette of the face.

VIEW 1

Degree of difficulty: 1

Position of the patient:
- Seated opposite the practitioner on a swivel stool with head and eyes facing straight ahead

Position of the assistant:
- Not applicable

Position of the practitioner:
- Seated on a wheeled swivel stool about 1.5 m (5 ft) in front of the patient

Camera settings:
- Camera held vertically
- Magnification ratio 1:8 to 1:10; aperture f/11
- Aiming point on the median line level with the lower orbital rims; focal point on the zygoma (Fig 11-3a)
- Flash units at the 3- and 9-o'clock positions (Fig 11-3b)

Type of cheek retractor:
- Not applicable

Type of mirror:
- Not applicable

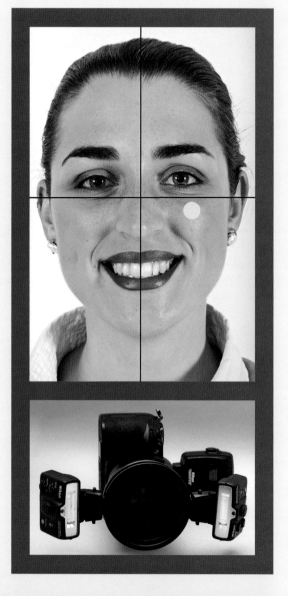

Fig 11-3a

Fig 11-3b

COMMENTS

The patient is seated on a wheeled swivel stool with thighs parallel to the floor, so that he or she can change position for the profile views without getting up. The practitioner is seated opposite on a wheeled stool for ease and rapidity of movement. The first frontal shot is taken with the camera in a vertical position, framing the face vertically from the top of the head to the base of the neck, and laterally from ear to ear. For the second shot, the operator asks the patient to smile.

Frontal Face, Smiling and with Lips Relaxed

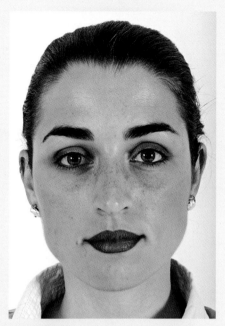

Fig 11-4
Frontal view of face with the lips relaxed.

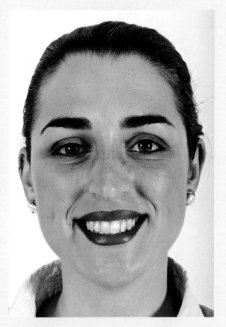

Fig 11-5
Frontal view of face while smiling.

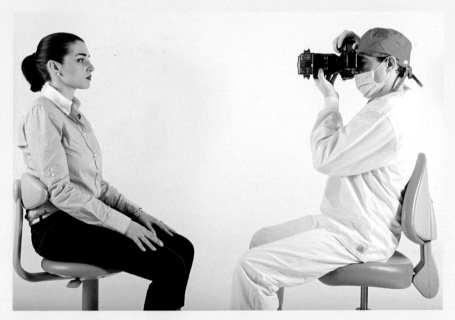

Fig 11-6
Correct position of patient and practitioner for this view.

VIEW 2

Degree of difficulty: 1

Position of the patient:
- Seated opposite the practitioner on a swivel stool, positioned 90 degrees away from the frontal view to the right or left; head and eyes facing straight ahead

Position of the assistant:
- Not applicable

Position of the practitioner:
- Seated on a wheeled swivel stool about 1.5 m (5 ft) lateral to the patient

Camera settings:
- Camera held vertically
- Magnification ratio 1:8 to 1:10; aperture f/11
- Aiming point posterior to the zygoma at the level of the lower orbital rim; focal point on the zygoma (Fig 11-7a)
- Flash units at the 3- and 9-o'clock positions (Fig 11-7b)

Type of cheek retractor:
- Not applicable

Type of mirror:
- Not applicable

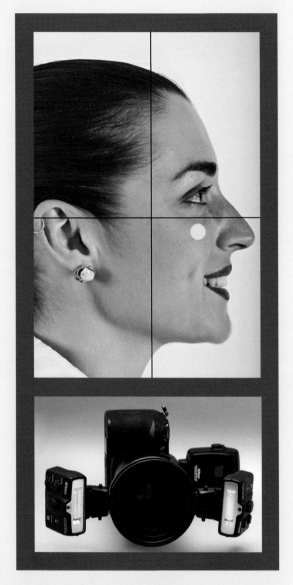

Fig 11-7a

Fig 11-7b

COMMENTS

The patient is seated on a wheeled swivel stool with thighs parallel to the floor, so that he or she can change position for the profile views without getting up. The practitioner is seated opposite on a wheeled chair for ease and rapidity of movement. The right and left lateral shots are taken with the camera in a vertical position, framing the face vertically from the top of the head to the base of the neck and laterally to include the ear. For the second shot, the operator asks the patient to smile. The lateral full-face photographs should be taken with the same magnification ratio selected for the frontal views, so that the two images will have the same dimensions. The magnification ratio value should be recorded to facilitate subsequent superimposable images.

Profile, Smiling and with Lips Relaxed

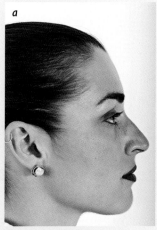 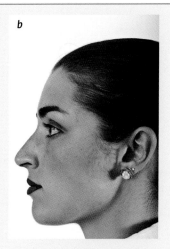

Fig 11-8
Right (a) and left (b) profile full-face views with the lips relaxed.

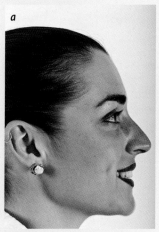 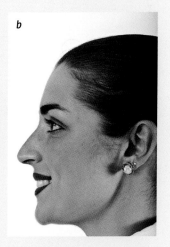

Fig 11-9
Right (a) and left (b) profile full-face views while smiling.

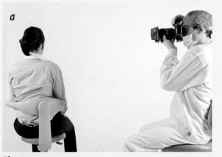 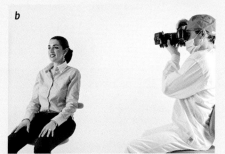

Fig 11-10
(a and b) Correct position of patient and practitioner for this view. The use of wheeled swivel stools expedites this procedure.

VIEW 3

Degree of difficulty: 1

Position of the patient:
- Seated opposite the practitioner on a swivel stool with head and eyes facing straight ahead

Position of the assistant:
- Not applicable

Position of the practitioner:
- Seated on a wheeled swivel stool about 50 cm (20 inches) away from the patient

Camera settings:
- Camera held horizontally about 40 cm (16 inches) from the focal point
- Magnification ratio 1:2; aperture f/32 (minimum aperture)
- Aiming point at the middle third of the central incisors; focal point at the level of contact between the lateral incisor and the canine (Fig 11-11a)
- Flash units at the 3- and 9-o'clock positions (Fit 11-11b)

Type of cheek retractor:
- Not applicable

Type of mirror:
- Not applicable

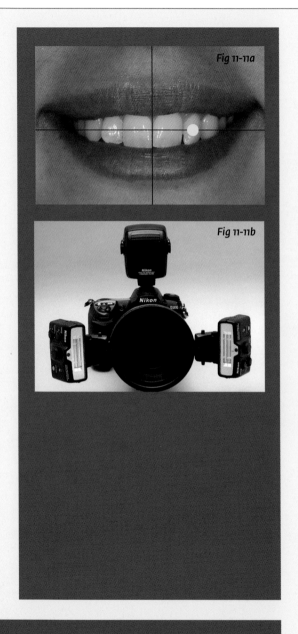

Fig 11-11a

Fig 11-11b

COMMENTS

The patient is seated on a wheeled swivel stool with the thighs parallel to the floor, so that he or she can change position for the profile views without getting up. The practitioner is seated opposite, on a wheeled chair for ease and rapidity of movement; he or she is closer to the patient because of the greater magnification ratio required. The operator asks the patient to smile three times: first, a slight, barely perceptible smile; second, an average smile; and third, a maximum or forced smile. With these three images, the practitioner can assess the esthetics of the smile and the lips.

Slight, Average, and Maximum Smiles

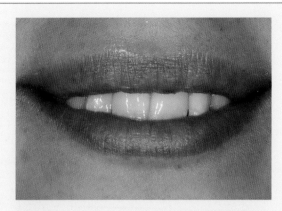

Fig 11-12a
Slight smile.

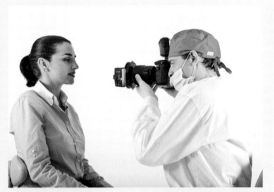

Fig 11-12b
Correct position for this view.

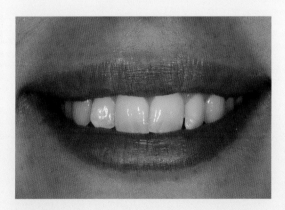

Fig 11-13a
Average smile.

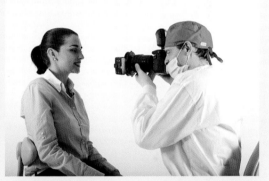

Fig 11-13b
Correct position for this view.

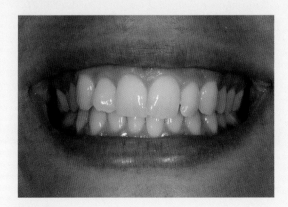

Fig 11-14a
Maximum smile.

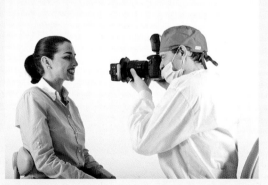

Fig 11-14b
Correct position for this view.

VIEW 4

Degree of difficulty: 1

Position of the patient:
- Seated opposite the practitioner on a swivel stool, positioned 90 degrees away from the frontal view to the right or left; head and eyes facing straight ahead

Position of the assistant:
- Not applicable

Position of the practitioner:
- Seated on a wheeled swivel stool about 50 cm (20 inches) away from the patient

Camera settings:
- Camera held horizontally about 40 cm (16 inches) from the focal point
- Magnification ratio 1:2; aperture f/32 (minimum aperture)
- Aiming point at the level of contact between the lateral incisor and the canine; focal point on the plane of the lateral incisor (Fig 11-15a)
- Flash units at the 3- and 9-o'clock positions (Fig 11-15b)

Type of cheek retractor:
- Not applicable

Type of mirror:
- Not applicable

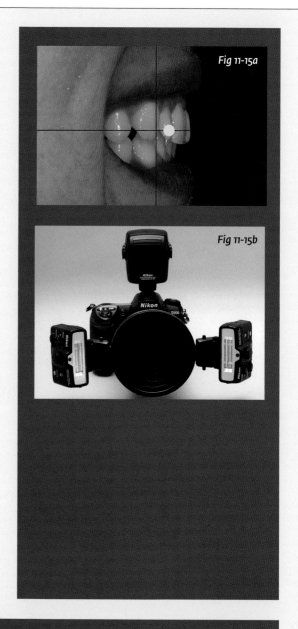

Fig 11-15a

Fig 11-15b

COMMENTS

The patient is seated on a wheeled swivel stool with thighs parallel to the floor, so that he or she can change position for the profile views without getting up. The practitioner is seated opposite, on a wheeled chair for ease and rapidity of movement; he or she is closer to the patient because of the greater magnification ratio required. The right and left lateral shots are taken with the camera in a horizontal position, and the patient is requested to smile while showing the teeth as much as possible.

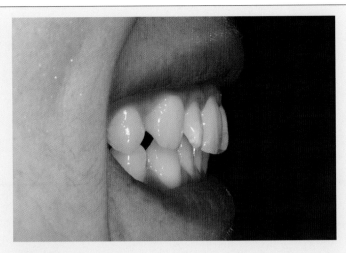

Fig 11-16a
Right lateral smile

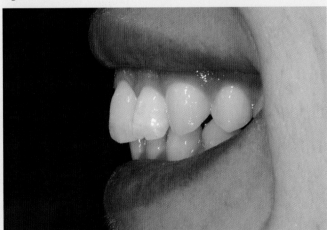

Fig 11-16b
Left lateral smile.

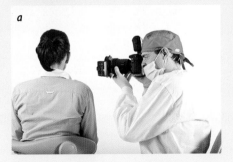 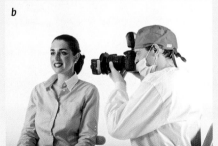

Fig 11-17
(a and b) *Correct position for this view.*

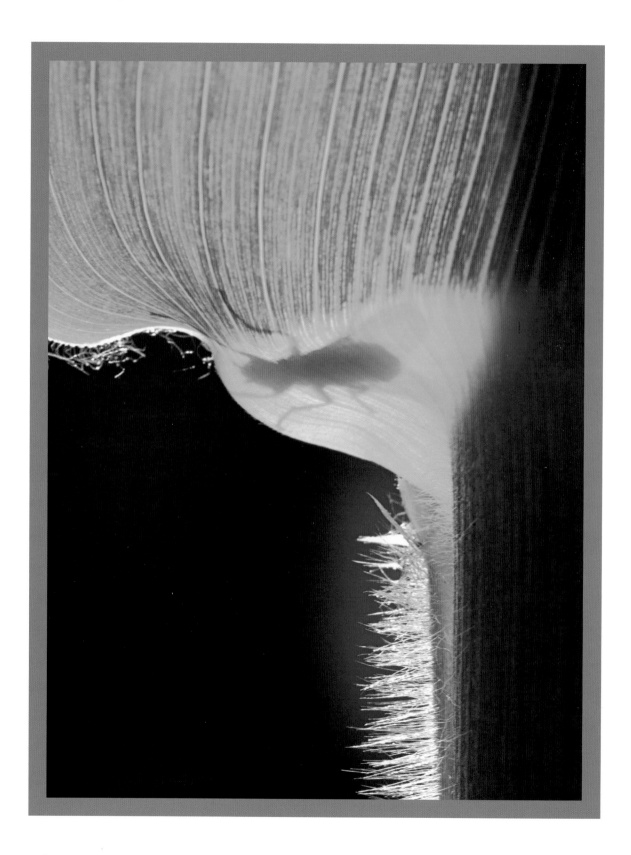

Chapter 12

Intraoral Series

Unlike the extraoral series, the intraoral series requires the assistant's help. Another difference is that the patient must be seated in the dental treatment chair.

An important consideration is that the mirrors should be warmed to prevent them from fogging. If necessary, the mirrors can be cleaned with a soft cloth to remove traces of saliva. Moreover, it is essential to keep the saliva ejector in the oral cavity.

Not all patients are easy subjects to photograph, for reasons relating to anatomy or character. Generally, it is more difficult to photograph the mandible because of the presence of saliva, which tends to collect in the back of the mouth. For maximum efficiency, the protocols that follow are grouped according to two criteria: the inclination of the dental chair and the type of accessories required.

All photographs are taken with the chair inclined in one of three positions: 110, 135, or 180 degrees. This allows the practitioner to quickly take all photographs in a certain position before adjusting the chair, avoiding unnecessary and tiresome movements.

For photographs taken at 110 degrees, which are not particularly taxing, the assistant can remain standing; the other two positions (135 and 180 degrees) require more engagement on the part of the assistant, who should be seated for greater stability.

The second priority is to limit how frequently the necessary accessories must be switched between shots. The shots are organized in a sequence that minimizes putting down and picking up accessories.

For example, for views of the posterior sextant, the maxillary right shots are taken, followed by the mandibular left, because they require the same accessories. Similarly, the maxillary left and mandibular right sextants are photographed together.

VIEW 5
Right overjet

VIEW 6
Left overjet

VIEW 7
Full arches in normal occlusion

VIEW 8
Anterior sextants in normal occlusion

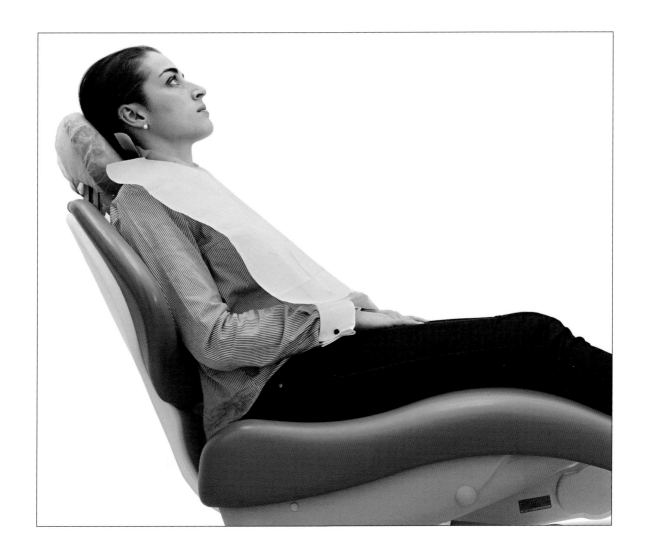

DENTAL CHAIR INCLINED AT 110 DEGREES

VIEW 5

Degree of difficulty: 2

Position of the patient:
- Backrest of the treatment chair inclined 110 degrees (Fig 12-1a)
- Patient's head and eyes facing straight ahead
- Teeth in normal occlusion

Position of the assistant:
- Standing at the 12-o'clock position (Figs 12-1a and 12-1b)
- Two cheek retractors are used by pulling the handles toward the cheeks, or
- A cheek retractor held in the right hand and a contrastor held in the left hand are used to retract the lips and cheeks

Position of the practitioner:
- Standing or seated at the 9-o'clock position (Figs 12-1a and 12-1b)

Camera settings:
- Camera held horizontally 35 cm (14 inches) from the focal point
- Magnification ratio 1:1.5; aperture f/32 (minimum aperture)
- Flash units at the 3- and 9-o'clock positions (Fig 12-1c)
- Aiming point at distal of the right central incisor; focal point on the plane of the right lateral incisor (Fig 12-1d)

Type of cheek retractor:
- Two handheld cheek retractors, or
- One cheek retractor and one contrastor

Type of mirror:
- Not applicable

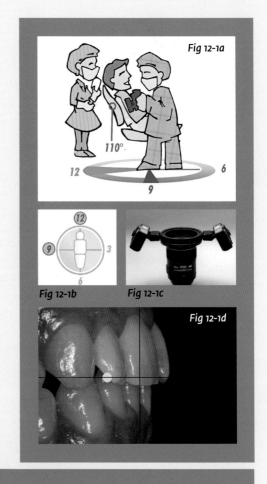

Fig 12-1a

Fig 12-1b   Fig 12-1c

Fig 12-1d

ACCESSORIES NEEDED

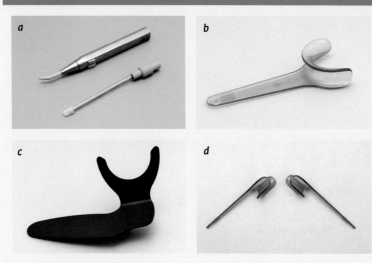

Fig 12-2a
Saliva ejector and air-water spray.

Fig 12-2b
Handheld cheek retractor.

Fig 12-2c
This contrastor is useful because it retracts the lip and creates an ideal dark background at the same time.

Fig 12-2d
The correct angle of the two cheek retractors, about 110 degrees, as seen from above.

Right Overjet

COMMENTS

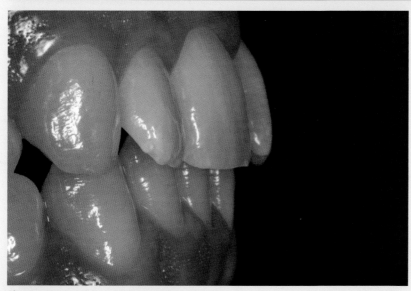

The anterior teeth are shown in intercuspal position from the patient's right side. It is important to maintain a homogeneous, and preferably dark, background to increase the contrast with the color of the teeth; the increased contrast highlights the anteroposterior distance between the maxillary and mandibular incisors. The metal contrastor has two functions, as a cheek retractor and as a dark background.

Fig 12-3
Right overjet.

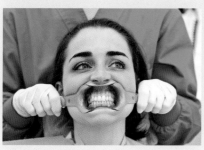

a

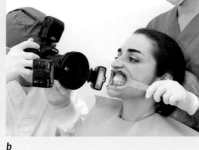

b

Fig 12-4a
The assistant's position when using two cheek retractors.

Fig 12-4b
This view shows the position of the practitioner when framing the shot. For this view, it is important to maintain a dark, uniform background.

ALTERNATIVE METHOD

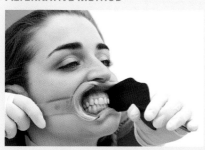

a

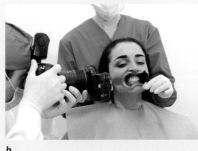

b

Fig 12-5a
The assistant's position when using one cheek retractor and one contrastor.

Fig 12-5b
This view shows the position of the practitioner when framing the shot.

VIEW 6

Degree of difficulty: 2

Position of the patient:

- Backrest of the treatment chair inclined 110 degrees (Fig 12-6a)
- Patient's head and eyes facing straight ahead
- Teeth in normal occlusion

Position of the assistant:

- Standing at the 12-o'clock position (Figs 12-6a and 12-6b)
- Two cheek retractors are used by pulling the handles toward the cheeks, or
- A cheek retractor held in the left hand and a contrastor held in the right hand are used to retract the lips and cheeks

Position of the practitioner:

- Standing or seated at the 3-o'clock position (Figs 12-6a and 12-6b)

Camera settings:

- Camera held horizontally 35 cm (14 inches) from the focal point
- Magnification ratio 1:1.5; aperture f/32 (minimum aperture)
- Flash units at the 3- and 9-o'clock positions (Fig 12-6c)
- Aiming point at distal of the left central incisor; focal point on the plane of the left lateral incisor (Fig 12-6d)

Type of cheek retractor:

- Two handheld cheek retractors, or
- One cheek retractor and one contrastor

Type of mirror:

- Not applicable

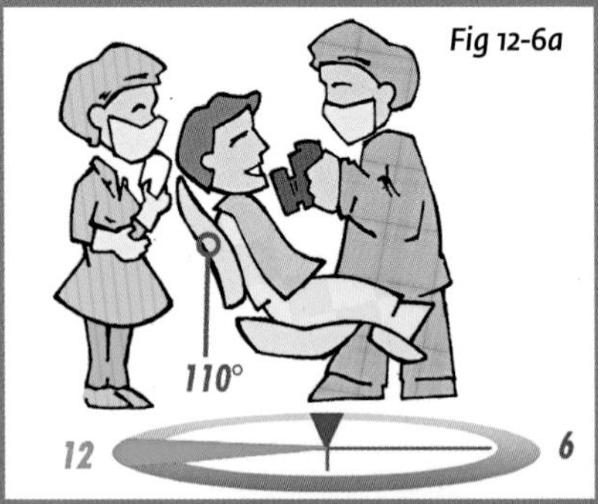

Fig 12-6a

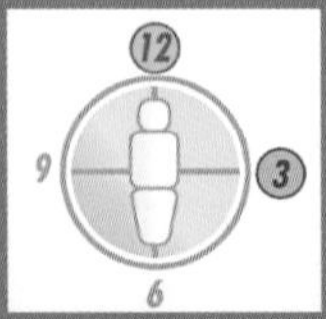

Fig 12-6b

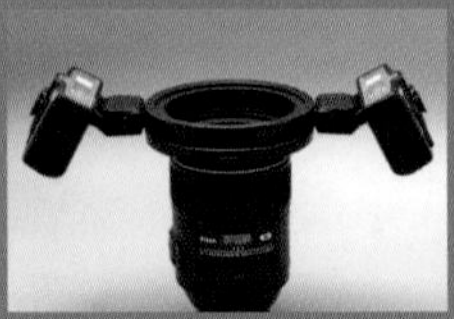

Fig 12-6c

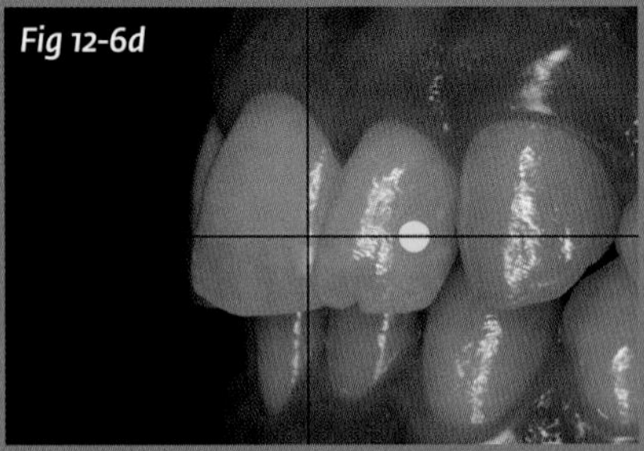

Fig 12-6d

ACCESSORIES NEEDED

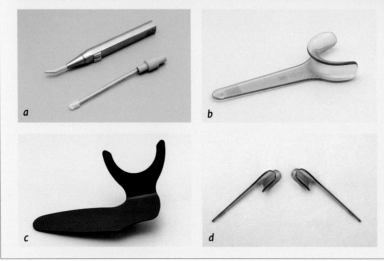

a

b

c

d

Fig 12-7a
Saliva ejector and air-water spray.

Fig 12-7b
Handheld cheek retractor.

Fig 12-7c
The contrastor is useful because it retracts the lip and also creates an ideal dark background.

Fig 12-7d
The correct angle of the two cheek retractors, about 110 degrees, as seen from above.

Left Overjet

The anterior teeth are shown in intercuspal position from the patient's left side. As in the previous shot, it is important to maintain a homogeneous, dark background to increase the contrast with the color of the teeth; the increased contrast highlights the anteroposterior distance between the maxillary and mandibular incisors. The metal contrastor functions as a cheek retractor and as a dark background.

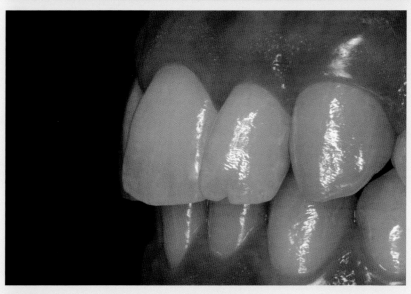

Fig 12-8
Left overjet.

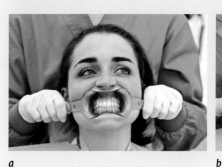

a

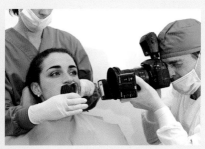

b

Fig 12-9a
The assistant's position when using two cheek retractors.

Fig 12-9b
This view shows the position of the practitioner when framing the shot. For this view, it is important to maintain a dark, uniform background.

ALTERNATIVE METHOD

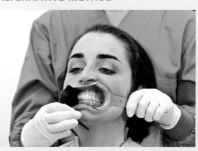

a

b

Fig 12-10a
The assistant's position when using one cheek retractor and one contrastor is shown.

Fig 12-10b
This view shows the position of the practitioner when framing the shot.

VIEW 7

Degree of difficulty: 2

Position of the patient:

- Backrest of the treatment chair inclined 110 degrees (Fig 12-11a)
- Patient's head and eyes facing straight ahead

Position of the assistant:

- Standing at the 3-o'clock position (Figs 12-11a and 12-11c); self-retracting cheek retractor is held at the center of the handle, or
- Standing at the 12-o'clock position (Figs 12-11b and 12-11d); two cheek retractors are used with the handles at an angle of 160 degrees

Position of the practitioner:

- Standing at the 7-o'clock position (Figs 12-11a to 12-11d)

Camera settings:

- Camera held horizontally 45 cm (18 inches) from the focal point
- Magnification ratio 1:2.7, aperture f/32 (minimum aperture)
- Flash units at the 3- and 9-o'clock positions (Fig 12-11e)
- Aiming point at the intersection of the median line and the occlusal plane; focal point on the plane of the distal canine (Fig 12-11f)

Type of cheek retractor:

- One self-retracting or two handheld cheek retractors

Type of mirror:

- Not applicable

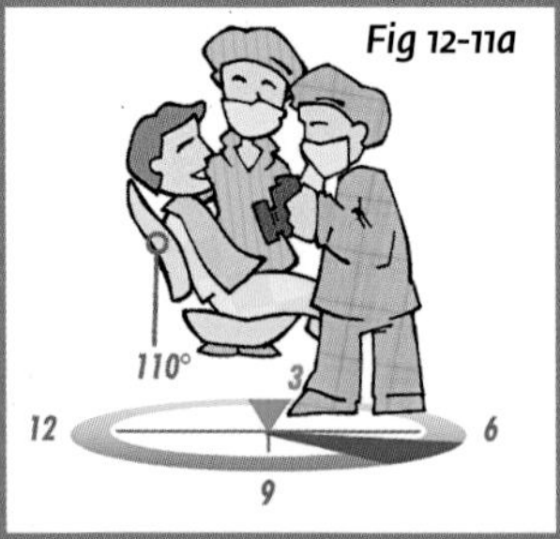

Fig 12-11a

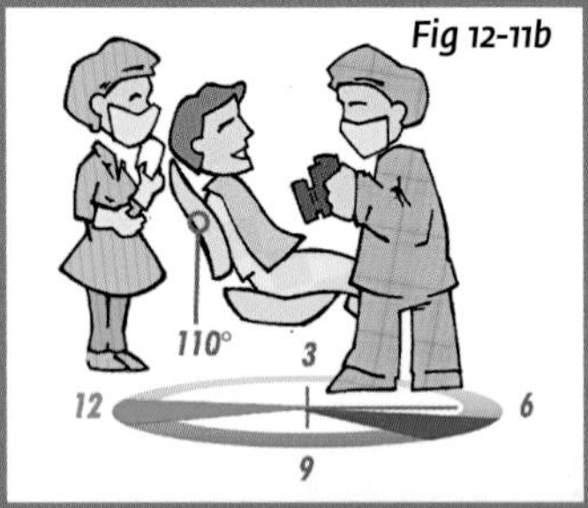

Fig 12-11b

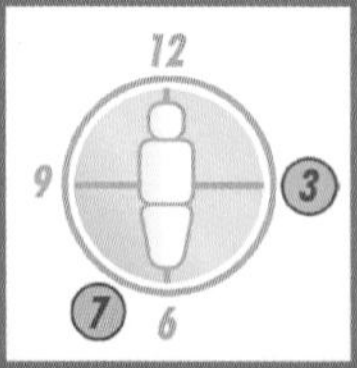

Fig 12-11c

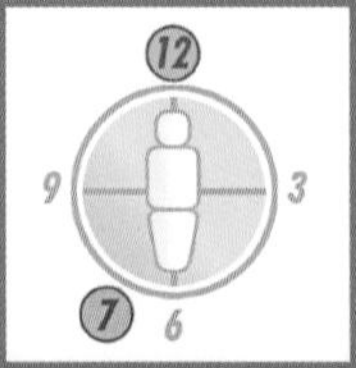

Fig 12-11d

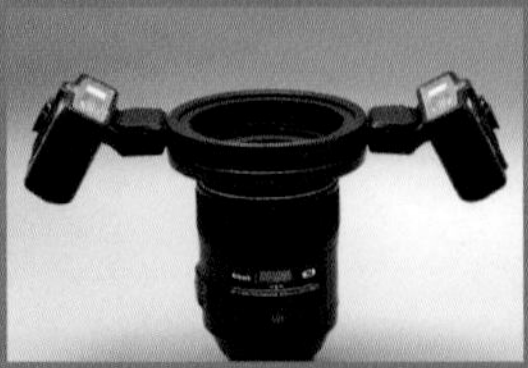

Fig 12-11e

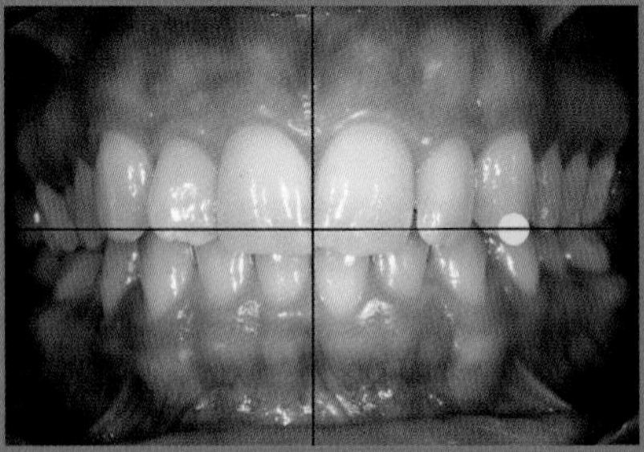

Fig 12-11f

ACCESSORIES NEEDED

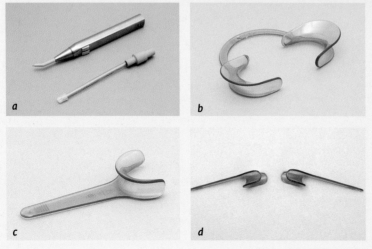

a

b

c

d

Fig 12-12a
Saliva ejector and air-water spray.

Fig 12-12b
Self-retracting cheek retractor.

Fig 12-12c
Handheld cheek retractor.

Fig 12-12d
The correct angle of the two cheek retractors to each other, about 160 degrees, as seen from above.

Full Arches in Normal Occlusion

COMMENTS

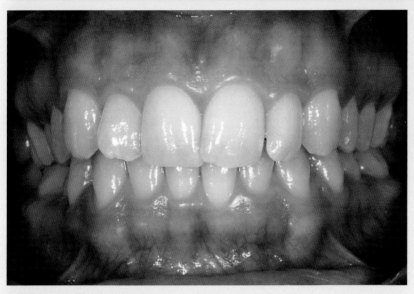

There are two methods of obtaining this image, using two handheld or one self-retracting cheek retractor. In the former method, the assistant stands at 12 o'clock, and the practitioner holds the saliva ejector. In the latter, the assistant is positioned at 3 o'clock and uses a free hand for the saliva ejector or air-water spray. For this shot, it is essential to use the grid on the viewfinder to correctly orient the camera to the planes of reference (the zero-coordinate rule) and obtain a well-centered photograph.

Fig 12-13
Full arches in normal occlusion.

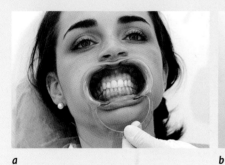

a

Fig 12-14a
Correct grasp of the handle of the self-retracting cheek retractor.

Fig 12-14b
The position of the practitioner when framing this view.

b

ALTERNATIVE METHOD

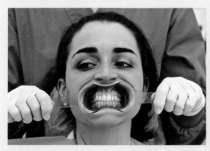

a

Fig 12-15a
Correct position and grasp of the handheld cheek retractors; unlike the overjet views, they are stretched outwards from the face.

Fig 12-15b
The position of the practitioner when framing this view.

b

VIEW 8

Degree of difficulty: 2

Position of the patient:
- Backrest of the treatment chair inclined 110 degrees (Fig 12-16a)
- Patient's head and eyes facing straight ahead

Position of the assistant:
- Standing at the 3-o'clock position (Figs 12-16a and 12-16c); self-retracting cheek retractor is held at the center of the handle, or
- Standing at the 12-o'clock position (Figs 12-16b and 12-16d); two handheld cheek retractors are used with the handles at an angle of 160 degrees

Position of the practitioner:
- Standing at the 7-o'clock position (Figs 12-16a to 12-16d)

Camera settings:
- Camera held horizontally 40 cm (16 inches) from the focal point
- Magnification ratio 1:2.2; aperture f/32 (minimum aperture)
- Flash units at the 3- and 9-o'clock positions (Fig 12-16e)
- Aiming point at the intersection of the median line and the occlusal plane; focal point on the plane of the lateral incisor (Fig 12-16f)

Type of cheek retractor:
- One self-retracting or two handheld cheek retractors

Type of mirror:
- Not applicable

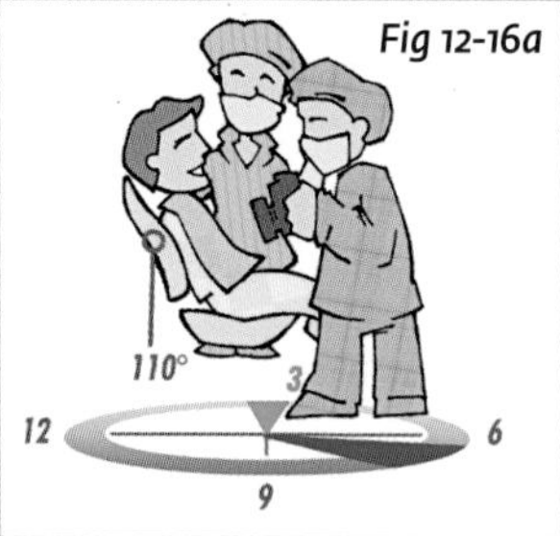

Fig 12-16a

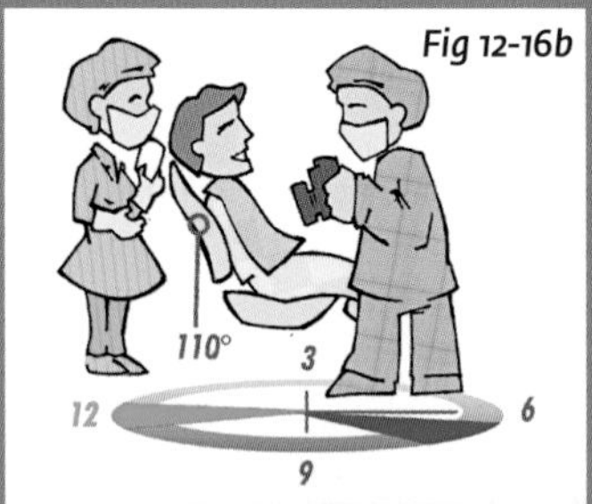

Fig 12-16b

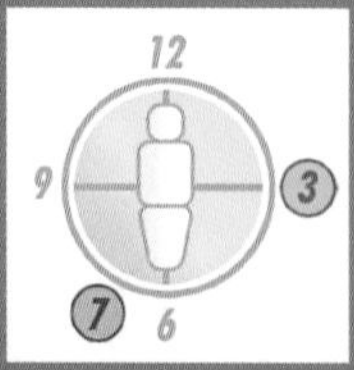

Fig 12-16c

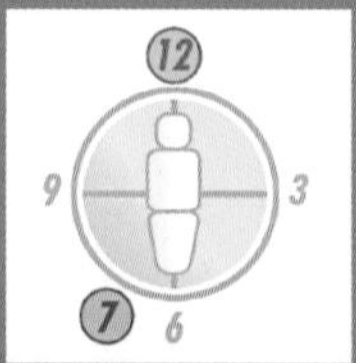

Fig 12-16d

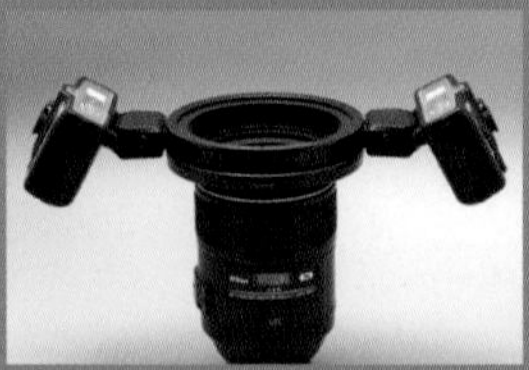

Fig 12-16e

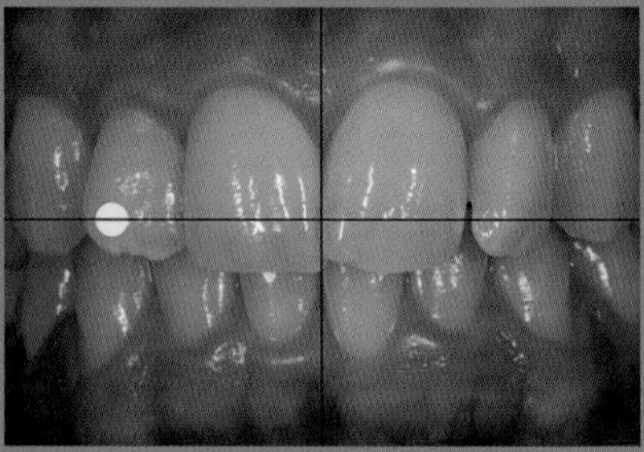

Fig 12-16f

ACCESSORIES NEEDED

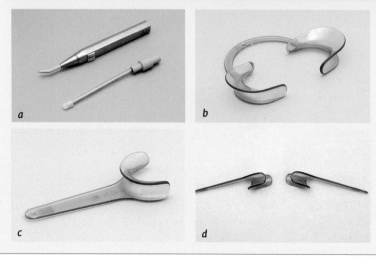

Fig 12-17a
Saliva ejector and air-water spray.

Fig 12-17b
Self-retracting cheek retractor.

Fig 12-17c
Handheld cheek retractor.

Fig 12-17d
The correct angle of the two cheek retractors to each other, about 160 degrees, as seen from above.

Anterior Sextants in Normal Occlusion

COMMENTS

This photograph is similar to view 7, the full-arch view, but the magnification ratio is greater. There are two methods of obtaining this image, using two handheld or one self-retracting cheek retractor. In the former method, the assistant stands at 12 o'clock, and the practitioner holds the saliva ejector. In the latter, the assistant is positioned at 3 o'clock and uses a free hand for the saliva ejector or air-water spray. For this shot, it is essential to use the grid on the viewfinder to correctly orient the camera to the planes of reference (the zero-coordinate rule) and obtain a well-aligned photograph.

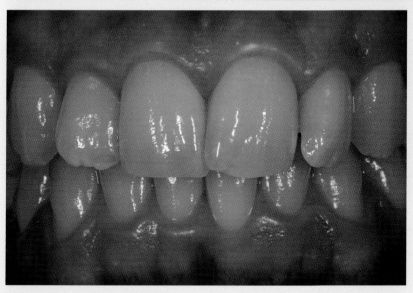

Fig 12-18
Anterior teeth in normal occlusion.

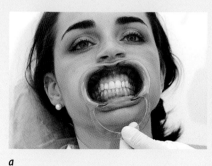

a

Fig 12-19a
Correct grasp of the handle of the self-retracting cheek retractor.

Fig 12-19b
The position of the practitioner when framing this view.

b

ALTERNATIVE METHOD

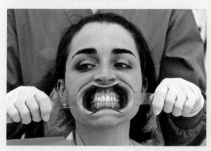

a

Fig 12-20a
Correct position and grasp of the handheld cheek retractors; unlike the overjet views, they are stretched outwards from the face.

Fig 12-20b
The position of the practitioner when framing this view.

b

VIEW 9
Right quadrants in occlusion

VIEW 10
Right posterior sextants in
occlusion

VIEW 11
Right quadrants in occlusion for
orthodontic documentation

VIEW 12
Left quadrants in occlusion

VIEW 13
Left posterior sextants in
occlusion

VIEW 14
Left quadrants in occlusion for
orthodontic documentation

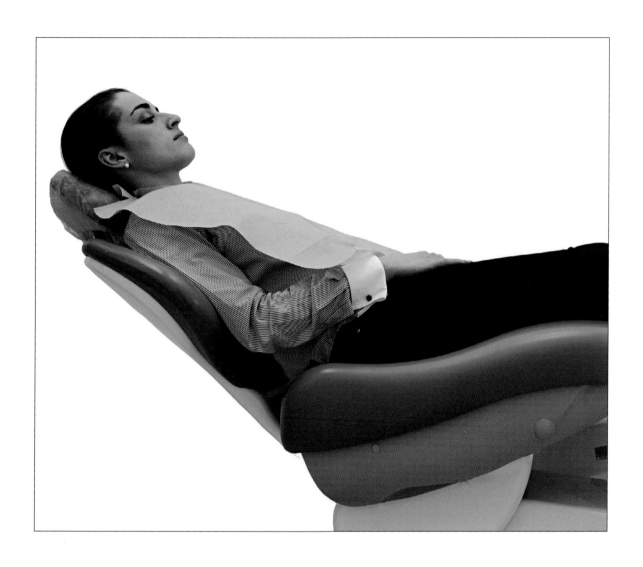

DENTAL CHAIR INCLINED AT 135 DEGREES

VIEW 9

Degree of difficulty: 5

Position of the patient:
- Backrest of the treatment chair inclined 135 degrees (Fig 12-21a)
- Head turned 70 degrees toward the practitioner

Position of the assistant:
- Seated at the 12-o'clock position (Figs 12-21a and 12-21b)
- Cheek retractor held in the left hand; mirror in the right hand

Position of the practitioner:
- Standing at the 7-o'clock position (Figs 12-21a and 12-21b)

Camera settings:
- Camera held horizontally 45 cm (18 inches) from the focal point
- Magnification ratio 1:2.7; aperture f/32 (minimum aperture)
- Flash units placed side by side at the 9-o'clock position (Fig 12-21c)
- Aiming point and focal point on the maxillary right first premolar (Fig 12-21d)

Type of cheek retractor:
- Handheld cheek retractor

Type of mirror:
- Bean-shaped mirror; tapered end used

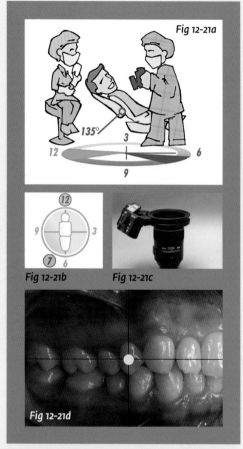

Fig 12-21a

Fig 12-21b

Fig 12-21c

Fig 12-21d

ACCESSORIES NEEDED

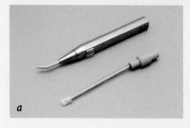

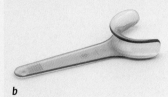

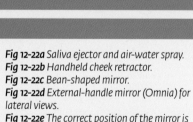

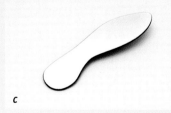

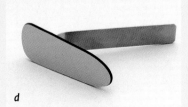

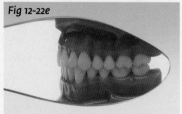

Fig 12-22a *Saliva ejector and air-water spray.*
Fig 12-22b *Handheld cheek retractor.*
Fig 12-22c *Bean-shaped mirror.*
Fig 12-22d *External-handle mirror (Omnia) for lateral views.*
Fig 12-22e *The correct position of the mirror is shown; the concave-convex edge of the tapered end is positioned above, with the convex one below.*

a

b

c

d

Fig 12-22e

Right Quadrants in Occlusion

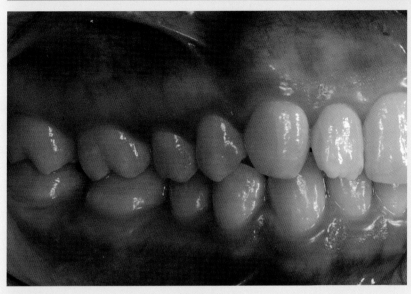

Fig 12-23
This image of the right quadrants in normal occlusion, from the central incisor to the second molar, is suitable for orthodontic documentation.

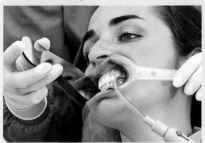

Fig 12-24a
The correct position of accessories and proper grasp of instruments.

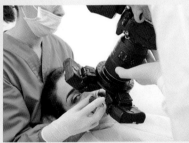

Fig 12-24b
The correct position of the practitioner and the flash units.

ALTERNATIVE METHOD

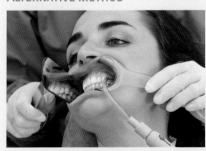

a   *b*

COMMENTS

The difficulty of this shot is that it is extremely hard, or even impossible, to view the teeth in occlusion as far back as the second molar while remaining perpendicular to the arches themselves; this shot often has an angulated perspective.

In this procedure, the assistant retracts the lips on the contralateral side using the retractor without excessive force. The drop-shaped end of the bean-shaped mirror is held in the right hand and inserted horizontally into the mouth until the tip reaches the distal of the second molar. At this point, the patient is asked to open widely, and the assistant pushes the mirror toward the cheek while rotating it 90 degrees, bringing the convex edge toward the maxillary vestibule. The patient is then asked to gently close the teeth without contracting the masseter muscle; this enables the assistant to bring the tip of the mirror, which at this point is distal to the second molars, outward toward the cheek. This procedure creates the maximum possible space between the teeth and mirror. If the inclination of the mirror is 50 degrees away from plane of the facial surfaces of the teeth, the photograph will conform to the zero-coordinate rule.

The assistant holds the mirror firmly without obstructing the light from the flash units, which should reflect onto the mirror to illuminate the entire frame. The practitioner should make an effort to keep the teeth dry with the saliva ejector and the air-water spray, asking the patient to move the tongue as far as possible from the teeth, toward the back of the throat.

Fig 12-2ga
Because this shot requires the assistant to apply a great deal of strength, a mirror with an external handle can be used.

Fig 12-25b
The correct position of the practitioner and the patient, whose head must be correctly rotated.

VIEW 10

Degree of difficulty: 5
Position of the patient:

- Backrest of the treatment chair inclined 135 degrees (Fig 12-26a)
- Head turned 70 degrees toward the practitioner

Position of the assistant:

- Seated at the 12-o'clock position (Figs 12-26a and 12-26b)
- Cheek retractor held in the left hand; mirror held in the right hand

Position of the practitioner:

- Standing at the 7-o'clock position (Figs 12-26a and 12-26b)

Camera settings:

- Camera held horizontally 35 cm (14 inches) from the focal point
- Magnification ratio 1:1.5; aperture f/32 (minimum aperture)
- Flash units placed side by side at the 9-o'clock position (Fig 12-26c)
- Aiming point and focal point on the mesiobuccal cusp of the maxillary right first molar (Fig 12-26d)

Type of cheek retractor:

- Handheld cheek retractor

Type of mirror:

- Bean-shaped mirror; tapered end used

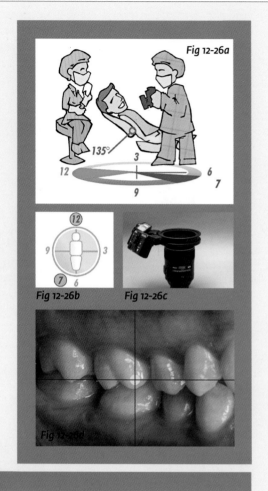

Fig 12-26a

Fig 12-26b   Fig 12-26c

Fig 12-26d

ACCESSORIES NEEDED

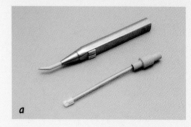

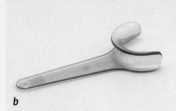

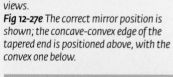

Fig 12-27a Saliva ejector and air-water spray.
Fig 12-27b Handheld cheek retractor.
Fig 12-27c Bean-shaped mirror.
Fig 12-27d External-handle mirror for lateral views.
Fig 12-27e The correct mirror position is shown; the concave-convex edge of the tapered end is positioned above, with the convex one below.

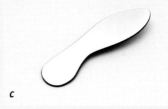

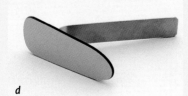

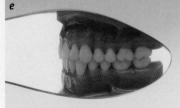

Right Posterior Sextants in Occlusion

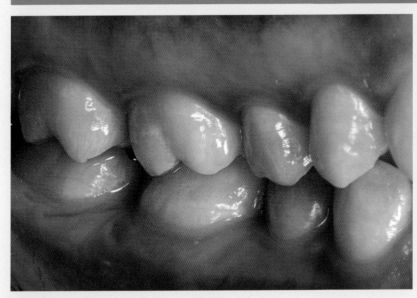

Fig 12-28
The right posterior teeth in occlusion.

This photograph is similar to view 9, the hemiarch view, but the magnification ratio is greater. This means that the practitioner must be closer to the patient. It is extremely hard, and even impossible, to view the teeth in occlusion as far back as the second molar while remaining perpendicular to the arches themselves; this shot often has an angulated perspective.

In this procedure, the assistant retracts the lips on the contralateral side using the retractor in the left hand without excessive traction. The drop-shaped end of the bean-shaped mirror is held in the right hand and inserted horizontally into the mouth until the tip reaches the distal of the second molars. At this point, the patient is asked to open widely, and the assistant pushes the mirror toward the cheek while rotating it 90 degrees, bringing the convex edge toward the maxillary vestibule. The patient is then asked to gently close the teeth without contracting the masseter muscle; this enables the assistant to bring the tip of the mirror, which at this point is distal to the second molars, outward toward the cheek. This procedure creates the maximum possible space between the teeth and mirror. If the inclination of the mirror is 50 degrees away from plane formed by the facial surfaces of the teeth, the photograph will conform to the zero-coordinate rule. The assistant holds the mirror firmly without obstructing the light from the flash units, which should reflect onto the mirror and illuminate the whole frame. The practitioner should make an effort to keep the teeth dry with the saliva ejector and the air-water spray, asking the patient to move the tongue as far as possible from the teeth, toward the back of the throat.

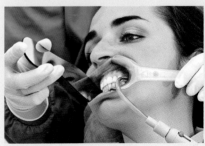

Fig 12-29a
The correct position of accessories and proper grasp of instruments.

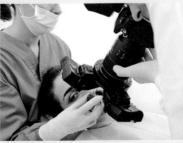

Fig 12-29b
The correct position of the practitioner and the flash units.

ALTERNATIVE METHOD

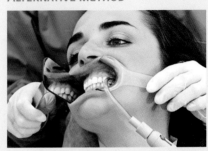

a

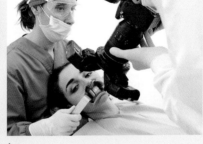

b

Fig 12-30a
Because this shot requires the assistant to apply a great deal of strength, a mirror with an external handle can be used.

Fig 12-30b
The correct position of the practitioner and the patient, whose head must be correctly rotated.

VIEW 11

Degree of difficulty: 2

Position of the patient:
- Backrest of the treatment chair inclined 135 degrees (Fig 12-31a)
- Head turned 70 degrees toward the practitioner

Position of the assistant:
- Seated at the 12-o'clock position (Figs 12-31a and 12-31b)
- Maxil cheek retractor held in the right hand; standard handheld retractor in the left hand

Position of the practitioner:
- Standing or sitting at the 9-o'clock position (Figs 12-31a and 12-31b)

Camera settings:
- Camera held horizontally 40 cm (16 inches) from the focal point
- Magnification ratio 1:2.2; aperture f/32 (minimum aperture)
- Flash units placed side by side at the 3-o'clock position (Fig 12-31c)
- Aiming point and focal point on the first premolars (Fig 12-31d)

Type of retractor:
- Maxil and standard handheld retractors

Type of mirror:
- Not applicable

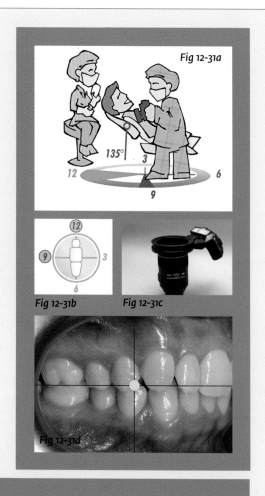

Fig 12-31a

Fig 12-31b

Fig 12-31c

Fig 12-31d

ACCESSORIES NEEDED

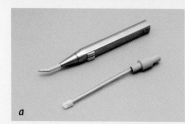

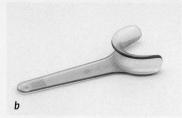

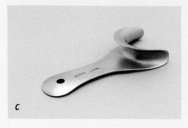

Fig 12-32a
Saliva ejector and air-water spray.

Fig 12-32b
Standard handheld cheek retractor.

Fig 12-32c
Maxil retractor.

Right Quadrants in Occlusion for Orthodontic Documentation

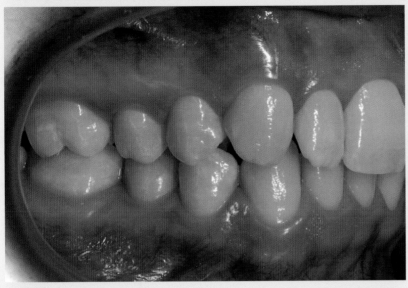

COMMENTS

This type of photo is suitable for the documentation of orthodontic cases in which the second molars have not yet erupted. A mirror is not used, but two different retractors are needed. The assistant is seated at the 12-o'clock position and holds the Maxil retractor with the right hand, firmly stretching it backwards. This retractor has a particularly pronounced concavity. At the same time, the assistant holds a standard handheld retractor in the left hand, which prevents the lips from collapsing onto the teeth, keeping the teeth in the frame for the shot. After carefully aspirating all traces of saliva, the practitioner is ready to take the shot. This view includes the teeth of the right quadrants from the mesial of the central incisor to the distal of the first molar.

Fig 12-33
This view of the right quadrants in normal occlusion from the central incisor to the mesial of the second molar is suitable for orthodontic documentation. A mirror is not used for this shot.

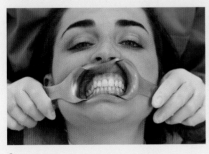

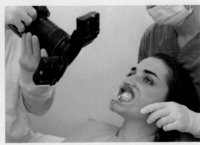

a   *b*

Fig 12-34a
The correct position of accessories and proper grasp of instruments.

Fig 12-34b
The correct position of the practitioner and the flash units.

VIEW 12

Degree of difficulty: 5

Position of the patient:
- Backrest of the treatment chair inclined 135 degrees (Fig 12-35a)
- Head turned 20 degrees toward the practitioner

Position of the assistant:
- Seated at the 12-o'clock position (Figs 12-35a and 12-35b)
- Cheek retractor held in the right hand; mirror held in the left hand

Position of the practitioner:
- Standing or seated at the 9-o'clock position (Figs 12-35a and 12-35b)

Camera settings:
- Camera held horizontally 45 cm (18 inches) from the focal point
- Magnification ratio 1:2.7; aperture f/32 (minimum aperture)
- Flash units placed side by side at the 3-o'clock position (Fig 12-35c)
- Aiming point and focal point on the maxillary left first premolar (Fig 12-35d)

Type of cheek retractor:
- Handheld cheek retractor

Type of mirror:
- Bean-shaped mirror; tapered end used

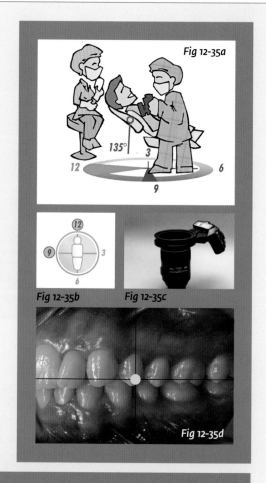

Fig 12-35a

Fig 12-35b   Fig 12-35c

Fig 12-35d

ACCESSORIES NEEDED

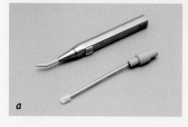

a

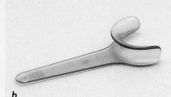

b

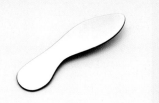

c

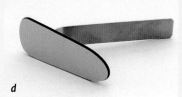

d

Fig 12-36a Saliva ejector and air-water spray.
Fig 12-36b Handheld cheek retractor.
Fig 12-36c Bean-shaped mirror.
Fig 12-36d Mirror with an external handle for lateral views.
Fig 12-36e The correct position of the mirror is shown; the concave-convex edge of the tapered end is positioned above, with the convex one below.

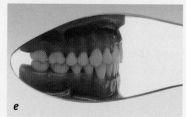

e

Left Quadrants in Occlusion

COMMENTS

The difficulty of this shot is that it is extremely hard to view the teeth in occlusion as far back as the second molar while remaining perpendicular to the arches themselves; this shot often has an angulated perspective.

In this procedure, the assistant retracts the lips on the contralateral side using the retractor without excessive force. The drop-shaped end of the bean-shaped mirror is held in the left hand and inserted horizontally into the mouth until the tip reaches the distal of the second molar. At this point, the patient is asked to open widely, and the assistant pushes the mirror toward the cheek while rotating it 90 degrees, bringing the convex edge toward the maxillary vestibule. The patient is then asked to gently close the teeth without contracting the masseter muscle; this enables the assistant to bring the tip of the mirror, which at this point is distal to the second molars, outward toward the cheek. This procedure creates the maximum possible space between the teeth and mirror. If the inclination of the mirror is 50 degrees away from the plane formed by the facial surfaces of the teeth, the photograph will conform to the zero-coordinate rule.

The assistant holds the mirror firmly without obstructing the light from the flash units, which should reflect onto the mirror to illuminate the entire frame. The practitioner should make an effort to keep the teeth dry with the saliva ejector and the air-water spray, asking the patient to move the tongue as far as possible from the teeth, toward the back of the throat.

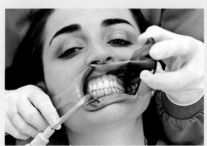

Fig 12-37 *This image of the left quadrants in normal occlusion, from the central incisor to the second molar, is suitable for orthodontic documentation.*

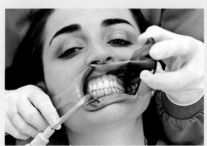

Fig 12-38a
The correct position of accessories and proper grasp of instruments.

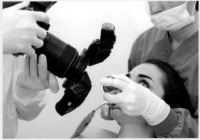

Fig 12-38b
The correct position of the practitioner and the flash units.

ALTERNATIVE METHOD

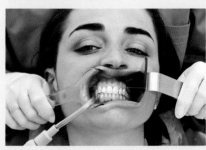

a

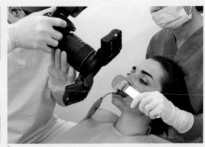

b

Fig 12-39a
Because this shot requires the assistant to apply a great deal of strength, a mirror with an external handle can be used.

Fig 12-39b
The correct position of the practitioner and the patient, whose head must be correctly rotated.

VIEW 13

Degree of difficulty: 5

Position of the patient:
- Backrest of the treatment chair inclined 135 degrees (Fig 12-40a)
- Head inclined toward the practitioner

Position of the assistant:
- Standing or seated at the 12-o'clock position (Figs 12-40a and 12-40b)
- Cheek retractor held in the right hand; mirror held in the left hand

Position of the practitioner:
- Standing or seated at the 9-o'clock position (Figs 12-40a and 12-40b)

Camera settings:
- Camera held horizontally 35 cm (14 inches) from the focal point
- Magnification ratio 1:1.5; aperture f/32 (minimum aperture)
- Flash units placed side by side at the 3-o'clock position (Fig 12-40c)
- Aiming point and focal point on the contact between the maxillary second premolar and first molar (Fig 12-40d)

Type of retractor:
- Handheld cheek retractor

Type of mirror:
- Bean-shaped mirror; tapered end used

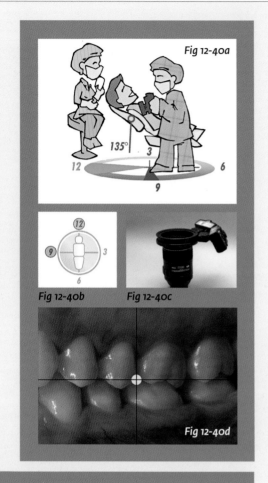

Fig 12-40a

Fig 12-40b   Fig 12-40c

Fig 12-40d

ACCESSORIES NEEDED

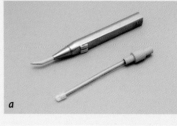

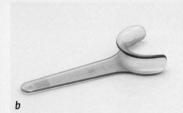

Fig 12-41a *Saliva ejector and air-water spray.*
Fig 12-41b *Handheld cheek retractor.*
Fig 12-41c *Bean-shaped mirror.*
Fig 12-41d *External-handle mirror for lateral views.*
Fig 12-41e *The correct mirror position is shown; the concave-convex edge of the tapered end is positioned above, with the convex one below.*

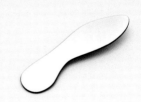

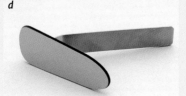

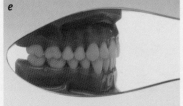

Left Posterior Sextants in Occlusion

COMMENTS

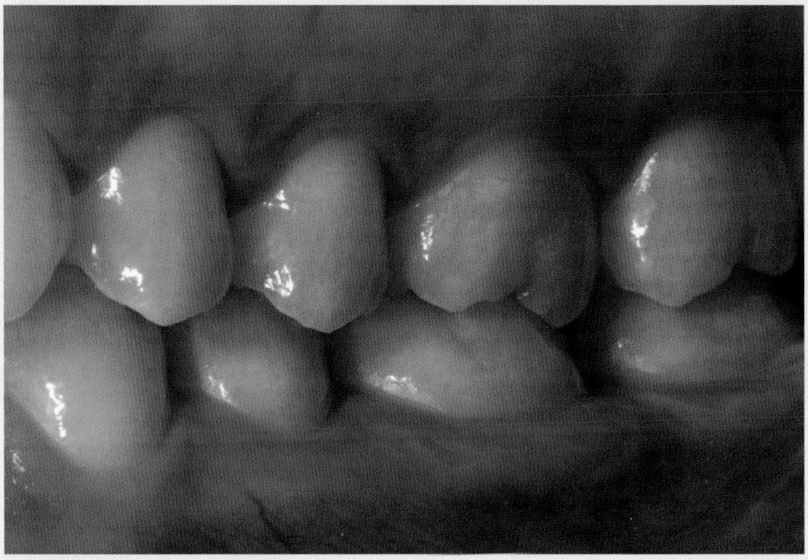

This photograph is similar to view 12, the hemiarch view, but the magnification ratio is greater. This means that the practitioner must be closer to the patient. It is extremely hard to view the teeth in occlusion as far back as the second molar while remaining perpendicular to the arches themselves; this shot often has an angulated perspective.

In this procedure, the assistant retracts the lips on the contralateral side using the retractor in the right hand without excessive traction. The drop-shaped end of the bean-shaped mirror is held in the left hand and inserted horizontally into the mouth until the tip reaches the distal of the second molars. At this point, the patient is asked to open widely, and the assistant pushes the mirror toward the cheek while rotating it 90 degrees, bringing the convex edge toward the maxillary vestibule. The patient is then asked to gently close the teeth without contracting the masseter muscle; this enables the assistant to bring the tip of the mirror, which at this point is distal to the second molars, outward toward the cheek. This procedure creates the maximum possible space between the teeth and mirror. If the inclination of the mirror is 50 degrees away from plane formed by the facial surfaces of the teeth, the photograph will conform to the zero-coordinate rule. The assistant holds the mirror firmly without obstructing the light from the flash units, which should reflect onto the mirror and illuminate the whole frame. The practitioner should make an effort to keep the teeth dry with the saliva ejector and the air-water spray, asking the patient to move the tongue as far as possible from the teeth, toward the back of the throat.

Fig 12-42
The left posterior teeth in occlusion.

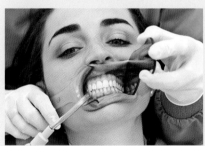

Fig 12-43a
The correct position of accessories and proper grasp of instruments.

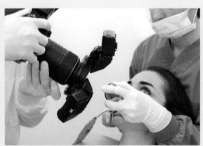

Fig 12-43b
The correct position of the practitioner and the flash units.

ALTERNATIVE METHOD

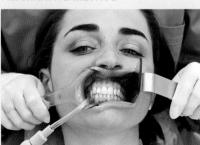

a

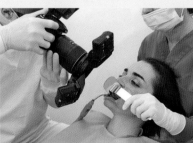

b

Fig 12-44a
Because this shot requires the assistant to apply a great deal of strength, a mirror with an external handle can be used.

Fig 12-44b
The correct position of the practitioner and the patient, whose head must be facing straight ahead.

VIEW 14

Degree of difficulty: 2

Position of the patient:
- Backrest of the treatment chair inclined 135 degrees (Fig 12-45a)
- Head turned 80 degrees toward the practitioner

Position of the assistant:
- Seated at the 12-o'clock position (Figs 12-45a and 12-45b)
- Maxil cheek retractor held in the left hand; standard handheld retractor in the right hand

Position of the practitioner:
- Standing or sitting at the 7-o'clock position (Figs 12-45a and 12-45b)

Camera settings:
- Camera held horizontally 40 cm (16 inches) from the focal point
- Magnification ratio 1:2.2; aperture f/32 (minimum aperture)
- Flash units placed side by side at the 9-o'clock position (Fig 12-45c)
- Aiming point and focal point on the maxillary first premolar (Fig 12-45d)

Type of retractor:
- Maxil and standard handheld retractors

Type of mirror:
- Not applicable

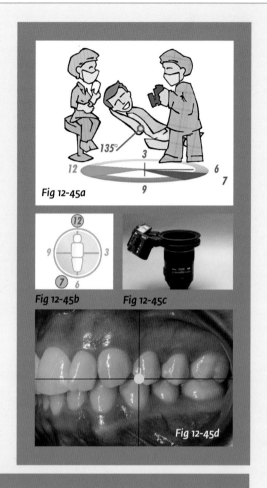

Fig 12-45a

Fig 12-45b

Fig 12-45c

Fig 12-45d

ACCESSORIES NEEDED

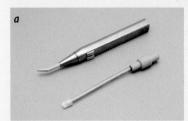

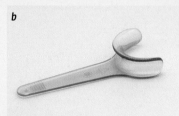

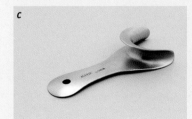

Fig 12-46a
Saliva ejector and air-water spray.

Fig 12-46b
Standard handheld cheek retractor.

Fig 12-46c
Maxil retractor.

Left Quadrants in Occlusion for Orthodontic Documentation

COMMENTS

This type of photo is suitable for the documentation of orthodontic cases in which the second molars have not yet erupted. A mirror is not used, but two different retractors are needed. The assistant is seated at the 12-o'clock position and holds the Maxil retractor with the left hand, firmly stretching it backwards. This retractor has a particularly pronounced concavity. At the same time, the assistant holds a standard handheld retractor in the right hand, which prevents the lips from collapsing onto the teeth, keeping the teeth in the frame for the shot. After carefully aspirating all traces of saliva, the practitioner is ready to take the shot. This view includes the teeth of the left quadrants from the mesial of the central incisor to the distal of the first molar.

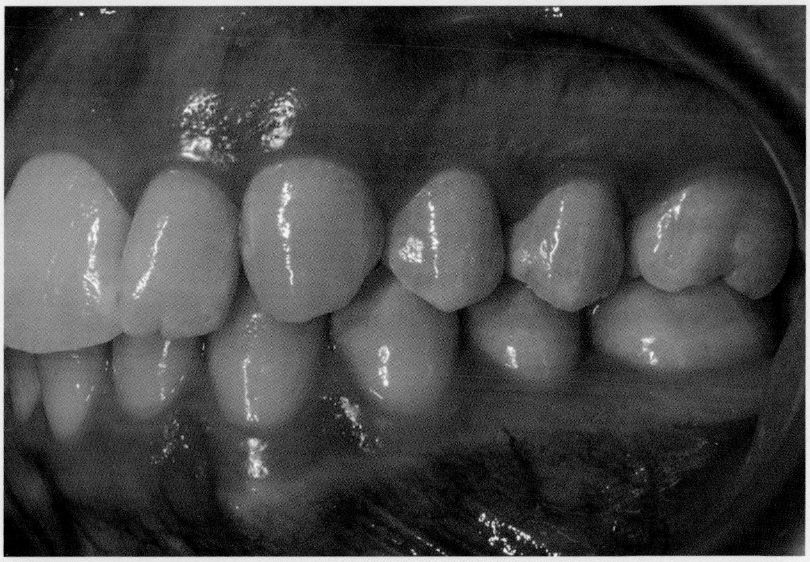

Fig 12-47
This view of the left quadrants in normal occlusion from the central incisor to the mesial of the second molar is suitable for orthodontic documentation. A mirror is not used for this shot.

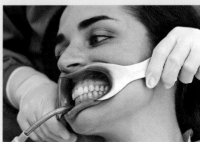

Fig 12-48a
The correct position of accessories and proper grasp of instruments.

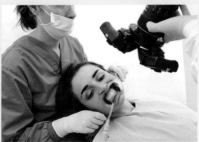

Fig 12-48b
The correct position of the practitioner and the flash units. The patient's head must be rotated toward the practitioner.

VIEW 15
Complete maxillary
dentition: occlusal view

VIEW 19
Complete mandibular
dentition: occlusal view

VIEW 23
Maxillary right posterior
sextant: occlusal view

VIEW 27
Maxillary left posterior
sextant: occlusal view

VIEW 16
Maxillary anterior sextant:
incisal view

VIEW 20
Mandibular anterior
sextant: incisal view

VIEW 24
Maxillary right posterior
sextant: palatal view

VIEW 28
Maxillary left posterior
sextant: palatal view

VIEW 17
Maxillary anterior sextant:
palatal view

VIEW 21
Mandibular anterior
sextant: lingual view

VIEW 25
Mandibular left posterior
sextant: occlusal view

VIEW 29
Mandibular right posterior
sextant: occlusal view

VIEW 18
Maxillary anterior sextant:
facial view

VIEW 22
Mandibular anterior
sextant: facial view

VIEW 26
Mandibular left posterior
sextant: lingual view

VIEW 30
Mandibular right posterior
sextant: lingual view

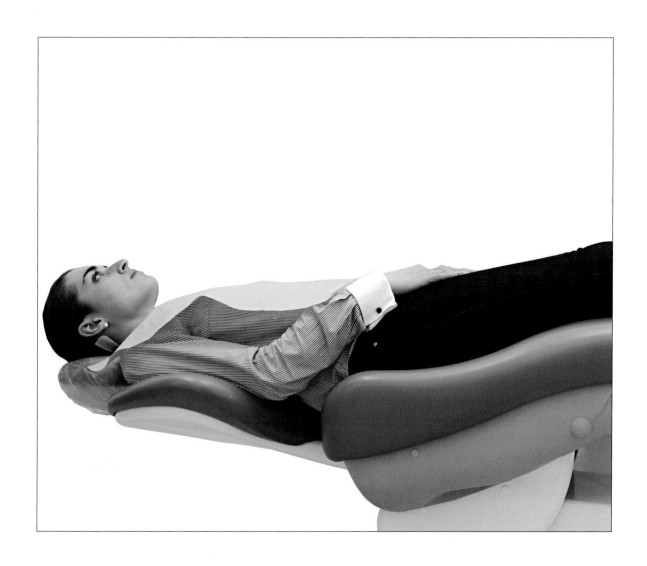

DENTAL CHAIR INCLINED AT 180 DEGREES

VIEW 15

Degree of difficulty: 4

Position of the patient:
- Backrest of the treatment chair inclined 180 degrees (Fig 12-49a)
- Head held straight with chin lifted slightly

Position of the assistant:
- Seated at the 3-o'clock position (Figs 12-49a and 12-49b)
- Retractor held in the right hand with handle toward the patient's nose; mirror held in the left hand

Position of the practitioner:
- Standing at the 12-o'clock position (Figs 12-49a and 12-49b)

Camera settings:
- Camera held horizontally 50 cm (20 inches) from the focal point
- Magnification ratio 1:3.3; aperture f/32 (minimum aperture)
- Flash units at the 3- and 9-o'clock positions (Fig 12-49c)
- Aiming point on the median line at the level of the premolars; focal point on the plane of the premolar papillae (Fig 12-49d)

Type of cheek retractor:
- Modified self-retracting cheek retractor

Type of mirror:
- Large figure eight–shaped mirror

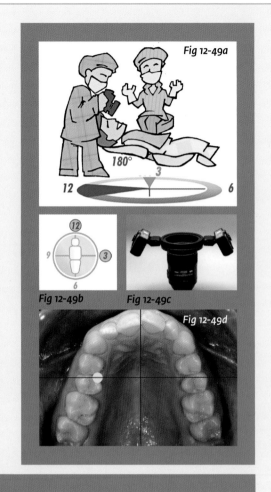

Fig 12-49a

Fig 12-49b

Fig 12-49c

Fig 12-49d

ACCESSORIES NEEDED

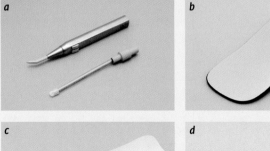

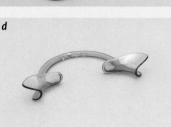

Fig 12-50a
Saliva ejector and air-water spray.

Fig 12-50b
Figure eight–shaped mirror.

Fig 12-50c
Figure eight–shaped mirror with handle (Omnia).

Fig 12-50d
Modified self-retracting cheek retractor.

Complete Maxillary Dentition: Occlusal View

COMMENTS

This is a reasonably difficult shot; it is particularly demanding for the assistant because it requires precision and a steady hand to hold the retractor and the mirror. The cheek retractor must be firmly stretched so that it cannot be seen in the frame. At the same time, the upper lip must be moved as far away as possible from the teeth, allowing for an optimum view of the vestibule. The wider end of the mirror should be inserted into the mouth almost to the throat so that the second molars can be seen; furthermore, the mirror should be pushed firmly against the mandibular teeth at an angle of about 40 degrees to the maxillary occlusal plane. Because the ideal position is unnatural and tiring, the assistant should ask the patient to relax the lips and cheeks and to open the mouth as wide as possible only at the moment of taking the shot. The practitioner should be positioned at 12 o'clock with the knee firmly against the headrest of the chair for greater stability. The camera settings are selected, and the positions of the mirror and the retractor are checked to eliminate any distracting elements in the frame. The image in the mirror should be perpendicular to the occlusal plane. When the practitioner is ready to take the shot, the assistant asks the patient to open the mouth as wide as possible and uses whatever strength is necessary to position the mirror without blocking the light from the flash. Because this procedure involves a great deal of stress for the patient and clinic staff, it should be done rapidly. The saliva ejector must remain in the oral cavity at all times to prevent the mirror from fogging.

Fig 12-51
Occlusal view of the complete maxillary dentition.

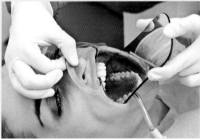

Fig 12-52a
The correct position of accessories and proper grasp of instruments.

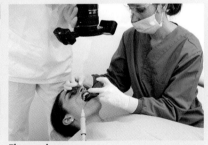

Fig 12-52b
The correct position of the practitioner, the camera, and the flash units. The knee is held against the headrest for stability.

ALTERNATIVE METHOD

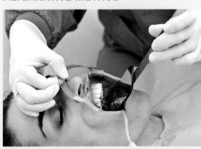

a

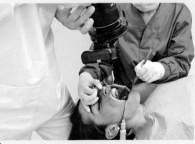

b

Figs 12-53a and 12-53b
This shot can be taken in an identical manner using a mirror with a handle.

VIEW 16

Degree of difficulty: 2

Position of the patient:
- Backrest of the treatment chair inclined 180 degrees (Fig 12-54a)
- Head held straight with chin lifted slightly

Position of the assistant:
- Seated at the 3-o'clock position (Figs 12-54a and 12-54b)
- Retractor held in the right hand with handle toward the patient's nose; mirror held in the left hand

Position of the practitioner:
- Standing at the 12-o'clock position (Figs 12-54a and 12-54b)

Camera settings:
- Camera held horizontally 40 cm (16 inches) from the focal point
- Magnification ratio 1:2.2; aperture f/32 (minimum aperture)
- Flash units at the 3- and 9-o'clock positions (Fig 12-54c)
- Aiming point at the incisive papilla; focal point on the plane of the papillae between the central and lateral incisors (Fig 12-54d)

Type of retractor:
- Modified self-retracting cheek retractor

Type of mirror:
- Large figure eight–shaped mirror

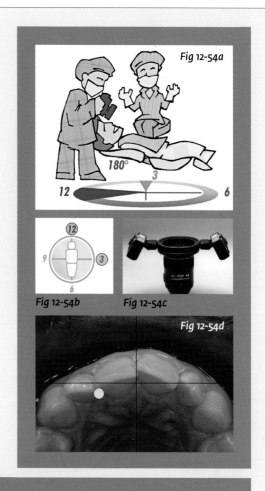

Fig 12-54a

Fig 12-54b

Fig 12-54c

Fig 12-54d

ACCESSORIES NEEDED

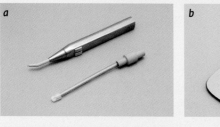

a

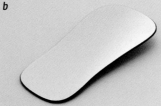

b

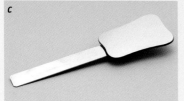

c

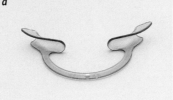

d

Fig 12-55a
Saliva ejector and air-water spray.

Fig 12-55b
Figure eight–shaped mirror.

Fig 12-55c
Figure eight–shaped mirror with handle.

Fig 12-55d
Modified self-retracting cheek retractor.

Maxillary Anterior Sextant: Incisal View

It is most efficient and ergonomic to take this shot immediately after the occlusal view of the complete maxillary dentition. The only movement required is partial removal of the mirror to the level of the first premolars. An excellent image can be taken without changing the position of the operators or the accessories. For this image, it is easier to position the retractor to reveal the vestibule. The assistant should reduce the angle of the mirror to the occlusal plane to 30 degrees while keeping it in contact with the mandibular teeth. After increasing the camera's magnification ratio by moving closer to the subject, the practitioner should steady himself or herself with a knee against the side of the headrest and ensure that the mirror is inclined to allow a symmetric view of the facial and palatal surfaces of the central incisors. The saliva ejector should remain inside the oral cavity at all times to prevent fogging of the mirrors.

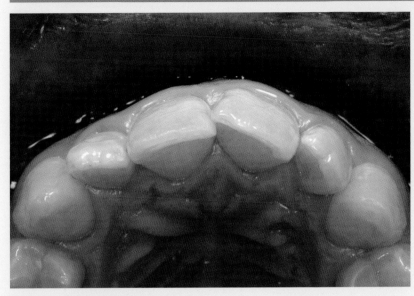

Fig 12-56
Incisal view of the maxillary anterior sextant.

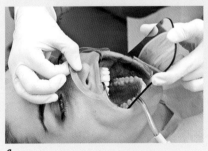

a

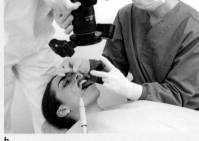

b

Fig 12-57a
The correct position of accessories and proper grasp of instruments.

Fig 12-57b
The correct position of the practitioner, the camera, and the flash units. A knee is used against the headrest for stability.

ALTERNATIVE METHOD

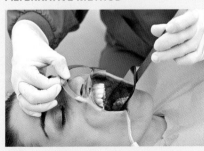

a

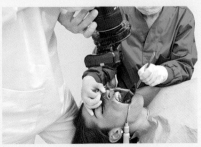

b

Fig 12-58
This shot can be taken in an identical manner using a mirror with a handle.

VIEW 17

Degree of difficulty: 2

Position of the patient:
- Backrest of the treatment chair inclined 180 degrees (Fig 12-59a)
- Head held straight with chin lifted slightly

Position of the assistant:
- Seated at the 3-o'clock position (Figs 12-59a and 12-59b)
- Mirror held in the left hand in contact with the mandibular teeth at an angle of 60 degrees to the maxillary occlusal plane

Position of the practitioner:
- Standing at the 12-o'clock position (Figs 12-59a and 12-59b)

Camera settings:
- Camera held horizontally 40 cm (16 inches) from the focal point
- Magnification ratio 1:2.2; aperture f/32 (minimum aperture)
- Flash units at the 3- and 9-o'clock positions (Fig 12-59c)
- Aiming point at the contact between central incisors; focal point on the plane of the gingiva of the lateral incisors (Fig 12-59d)

Type of retractor:
- Not applicable

Type of mirror:
- Large figure eight–shaped mirror

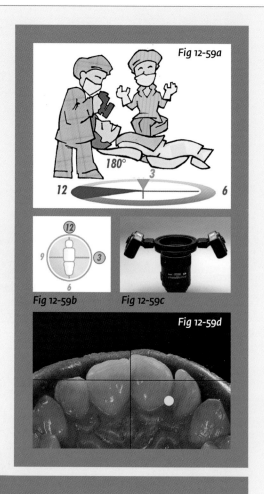

Fig 12-59a

Fig 12-59b   Fig 12-59c

Fig 12-59d

ACCESSORIES NEEDED

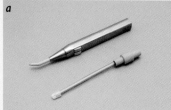

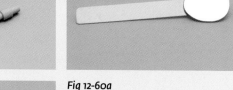

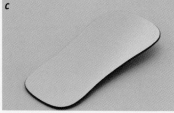

Fig 12-60a
Saliva ejector and air-water spray.

Fig 12-60b
Drop-shaped mirror with handle (Omnia).

Fig 12-60c *Large figure eight–shaped mirror.*

Maxillary Anterior Sextant: Palatal View

COMMENTS

It is most efficient and ergonomic to take this shot immediately after the incisal view of the maxillary anterior sextant. The only movements required are removing the retractor and inclining the mirror 60 degrees away from the maxillary occlusal plane, which gives a good view of the palatal surfaces of the anterior teeth. This position of the mirror creates a dark background without the aid of a contrastor and eliminates the nose from the frame. To remove the upper lip from the image, the bent, concave end of a metallic contrastor (see Fig 10-6a) is inserted into the mouth and rests at the base of the teeth. When the lip is removed from the image in this way, the exact contour of the incisal edges is easily perceived against the black background. After verifying that the mirror is positioned so that the view is perpendicular to the palatal plane, the shot is taken. The saliva ejector should remain inside the oral cavity at all times to prevent fogging of the mirrors.

Fig 12-61
Palatal view of the maxillary anterior sextant.

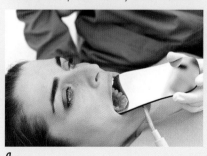

a

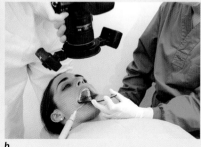

b

Fig 12-62a
The correct position of accessories and proper grasp of instruments for the palatal view.

Fig 12-62b
The correct position of the practitioner, the camera, and the flash units.

ALTERNATIVE METHOD

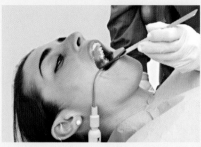

a

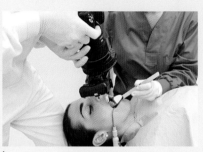

b

Figs 12-63a and 12-63b
This shot can be taken in an identical manner using a drop-shaped mirror with a handle.

VIEW 18

Degree of difficulty: 2

Position of the patient:
- Backrest of the treatment chair inclined 180 degrees (Fig 12-64a)
- Head held straight, looking ahead

Position of the assistant:
- Seated at the 3-o'clock position (Figs 12-64a and 12-64b)
- Cheek retractor held in the right hand; contrastor held in the left

Position of the practitioner:
- Standing at the 12-o'clock position (Figs 12-64a and 12-64b)

Camera settings:
- Camera held horizontally 40 cm (16 inches) from the focal point
- Magnification ratio 1:2.2; aperture f/32 (minimum aperture)
- Flash units at the 3- and 9-o'clock positions (Fig 12-64c)
- Aiming point at the contact between central incisors; focal point on the plane of the lateral incisors (Fig 12-64d)

Type of retractor:
- Modified self-retracting cheek retractor

Type of mirror:
- Not applicable

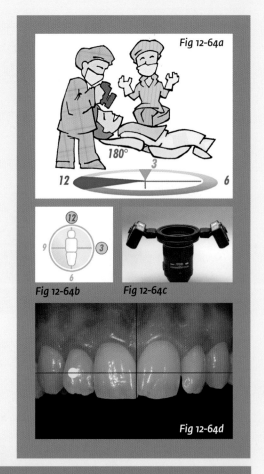

Fig 12-64a

Fig 12-64b   Fig 12-64c

Fig 12-64d

ACCESSORIES NEEDED

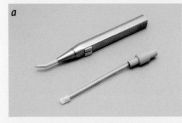

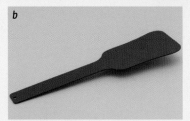

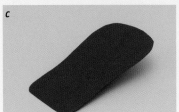

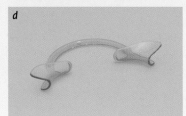

Fig 12-65a
Saliva ejector and air-water spray.

Fig 12-65b
Spade-shaped metal contrastor (Nike).

Fig 12-65c
Disposable black cardboard contrastor, an alternative to the metal contrastor.

Fig 12-65d
Modified self-retracting cheek retractor.

Maxillary Anterior Sextant: Facial View

COMMENTS

The assistant inserts the modified self-retracting cheek retractor, with the handle toward the patient's nose, and a contrastor to obtain the dark background that is useful for better perception of the characteristics of the teeth. The contrastor should be held as far away from the teeth as possible, so that its presence is not made obvious by the flash, and it is not in focus in the photograph. If black cardboard is used, it should be folded in half so that it forms a concavity towards the camera.

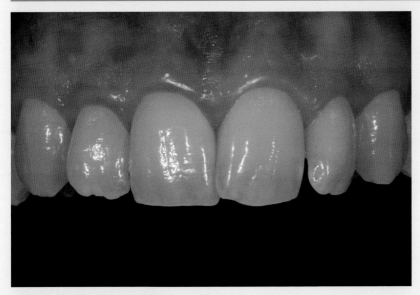

Fig 12-66
Facial view of the maxillary anterior sextant.

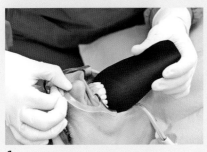

a

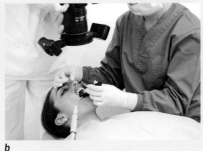

b

Fig 12-67a
The correct position of the accessories held by the assistant. The disposable black cardboard is held in a curved position to prevent reflection, which would not produce a uniformly black background.

Fig 12-67b
Correct position of assistant and practitioner.

ALTERNATIVE METHOD

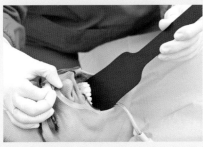

a

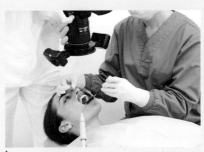

b

Fig 12-68a
The same image can be obtained with a spade-shaped metal contrastor.

Fig 12-68b
The correct position of the practitioner, the camera, and the flash units.

VIEW 19

Degree of difficulty: 5

Position of the patient:
- Backrest of the treatment chair inclined 180 degrees (Fig 12-69a)
- Head turned toward the practitioner with chin lifted slightly

Position of the assistant:
- Seated at the 3-o'clock position (Figs 12-69a and 12-69b)
- Retractor held in the left hand with handle toward the patient's chin; mirror held in the right hand

Position of the practitioner:
- Standing at the 7-o'clock position (Figs 12-69a and 12-69b)

Camera settings:
- Camera held horizontally 50 cm (20 inches) from the focal point
- Magnification ratio 1:3.3; aperture f/32 (minimum aperture)
- Flash units at the 3- and 9-o'clock positions (Fig 12-69c)
- Aiming point on the median line at the level of the premolars; focal point on the plane of the premolar papillae (Fig 12-69d)

Type of retractor:
- Modified self-retracting cheek retractor

Type of mirror:
- Large figure eight–shaped mirror

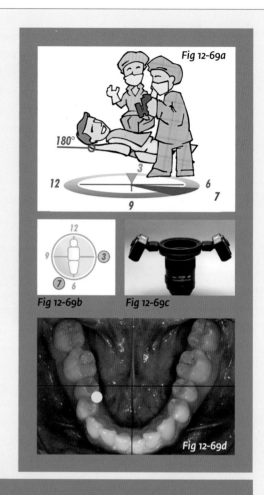

Fig 12-69a

Fig 12-69b   Fig 12-69c

Fig 12-69d

ACCESSORIES NEEDED

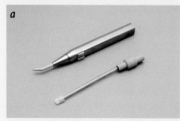

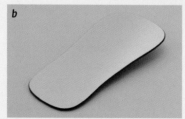

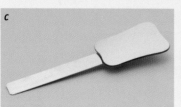

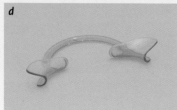

Fig 12-70a
Saliva ejector and air-water spray.

Fig 12-70b
Figure eight–shaped mirror.

Fig 12-70c
Figure eight–shaped mirror with handle.

Fig 12-70d
Modified self-retracting cheek retractor.

Complete Mandibular Dentition: Occlusal View

COMMENTS

Taking this shot can be complex because of the difficulty in positioning the tongue correctly, especially in the presence of a short lingual frenulum. The frenulum must stretch so that the tongue is between the palate and upper surface of the mirror and the floor of the mouth is visible in the mirror. Furthermore, when the patient opens the mouth extremely wide, the assistant may be prevented from retracting the lower lip a satisfactory distance away from the facial surfaces of the anterior teeth. The figure eight–shaped mirror is appropriate for this shot, and the wider part should be inserted until the mandibular second molars are visible. The assistant is seated at 3 o'clock and holds the modified cheek retractor, handle facing toward the chin, with the left hand and the mirror with the right hand. The mirror should positioned as far as possible from the occlusal surfaces of the mandibular teeth and pushed firmly against the maxillary teeth at an angle of about 40 degrees to the mandibular occlusal plane. The practitioner uses the air-water spray and the saliva ejector, positioned behind the mirror, to keep its surface clean. The assistant asks the patient to open the mouth as wide as possible while keeping the lower lip relaxed, and the practitioner takes the shot rapidly to avoid any unnecessary discomfort for the patient from the position of the tongue.

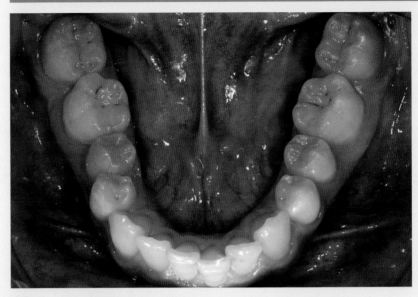

Fig 12-71
Occlusal view of the complete mandibular dentition.

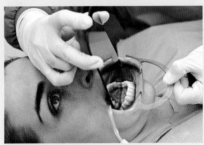

Fig 12-72a
The correct position of accessories and proper grasp of instruments.

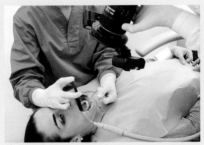

Fig 12-72b
The correct position of the camera and the flash units.

ALTERNATIVE METHOD

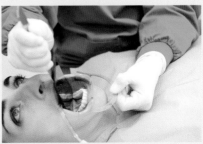

a

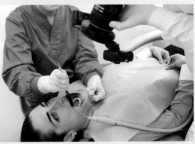

b

Figs 12-73a and 12-73b
This shot can be taken in an identical manner using a mirror with a handle.

285

VIEW 20

Degree of difficulty: 3

Position of the patient:
- Backrest of the treatment chair inclined 180 degrees (Fig 12-74a)
- Head turned toward the practitioner with chin lifted

Position of the assistant:
- Seated at the 3-o'clock position (Figs 12-74a and 12-74b)
- Retractor held in the left hand with handle toward the patient's chin; mirror held in the right hand

Position of the practitioner:
- Standing at the 7-o'clock position (Figs 12-74a and 12-74b)

Camera settings:
- Camera held horizontally 35 cm (14 inches) from the focal point
- Magnification ratio 1:1.5; aperture f/32 (minimum aperture)
- Flash units at the 3- and 9-o'clock positions (Fig 12-74c)
- Aiming point at the intercisive papilla; focal point on the plane of the papilla between the central and lateral incisors (Fig 12-74d)

Type of retractor:
- Modified self-retracting cheek retractor

Type of mirror:
- Large figure eight–shaped mirror

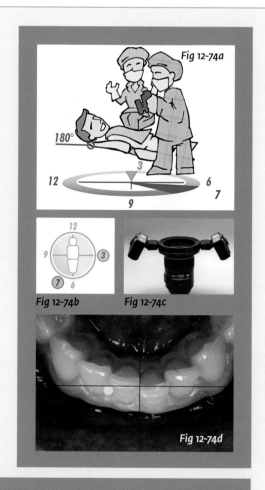

Fig 12-74a

Fig 12-74b

Fig 12-74c

Fig 12-74d

ACCESSORIES NEEDED

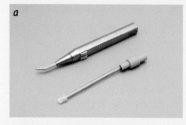

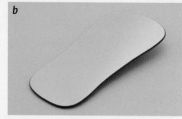

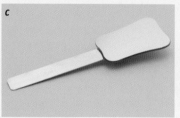

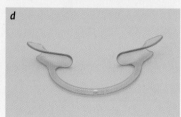

Fig 12-75a
Saliva ejector and air-water spray.

Fig 12-75b
Figure eight–shaped mirror.

Fig 12-75c
Figure eight–shaped mirror with handle.

Fig 12-75d
Modified self-retracting cheek retractor.

Mandibular Anterior Sextant: Incisal View

COMMENTS

It is most efficient and ergonomic to take this shot immediately after the occlusal view of the complete mandibular dentition. The only difference is the greater magnification ratio. The mirror is partially removed, and its inclination is adjusted to an angle of 30 degrees from the mandibular occlusal plane. The image will include the anterior teeth from canine to canine; the incisors should be symmetric on the image in the facio-lingual dimension. The assistant, seated at 3 o'clock, holds the modified retractor in the left hand, inserted with the handle toward the chin. The retractor should be grasped at the center of the handle and stretched outward to retract the lower lips, revealing the vestibule. It is always a good idea to avoid the appearance of this accessory in the frame. The figure eight–shaped mirror should be held with the right hand and inserted, widest end first, to the level of the first premolars. The practitioner stands at 7 o'clock with a knee against the side of the headrest for stability. Because the greatest complication is saliva, which tends to collect in the floor of the oral cavity, the saliva ejector should always be positioned behind the mirror. The practitioner can use the air-water spray to keep the mirror clean while waiting for the right moment to take the shot. This shot is easier than the full-arch view, even with patients who have a short lingual frenulum.

Fig 12-76
Incisal view of the mandibular anterior sextant.

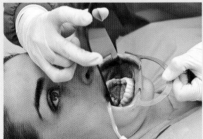

Fig 12-77a
The correct position of accessories and proper grasp of instruments.

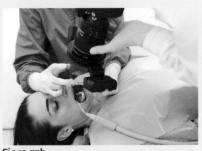

Fig 12-77b
The correct position of the camera and the flash units.

ALTERNATIVE METHOD

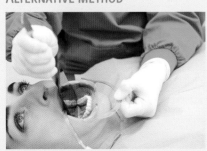

a

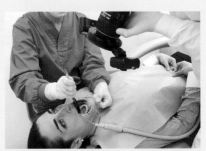

b

Figs 12-78a and 12-78b
This shot can be taken in an identical manner using a mirror with a handle.

VIEW 21

Degree of difficulty: 3

Position of the patient:
- Backrest of the treatment chair inclined 180 degrees (Fig 12-79a)
- Head turned toward the practitioner with chin lifted

Position of the assistant:
- Seated at the 3-o'clock position (Figs 12-79a and 12-79b)
- Mirror held in the right hand; contrastor held in the left hand

Position of the practitioner:
- Standing at the 7-o'clock position (Figs 12-79a and 12-79b)

Camera settings:
- Camera held horizontally 35 cm (14 inches) from the focal point
- Magnification ratio 1:1.5; aperture f/32 (minimum aperture)
- Flash units at the 3- and 9-o'clock positions (Fig 12-79c)
- Aiming point at the contact between the central incisors; focal point on the plane of the papillae between the central and lateral incisors (Fig 12-79d)

Type of retractor:
- Not applicable

Type of mirror:
- Large figure eight–shaped mirror

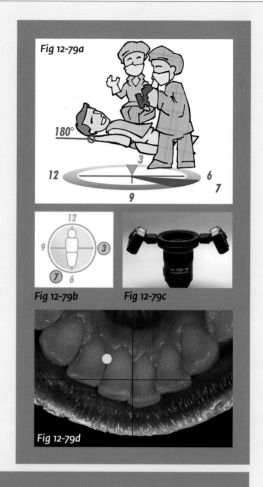

Fig 12-79a

Fig 12-79b   Fig 12-79c

Fig 12-79d

ACCESSORIES NEEDED

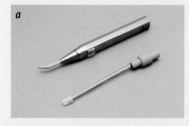

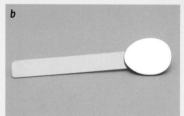

Fig 12-80a Saliva ejector and air-water spray.
Fig 12-80b Drop-shaped mirror with handle.
Fig 12-80c Disposable black cardboard contrastor.
Fig 12-80d Large figure eight–shaped mirror.
Fig 12-80e Spade-shaped metal contrastor.

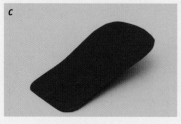

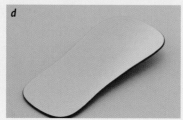

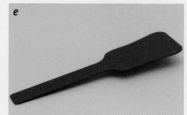

Mandibular Anterior Sextant: Lingual View

COMMENTS

Similar to the maxillary version of this shot, the assistant removes the cheek retractor and increases the inclination of the mirror to 60 degrees from the mandibular occlusal plane; the black cardboard contrastor is held with the left hand about 10 cm (4 inches) below the patient's chin to create an adequate black background.

Because the greatest complication is saliva, which tends to collect in the floor of the oral cavity, the saliva ejector should always be positioned behind the mirror.

The practitioner stands at 7 o'clock, using a knee against the side of the headrest for stability. The practitioner can use the air-water spray to keep the mirror clean while waiting for the right moment to take the shot.

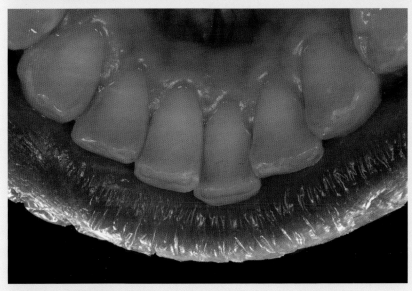

Fig 12-81
Lingual view of the mandibular anterior sextant.

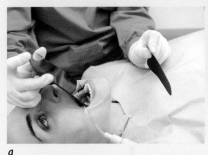

a

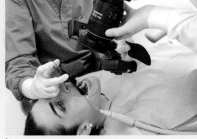

b

Fig 12-82a
The correct position of accessories and proper grasp of instruments.

Fig 12-82b
The correct position of the camera and the flash units.

ALTERNATIVE METHOD

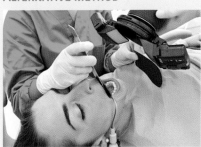

a

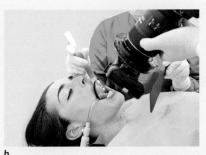

b

Fig 12-83a
This shot can be taken in an identical manner using a mirror with a handle.

Fig 12-83b
The spade-shaped metal contrastor can be substituted for the cardboard constrastor.

VIEW 22

Degree of difficulty: 2

Position of the patient:
- Backrest of the treatment chair inclined 180 degrees (Fig 12-84a)
- Head turned toward the practitioner with chin lifted

Position of the assistant:
- Seated at the 3-o'clock position (Figs 12-84a and 12-84b)
- Modified self-retracting cheek retractor held in left hand; contrastor held in the right hand

Position of the practitioner:
- Standing at the 7-o'clock position (Figs 12-84a and 12-84b)

Camera settings:
- Camera held horizontally 35 cm (14 inches) from the focal point
- Magnification ratio 1:1.5; aperture f/32 (minimum aperture)
- Flash units at the 3- and 9-o'clock positions (Fig 12-84c)
- Aiming point at the contact between the central incisors; focal point on the plane of the lateral incisors (Fig 12-84d)

Type of retractor:
- Modified self-retracting cheek retractor

Type of mirror:
- Not applicable

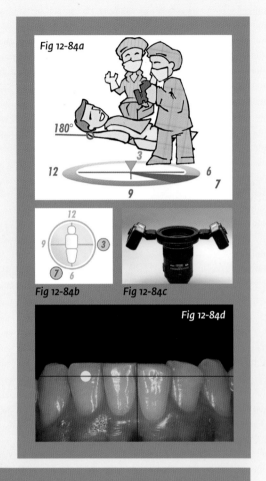

Fig 12-84a

Fig 12-84b   Fig 12-84c

Fig 12-84d

ACCESSORIES NEEDED

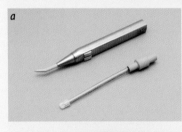

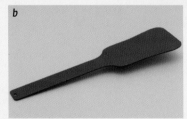

Fig 12-85a
Saliva ejector and air-water spray.

Fig 12-85b
Spade-shaped metal contrastor.

Fig 12-85c
Disposable black cardboard contrastor.

Fig 12-85d
Modified self-retracting cheek retractor.

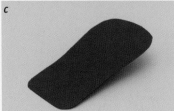

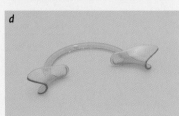

Mandibular Anterior Sextant: Facial View

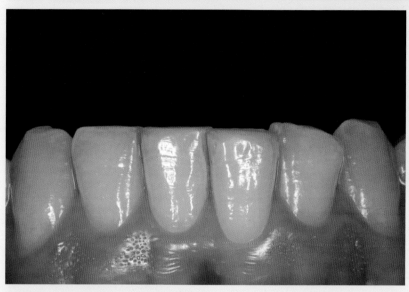

Fig 12-86
Facial view of the mandibular anterior sextant.

COMMENTS

With the handle toward the chin, the modified retractor is used to reveal the mucogingival line; this landmark is valuable for periodontal and esthetic assessment. If a disposable black cardboard contrastor is used, it is important that the assistant should curve it and hold it as far away from the anterior teeth as possible to obtain a uniformly dark background. The operator stands at 7 o'clock, using the knee against the side of the headrest for stability.

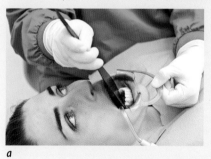

a

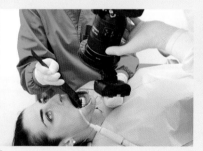

b

Fig 12-87a
The correct position of accessories and proper grasp of instruments. Here, the assistant is using the spade-shaped contrastor.

Fig 12-87b
The correct position of the camera and the flash units.

ALTERNATIVE METHOD

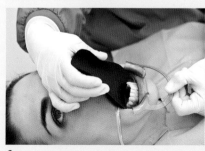

a

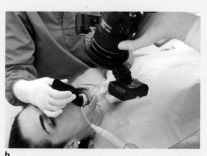

b

Figs 12-88a and 12-88b
This shot can also be taken with a disposable black cardboard, curved to avoid reflection of the light from the flash unit.

VIEW 23

Degree of difficulty: 3

Position of the patient:
- Backrest of the treatment chair inclined 180 degrees (Fig 12-89a)
- Head turned toward the practitioner

Position of the assistant:
- Seated at the 3-o'clock position (Figs 12-89a and 12-89b)
- Retractor held in right hand; mirror held in the left hand

Position of the practitioner:
- Standing at the 9-o'clock position (Figs 12-89a and 12-89b)

Camera settings:
- Camera held horizontally 37 cm (14.5 inches) from the focal point
- Magnification ratio 1:1.8; aperture f/32 (minimum aperture)
- Flash units side by side at the 3-o'clock position (Fig 12-89c)
- Aiming point at mesial fossa of the first molar; focal point on the plane of the gingival papilla between the second premolar and first molar (Fig 12-89d)

Type of retractor:
- Retractor modified for the maxillary right and mandibular left sextants

Type of mirror:
- Bean-shaped mirror, drop-shaped end

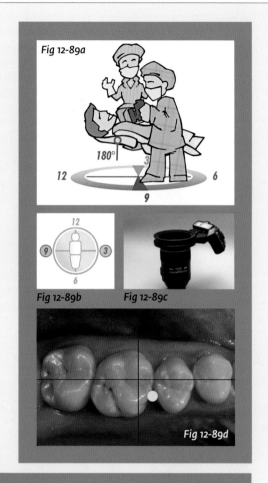

Fig 12-89a

Fig 12-89b

Fig 12-89c

Fig 12-89d

ACCESSORIES NEEDED

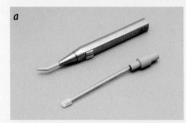

a

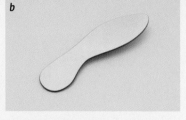

b

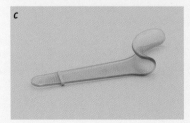

c

Fig 12-90a
Saliva ejector and air-water spray.

Fig 12-90b
Bean-shaped mirror.

Fig 12-90c
Retractor modified for the maxillary right and mandibular left sextants.

Maxillary Right Posterior Sextant: Occlusal View

COMMENTS

This series of views uses a retractor with the wing modified for the maxillary right and mandibular left sextants. This tool is ideal for eliminating the right upper lip from view. The retractor is held with the edge of the intact wing at the right labial commissure; with the right hand, the lip is stretched superiorly and laterally, with the handle against the cheek. The modified edge of the retractor should be as far away as possible from the teeth so that the retractor is not visible in the image and the light from the flash units completely illuminates the scene. For the same reason, the assistant's grasp of the mirror must be minimal. To prevent the cheek from collapsing onto the teeth, and to give a complete view of the vestibule distal to the second molar, the mirror should be held with the left hand at the tip of the tapered end and inserted horizontally into the mouth, with the more convex part of the drop-shaped end positioned toward the cheek. The mirror should be firmly resting against the mandibular teeth at an inclination of about 45 degrees from the maxillary occlusal plane and must not overlap the cheek retractor. Before taking the shot, the operator should check the position of the mirror to make sure that the image is perfectly aligned and includes the area between the mesial aspect of the first premolar and the distal aspect of the second molar.

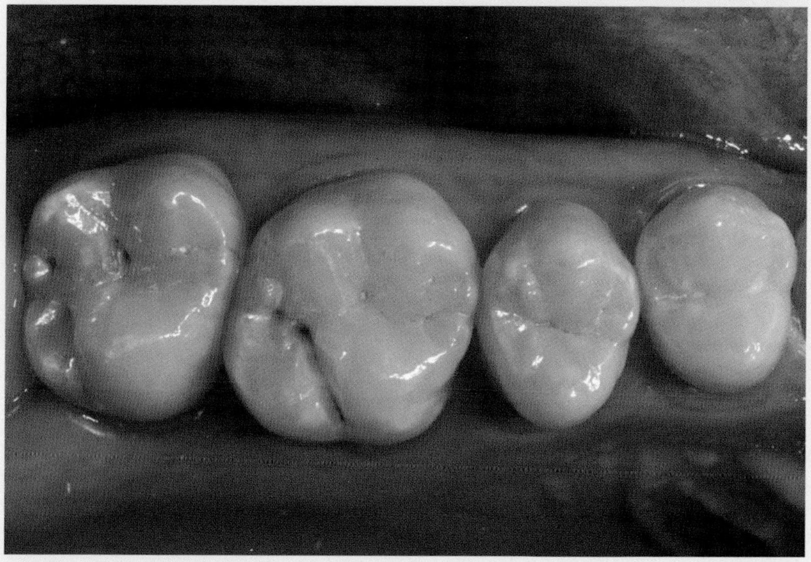

Fig 12-91
Occlusal view of the maxillary right posterior sextant.

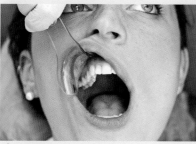

Fig 12-92a
The correct position and proper grasp of the retractor.

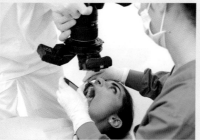

Fig 12-92b
The correct position of the camera and the flash units.

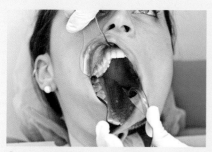

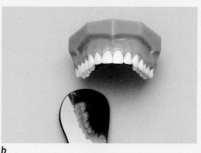

a   *b*

Fig 12-93a
Correct position and proper grasp of the retractor and mirror. The cheek retractor is positioned with the edge of the intact wing at the right labial commissure; the modified edge, near the incisors, is stretched outward.

Fig 12-93b
The convex edge of the drop-shaped end of the mirror is turned toward the cheek.

VIEW 24

Degree of difficulty: 3

Position of the patient:
- Backrest of the treatment chair inclined 180 degrees (Fig 12-94a)
- Head held straight, looking directly ahead

Position of the assistant:
- Seated at the 12-o'clock position (Figs 12-94a and 12-94b)
- Retractor held in right hand; mirror held in the left hand

Position of the practitioner:
- Standing at the 7-o'clock position (Figs 12-94a and 12-94b)

Camera settings:
- Camera held horizontally 37 cm (14.5 inches) from the focal point
- Magnification ratio 1:1.8; aperture f/32 (minimum aperture)
- Flash units side by side at the 3-o'clock position (Fig 12-94c)
- Aiming and focal points at the mesiolingual groove of the first molar (Fig 12-94d)

Type of retractor:
- Retractor modified for the maxillary right and mandibular left sextants

Type of mirror:
- Bean-shaped mirror, drop-shaped end

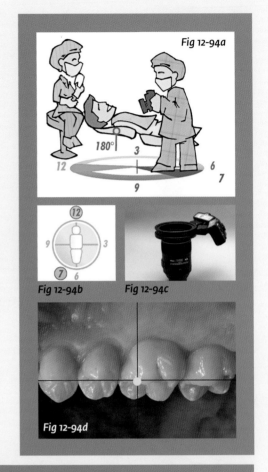

Fig 12-94a

Fig 12-94b   Fig 12-94c

Fig 12-94d

ACCESSORIES NEEDED

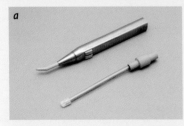

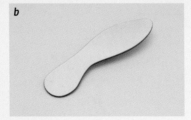

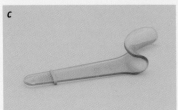

Fig 12-95a
Saliva ejector and air-water spray.

Fig 12-95b
Bean-shaped mirror.

Fig 12-95c
Handheld retractor modified for the maxillary right and mandibular left sextants.

Maxillary Right Posterior Sextant: Palatal View

COMMENTS

It is most efficient and ergonomic to take this shot immediately after the occlusal view of the maxillary right posterior sextant; the assistant uses the same accessories in a similar way. The retractor should be moved downwards until the modified edge of the wing rests at the right labial commissure. This position will prevent the retractor from appearing in the image; to achieve this result, the assistant needs to retract the cheek as far away as possible from the teeth.

The position of the mirror is similar to view 23, but the convex edge of the drop-shaped end faces the palate instead of the cheek; the concave edge between the two ends of the mirror should rest between the contralateral canine and first premolar. As previously, the assistant will have a minimal grasp on the mirror, as far away from the frame as possible, to prevent obstructing the light from the flash. The mirror should be inclined about 45 degrees from the mesiodistal plane and about 10 degrees away from the long axis of the teeth. It is essential that the mirror be positioned as far away as possible from the teeth to obtain a good view, especially at the level of the premolars. After having adjusted the position of the camera and accessories, the practitioner takes the shot.

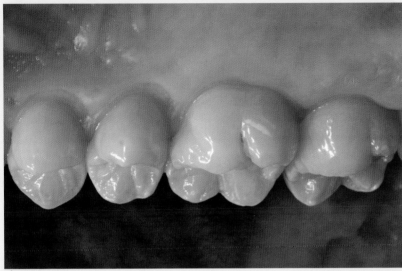

Fig 12-96
Palatal view of the maxillary right posterior sextant.

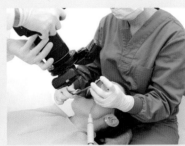

Fig 12-97a
The correct position and proper grasp of the retractor and mirror.

Fig 12-97b
The correct position of the camera and the flash units.

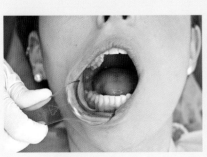

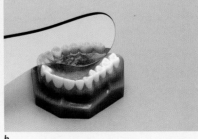

a

b

Fig 12-98a
The cheek retractor is positioned with the modified edge of the wing at the right labial commissure; the intact edge, near the mandibular incisors, is stretched outwards.

Fig 12-98b
The convex edge of the drop-shaped end of the mirror is turned toward the palate, and the mirror is inclined away from the molars. The edge of the isthmus between the mirror's two ends is positioned between the contralateral canine and first premolar.

VIEW 25

Degree of difficulty: 4

Position of the patient:
- Backrest of the treatment chair inclined 180 degrees (Fig 12-99a)
- Head held straight with chin lifted slightly, looking directly ahead

Position of the assistant:
- Seated at the 3-o'clock position (Figs 12-99a and 12-99b)
- Retractor held in the left hand; mirror held in the right hand

Position of the practitioner:
- Standing at the 9-o'clock position (Figs 12-99a and 12-99b)

Camera settings:
- Camera held horizontally 37 cm (14.5 inches) from the focal point
- Magnification ratio 1:1.8; aperture f/32 (minimum aperture)
- Flash units side by side at the 9-o'clock position (Fig 12-99c)
- Aiming point at mesial fossa of the first molar; focal point on the plane of the gingival papilla between the second premolar and first molar (Fig 12-99d)

Type of retractor:
- Retractor modified for the maxillary right and mandibular left sextants

Type of mirror:
- Bean-shaped mirror, drop-shaped end

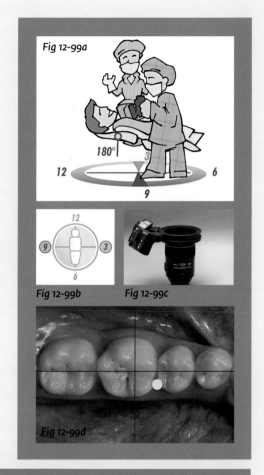

Fig 12-99a

Fig 12-99b   Fig 12-99c

Fig 12-99d

ACCESSORIES NEEDED

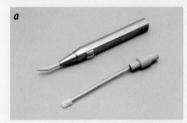

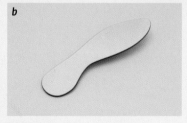

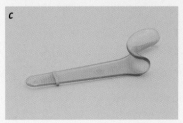

Fig 12-100a
Saliva ejector and air-water spray.
Fig 12-100b
Bean-shaped mirror.
Fig 12-100c
Retractor modified for the maxillary right and mandibular left sextants.

Mandibular Left Posterior Sextant: Occlusal View

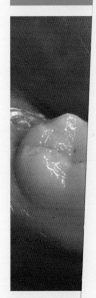

Fig 12-106
Lingual view of t

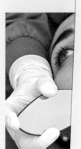

Fig 12-107a
The correct posi
retractor and m

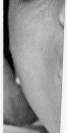

a

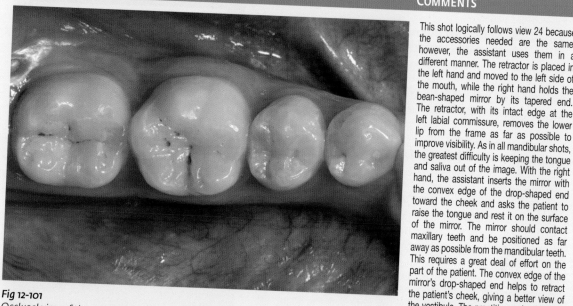

Fig 12-101
Occlusal view of the mandibular left posterior sextant.

COMMENTS

This shot logically follows view 24 because the accessories needed are the same; however, the assistant uses them in a different manner. The retractor is placed in the left hand and moved to the left side of the mouth, while the right hand holds the bean-shaped mirror by its tapered end. The retractor, with its intact edge at the left labial commissure, removes the lower lip from the frame as far as possible to improve visibility. As in all mandibular shots, the greatest difficulty is keeping the tongue and saliva out of the image. With the right hand, the assistant inserts the mirror with the convex edge of the drop-shaped end toward the cheek and asks the patient to raise the tongue and rest it on the surface of the mirror. The mirror should contact maxillary teeth and be positioned as far away as possible from the mandibular teeth. This requires a great deal of effort on the part of the patient. The convex edge of the mirror's drop-shaped end helps to retract the patient's cheek, giving a better view of the vestibule. The practitioner should make sure the teeth are kept dry with the saliva ejector or the air-water spray, and he or she should ask the patient to keep the tongue as far away as possible from the teeth by pushing it towards the back of the throat. This image includes the mesial of the first premolar to the distal of the second molar.

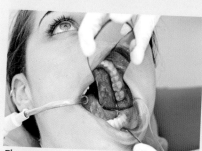

Fig 12-102a
The correct position and proper grasp of the retractor and mirror.

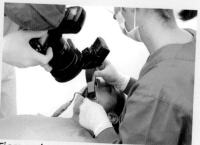
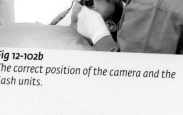

Fig 12-102b
The correct position of the camera and the flash units.

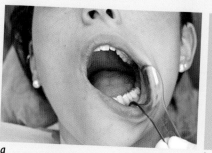

a

Fig 12-103a
The cheek retractor is positioned with the intact edge of the wing at the left labial commissure; the modified edge, near the mandibular incisors, is stretched outward.

Fig 12-103b The convex edge of the drop-shaped end of the mirror is turned toward the cheek.

b

VIEW 27

Degree of difficulty: 3

Position of the patient:
- Backrest of the treatment chair inclined 180 degrees (Fig 12-109a)
- Head held straight, looking directly ahead

Position of the assistant:
- Seated at the 12-o'clock position (Figs 12-109a and 12-109b)
- Retractor held in the left hand; mirror held in the right hand

Position of the practitioner:
- Standing at the 9-o'clock position (Figs 12-109a and 12-109b)

Camera settings:
- Camera held horizontally 37 cm (14.5 inches) from the focal point
- Magnification ratio 1:1.8; aperture f/32 (minimum aperture)
- Flash units side by side at the 3-o'clock position (Fig 12-109c)
- Aiming point at mesial fossa of the first molar; focal point on the plane of the gingival papilla between the second premolar and first molar (Fig 12-109d)

Type of retractor:
- Retractor modified for the maxillary left and mandibular right sextants

Type of mirror:
- Bean-shaped mirror, drop-shaped end

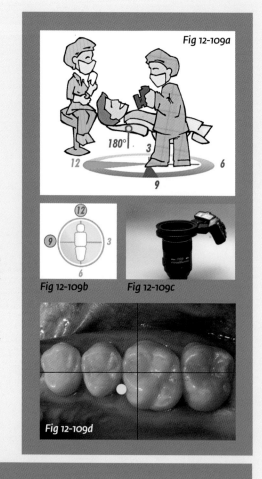

Fig 12-109a

Fig 12-109b   Fig 12-109c

Fig 12-109d

ACCESSORIES NEEDED

a

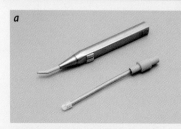

b

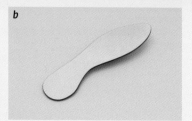

c

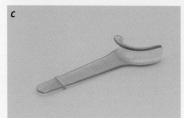

Fig 12-110a
Saliva ejector and air-water spray.
Fig 12-110b
Bean-shaped mirror.
Fig 12-110c
Retractor modified for the maxillary left and mandibular right sextants.

Photography in

VIEW 26

Degree of diffi
Position of the
- Backrest
- Head turn

Position of th
- Seated at
- Retracto

Position of th
- Standing

Camera setti
- Camera
- Magnifi
- Flash un
- Aiming
  (Fig 12-1

Type of retr
- Retract
  sextant

Type of mir
- Bean-s

ACCESSO

a

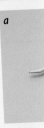

c

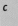

Maxillary Left Posterior Sextant: Occlusal View

This shot and the three that follow use a handheld retractor modified for the maxillary left and mandibular right sextants. This accessory is ideal for removing the left upper lip from the frame. With the edge of the intact wing at the left labial commissure and the handle pressed against the cheek, the retractor is held in the left hand and stretched upward and laterally so that the modified edge is moved as far away as possible from the teeth. This position removes the retractor from the frame and allows the flash units to fully illuminate the frame; for the same reason, the assistant's grasp on the mirror must be minimal. To prevent the cheek from collapsing onto the teeth and to allow for a complete view of the vestibule distal to the second molar, the mirror should be held with the right hand at the tip of the tapered end and inserted horizontally into the mouth, with the more convex part of the drop-shaped end positioned toward the cheek. The mirror should rest firmly against the mandibular teeth at an inclination of about 45 degrees to the maxillary occlusal plane and must not overlap the cheek retractor. Before taking the shot, the practitioner should check the position of the mirror to ensure that the image is perfectly aligned and includes the area between the mesial aspect of the first premolar and the distal border of the second molar.

Fig 12-111
Occlusal view of the maxillary left posterior sextant.

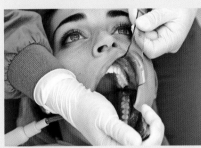

Fig 12-112a
The correct position and proper grasp of the retractor and mirror.

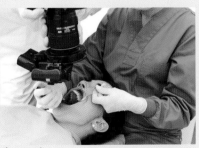

Fig 12-112b
The correct position of the camera and the flash units.

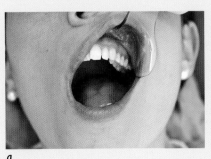

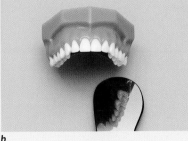

Fig 12-113a
The cheek retractor is positioned with the intact edge of the wing at the left labial commissure; the modified edge, near the maxillary incisors, is stretched outward.

Fig 12-113b
The convex edge of the drop-shaped end of the mirror is turned toward the cheek.

a

b

VIEW 28

Degree of difficulty: 3

Position of the patient:
- Backrest of the treatment chair inclined 180 degrees (Fig 12-114a)
- Head turned toward the practitioner

Position of the assistant:
- Seated at the 12-o'clock position (Figs 12-114a and 12-114b)
- Retractor held in the left hand; mirror held in the right hand

Position of the practitioner:
- Standing at the 7-o'clock position (Figs 12-114a and 12-114b)

Camera settings:
- Camera held horizontally 37 cm (14.5 inches) from the focal point
- Magnification ratio 1:1.8; aperture f/32 (minimum aperture)
- Flash units side by side at the 9-o'clock position (Fig 12-114c)
- Aiming and focal points at the mesiolingual groove of the first molar (Fig 12-114d)

Type of retractor:
- Retractor modified for the maxillary left and mandibular right sextants

Type of mirror:
- Bean-shaped mirror, drop-shaped end

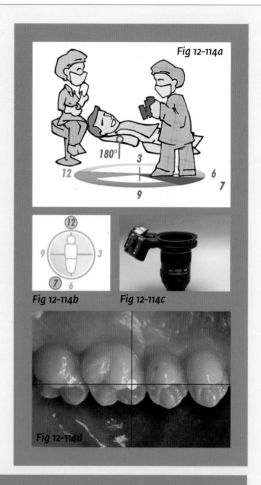

Fig 12-114a

Fig 12-114b

Fig 12-114c

Fig 12-114d

ACCESSORIES NEEDED

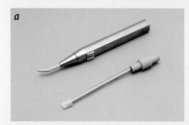

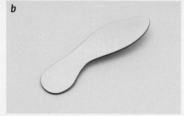

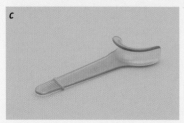

Fig 12-115a
Saliva ejector and air-water spray.
Fig 12-115b
Bean-shaped mirror.
Fig 12-115c
Retractor modified for the maxillary left and mandibular right sextants.

Maxillary Left Posterior Sextant: Palatal View

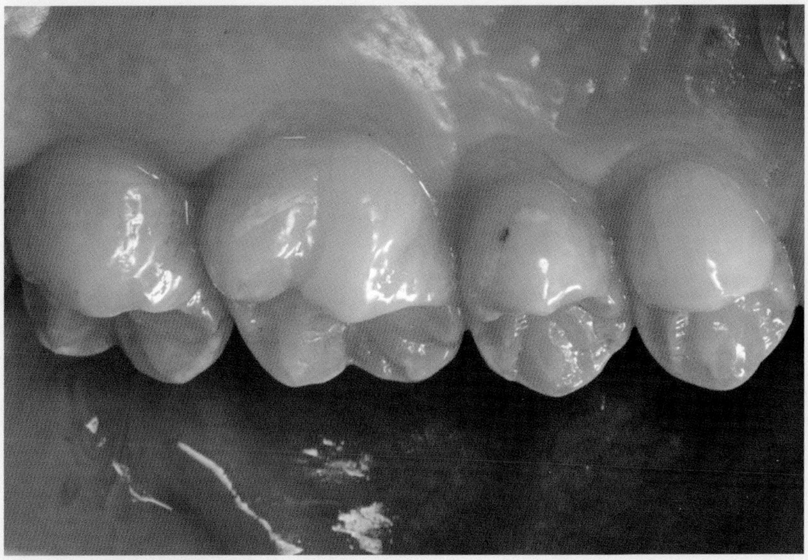

It is most efficient and ergonomic to take this shot immediately after the occlusal view of the maxillary left posterior sextant because the assistant uses the same accessories. The retractor, held in the left hand, is moved down until the modified edge of the wing rests at the left labial commissure. This will prevent the retractor from appearing in the image; to achieve this result, the assistant must retract the cheek as far as possible from the teeth. The mirror is held in the right hand and inserted with the convex edge of the drop-shaped end toward the palate; the edge at the narrowest part of the mirror should be resting between the contralateral canine and the first premolar. As previously, the assistant should have a minimal grasp on the mirror, and it should be as far away from the frame as possible so that the light from the flash can fully illuminate the frame. The mirror should be inclined about 45 degrees from the mesiodistal plane and about 10 degrees away from the long axis of the teeth. It is essential that the mirror should be held as far as possible from the teeth to gain a good view, especially at the level of the premolars. After having adjusted the position of the camera and accessories, the practitioner takes the shot.

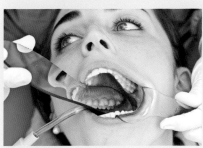

Fig 12-116
Palatal view of the maxillary left posterior sextant.

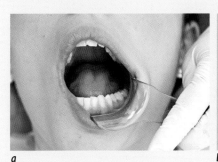

Fig 12-117a
The correct position and proper grasp of the retractor and mirror.

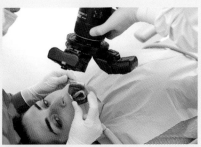

Fig 12-117b
The correct position of the camera and the flash units.

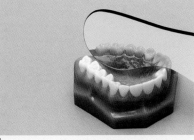

a

b

Fig 12-118a *The cheek retractor is positioned with the intact edge near the mandibular incisors; the modified edge of the wing, at the left labial commissure, is stretched outward.*
Fig 12-118b *The convex edge of the drop-shaped end of the mirror is turned toward the palate. The edge at the narrowest part is positioned between the contralateral canine and the first premolar.*

VIEW 29

Degree of difficulty: 4

Position of the patient:
- Backrest of the treatment chair inclined 180 degrees (Fig 12-119a)
- Head straight, chin slightly lifted, looking directly ahead

Assistant's position:
- Seated at the 12-o'clock position (Figs 12-119a and 12-119b)
- Retractor held in the right hand; mirror held in the left hand

Position of the practitioner:
- Standing at the 9-o'clock position (Figs 12-119a and 12-119b)

Camera settings:
- Camera held horizontally 37 cm (14.5 inches) from the focal point
- Magnification ratio 1:1.8; aperture f/32 (minimum aperture)
- Flash units side by side at the 9-o'clock position (Fig 12-119c)
- Aiming point at mesial fossa of the first molar; focal point on the plane of the gingival papilla between the second premolar and first molar (Fig 12-119d)

Type of retractor:
- Retractor modified for the maxillary left and mandibular right sextants

Type of mirror:
- Bean-shaped mirror, drop-shaped end

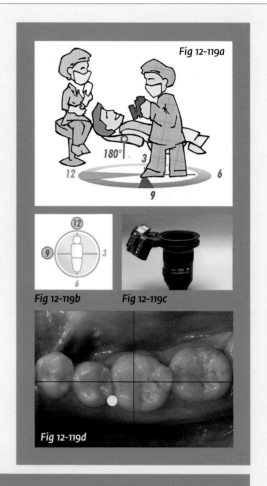

Fig 12-119a

Fig 12-119b

Fig 12-119c

Fig 12-119d

ACCESSORIES NEEDED

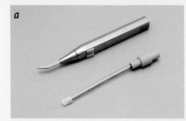

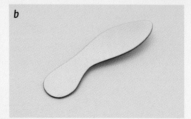

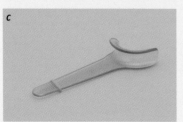

Fig 12-120a Saliva ejector and air-water spray.
Fig 12-120b Bean-shaped mirror.
Fig 12-120c Retractor modified for the maxillary left and mandibular right sextants.

Mandibular Right Posterior Sextant: Occlusal View

COMMENTS

This shot logically follows view 28 because the accessories needed are the same; however, the assistant uses them in a different manner. The retractor is placed in the right hand and moved to the right side of the mouth, while the left hand holds the bean-shaped mirror by its tapered end. The retractor, with its intact edge at the right labial commissure, retracts the lower lip away from the frame as far as possible to improve visibility. As in all mandibular shots, the greatest difficulty is keeping the tongue and saliva out of the image. With the left hand, the assistant inserts the mirror with the convex edge of the drop-shaped end toward the cheek and asks the patient to raise the tongue and rest it on the surface of the mirror. The mirror should contact maxillary teeth and be positioned as far away as possible from the mandibular teeth. This requires a great deal of effort on the part of the patient. The convex edge of the mirror's drop-shaped end helps to retract the patient's cheek, giving a better view of the vestibule. The practitioner should make sure the teeth are kept dry with the saliva ejector or the air-water spray, and he or she should ask the patient to keep the tongue as far away as possible from the teeth by pushing it toward the back of the throat. This image includes the mesial of the first premolar to the distal of the second molar.

Fig 12-121
Occlusal view of the mandibular right posterior sextant.

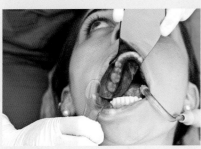

Fig 12-122a
The correct position and proper grasp of the retractor and mirror.

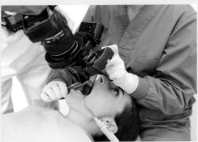

Fig 12-122b
The correct position of the camera and the flash units.

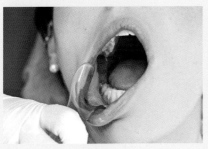

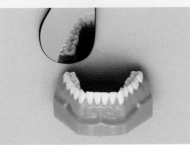

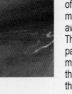

Fig 12-123a
The cheek retractor is positioned with the intact edge at the right labial commissure; the modified edge of the wing, near the mandibular incisors, is stretched outward.

Fig 12-123b
The convex edge of the drop-shaped end of the mirror is turned toward the cheek.

a

b

VIEW 30

Degree of difficulty: 4

Position of the patient:
- Backrest of the treatment chair inclined 180 degrees (Fig 12-124a)
- Head straight, looking directly ahead

Assistant's position:
- Seated at the 12-o'clock position (Figs 12-124a and 12-124b)
- Retractor held in the right hand; mirror held in the left hand

Position of the practitioner:
- Standing at the 9-o'clock position (Figs 12-124a and 12-124b)

Camera settings:
- Camera held horizontally 37 cm (14.5 inches) from the focal point
- Magnification ratio 1:1.8; aperture f/32 (minimum aperture)
- Flash units side by side at the 3-o'clock position (Fig 12-124c)
- Aiming and focal points at the mesial fossa of the first molar (Fig 12-124d)

Type of retractor:
- Retractor modified for the maxillary left and mandibular right sextants

Type of mirror:
- Bean-shaped mirror, drop-shaped end

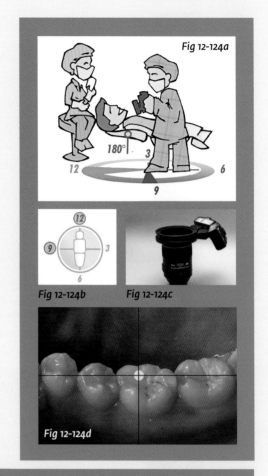

Fig 12-124a

Fig 12-124b   Fig 12-124c

Fig 12-124d

ACCESSORIES NEEDED

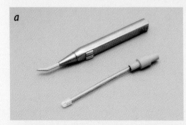

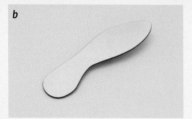

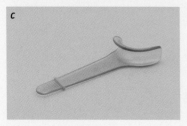

Fig 12-125a
Saliva ejector and air-water spray.

Fig 12-125b
Bean-shaped mirror.

Fig 12-125c
Retractor modified for the maxillary left and mandibular right sextants.

Mandibular Right Posterior Sextant: Lingual View

COMMENTS

This shot logically follows view 29 because the accessories needed are the same, and the assistant uses them in a similar manner. With the right hand, the retractor is moved upward until its modified edge is at the right labial commissure. It is used to retract the right upper lip to obtain a good visual field; at the same time, the retractor should be excluded from the frame. With the left hand, the mirror is inserted horizontally into the mouth and then rotated so that the more convex edge of the drop-shaped end faces the floor of the oral cavity. The assistant asks the patient to contract the lower lip downward to improve the visual field and to keep the tongue relaxed. The assistant uses the mirror to retract the tongue from the frame. The mirror should be inclined about 45 degrees from the mesiodistal plane and about 10 degrees away from the long axis of the teeth. The grasp on the mirror must, as usual, be minimal; this shot is demanding, especially with patients whose tongue is hypertrophic and strong. The practitioner should ensure the teeth are kept dry with the saliva ejector before taking the shot, which should include the mesial of the first premolar to the distal of the second molar.

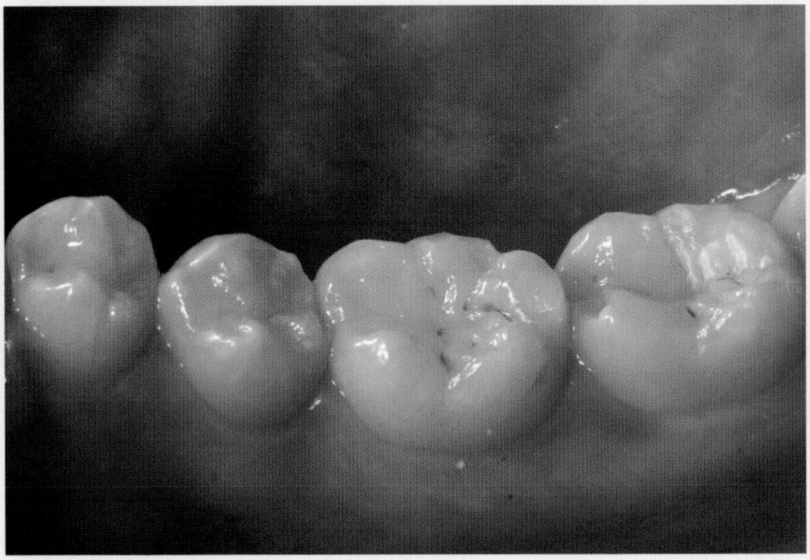

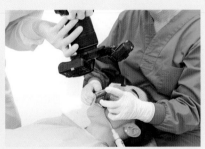

Fig 12-126
Lingual view of the mandibular right posterior sextant.

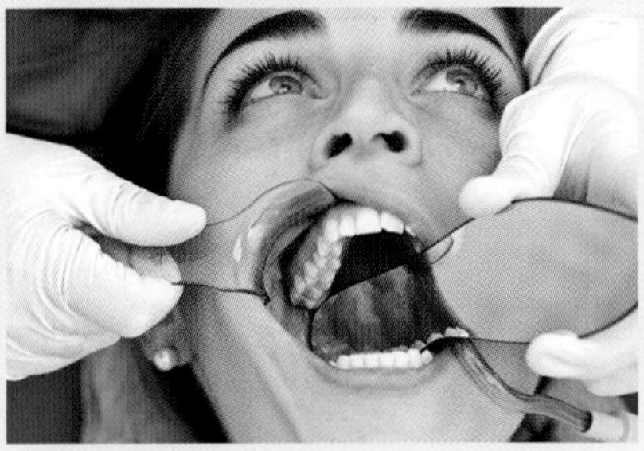

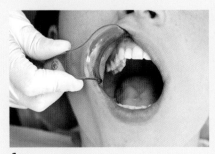

Fig 12-127a
The correct position and proper grasp of the retractor and mirror.

Fig 12-127b
The correct position of the camera and the flash units.

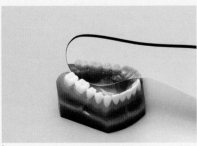

Fig 12-128a *The cheek retractor is positioned with the intact edge of the wing near the maxillary incisors; the modified edge, at the right labial commissure, is stretched outward.*
Fig 12-128b *The convex edge of the drop-shaped end of the mirror is turned toward the floor of the mouth, and its edge at the narrowest part rests between the contralateral canine and first premolar.*

a

b

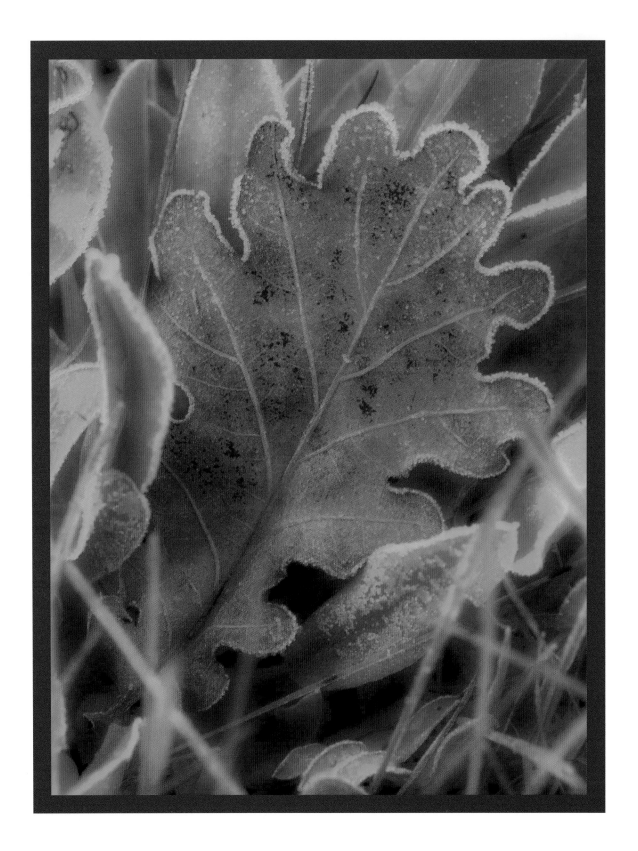

Chapter 13

Photographic
Documentation

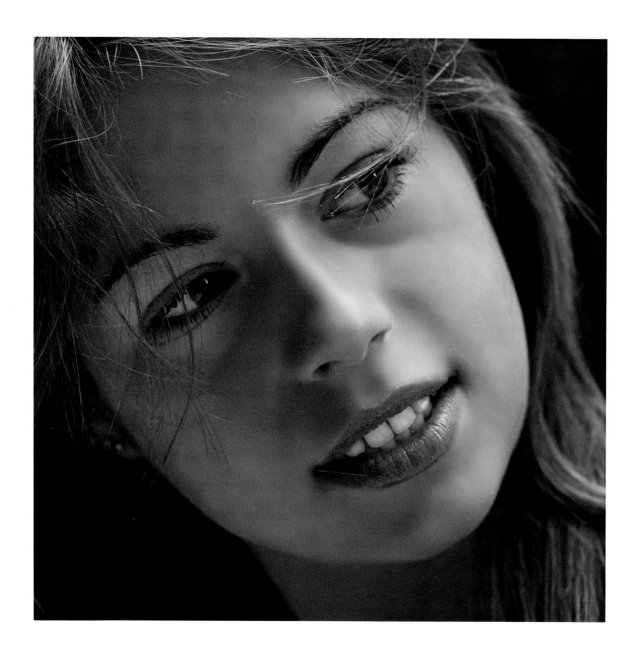

The various dental disciplines have specific documentary requirements; for this reason, it is not always necessary to record every view presented in chapters 11 and 12. For example, documentation of orthodontic cases does not require multiple images of the posterior regions of the mouth; similarly, documentation of a periodontal patient does not require occlusal views of the posterior teeth.

Only certain scientific societies or academies publish guidelines regarding photographic documentation. For example, in its 2007 guidelines, the Accademia Italiana di Conservativa listed a specific set of photographs for all presentations:

- Pretreatment: frontal, lateral, and occlusal
- Specific area to be treated, with and without rubber dam
- Sequential steps of tooth preparation
- Operative stages of reconstruction, according to the type of technique
- Completed and polished restoration with rubber dam, highlighting the correct integration of the restorations with the marginal tissues

It is clear that there are no well-defined criteria for either the number or type of photographs necessary for a presentation, so this situation remains vague and subject to interpretation. However, recommendations exist for standardized, repeatable documentation for each of the most common dental disciplines. The suggested photographic documentation is not identical to that needed to comply with specific academies or scientific societies, but it may prove useful in creating personal photographic files, complete with the practitioner's own clinical cases. Among the dental disciplines, prosthetic dentistry is likely the one that requires the greatest number of images. In fact, correct documentation of full-mouth rehabilitation requires all extraoral and intraoral shots previously described. Furthermore, it may also be necessary to document details considered significant during the operative stages of treatment; these images will only differ from the pretreatment series in the greater magnification ratio required.

Orthodontic Documentation

The orthodontic image series is undoubtedly the simplest to accomplish, and it is for this reason that orthodontists probably document their clinical cases the most often.

There are 14 photographs required for correct orthodontic documentation:

Extraoral views
- Frontal face, smiling and with lips relaxed
- Right profile, smiling and with lips relaxed
- Left profile, smiling and with lips relaxed
- Three-quarter profile, smiling

Intraoral views (Fig 13-1)
- Right and left overjet
- Full arches in occlusion
- Right quadrants in occlusion
- Left quadrants in occlusion
- Complete maxillary dentition, occlusal view
- Complete mandibular dentition, occlusal view

ORTHODONTIC

Fig 13-1a
Right overjet.

Fig 13-1b
Complete maxillary dentition, occlusal view.

Fig 13-1c
Left overjet.

Fig 13-1d
Right quadrants in occlusion for orthodontic documentation.

Fig 13-1e
Full arches in normal occlusion.

Fig 13-1f
Left quadrants in occlusion for orthodontic documentation.

Fig 13-1g
Right quadrants in occlusion.

Fig 13-1h
Complete mandibular dentition, occlusal view.

Fig 13-1i
Left quadrants in occlusion.

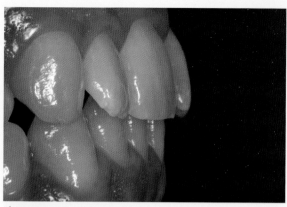

Fig 13-1a

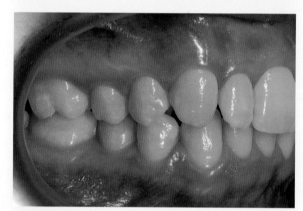

Fig 13-1d

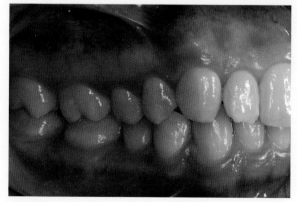

Fig 13-1g

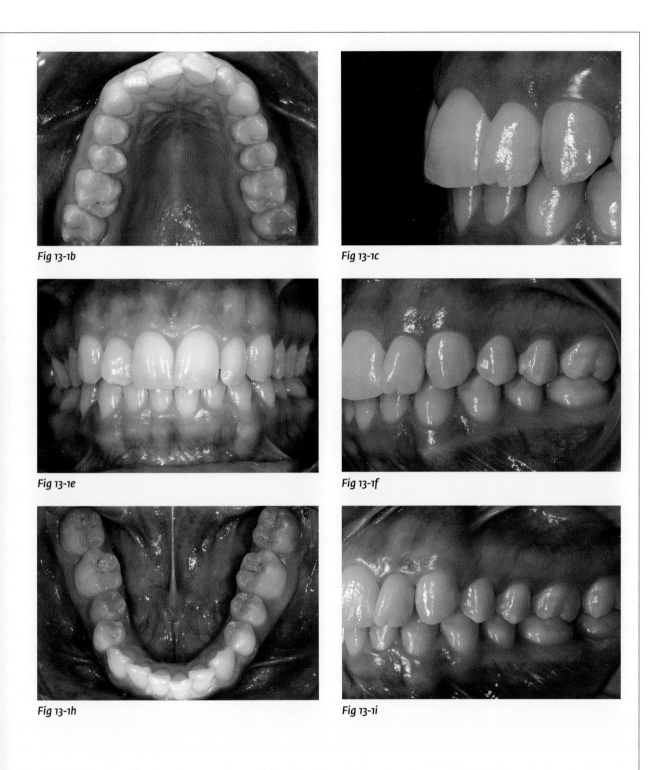

Fig 13-1b

Fig 13-1c

Fig 13-1e

Fig 13-1f

Fig 13-1h

Fig 13-1i

Periodontal Documentation

Photography of periodontal patients can be diverse. Presenters at medical conferences often demonstrate therapeutic steps with photographs of the tissues rather than the teeth because the tissues reveal more information about the patient's periodontal status.

For example, mucogingival therapy is often documented with buccal views of the posterior quadrants in which the aiming point is moved toward the mucogingival line because this is the anatomical landmark of significance in assessing the final result. These images have not been included in chapter 12, but the positions of the patient, assistant, and practitioner are identical; only the aiming point varies. The following views should be recorded before and after treatment:

Extraoral views
- Frontal face, smiling and with lips relaxed
- Right profile, smiling and with lips relaxed
- Left profile, smiling and with lips relaxed
- Right lateral smile
- Left lateral smile
- Slight, average, and maximum smiles

Intraoral views (Fig 13-2)
- Full arches in occlusion
- Anterior sextants in occlusion
- Right quadrants in occlusion
- Left quadrants in occlusion
- Complete maxillary dentition, occlusal view
- Complete mandibular dentition, occlusal view
- Maxillary right posterior sextant, palatal view
- Maxillary anterior sextant, palatal view
- Maxillary left posterior sextant, palatal view
- Mandibular left posterior sextant, lingual view
- Mandibular anterior sextant, lingual view
- Mandibular right posterior sextant, lingual view

This set of images is also appropriate for documentation of oral hygiene status by the hygienist.

PERIODONTAL

Fig 13-2a
Maxillary right posterior sextant, palatal view.

Fig 13-2b
Maxillary anterior sextant, palatal view.

Fig 13-2c
Maxillary left posterior sextant, palatal view.

Fig 13-2d
Right posterior sextants in occlusion.

Fig 13-2e
Anterior sextants in normal occlusion.

Fig 13-2f
Left posterior sextants in occlusion.

Fig 13-2g
Mandibular right posterior sextant, lingual view.

Fig 13-2h
Mandibular anterior sextant, lingual view.

Fig 13-2i
Mandibular left posterior sextant, lingual view.

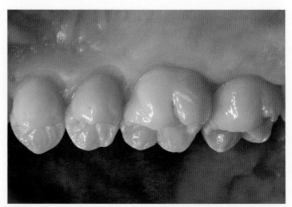

Fig 13-2a

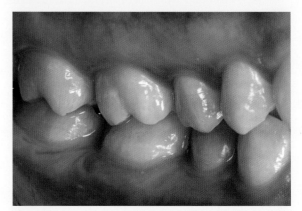

Fig 13-2d

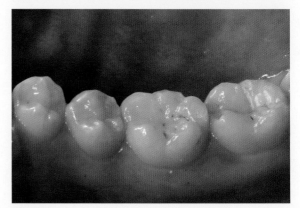

Fig 13-2g

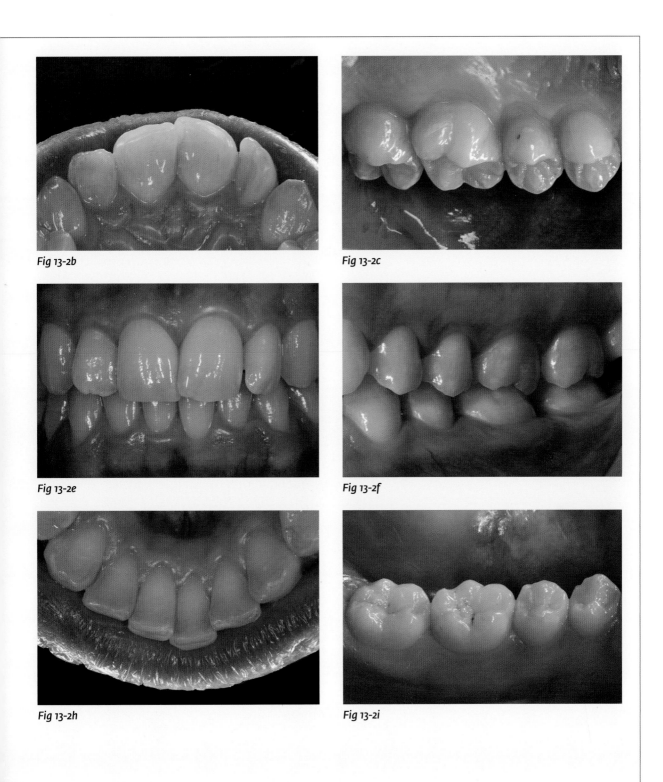

Fig 13-2b

Fig 13-2c

Fig 13-2e

Fig 13-2f

Fig 13-2h

Fig 13-2i

Prosthetic Documentation

As previously mentioned, correct documentation of prosthetic rehabilitation requires the complete set of extraoral and intraoral images. It is important to record any treatment previously completed by other dentists or specialists when documenting planned permanent prostheses. This includes implant placement, endodontic therapy, periodontal therapy, and orthodontic treatment. Furthermore, good documentation requires a complete set of photographs because information regarding every aspect of the tooth surface is necessary.

In addition to pre- and posttreatment images, photographs against a background that provides significant contrast are recommended to highlight the nuances of surface color and texture, especially in anterior regions with high esthetic value. A black background best distinguishes the details both of the teeth and the soft tissue. The following complete set of images is recommended:

Extraoral views
- Frontal face, smiling and with lips relaxed
- Right profile, smiling and with lips relaxed
- Left profile, smiling and with lips relaxed
- Right lateral smile
- Left lateral smile
- Slight, average, and maximum smiles

Intraoral views (Fig 13-3)
- Right and left overjet
- Full arches in occlusion
- Anterior sextants in occlusion
- Right quadrants in occlusion
- Left quadrants in occlusion
- Complete maxillary dentition, occlusal view
- Complete mandibular dentition, occlusal view
- Maxillary right posterior sextant, occlusal view
- Maxillary right posterior sextant, palatal view
- Maxillary anterior sextant, facial view
- Maxillary anterior sextant, incisal view
- Maxillary anterior sextant, palatal view
- Maxillary left posterior sextant, occlusal view
- Maxillary left posterior sextant, palatal view
- Mandibular left posterior sextant, occlusal view
- Mandibular left posterior sextant, lingual view
- Mandibular anterior sextant, facial view
- Mandibular anterior sextant, incisal view
- Mandibular anterior sextant, lingual view
- Mandibular right posterior sextant, occlusal view
- Mandibular right posterior sextant, lingual view

Conservative Dentistry Documentation

This list of required images is very similar to those listed for prosthetic patients. Because both direct and indirect restorations, such as inlays, may be placed, it is always necessary to document the patient's condition before and after treatment. The required photos are:

Extraoral views
- Frontal face, smiling and with lips relaxed
- Right profile, smiling and with lips relaxed
- Left profile, smiling and with lips relaxed
- Right lateral smile
- Left lateral smile
- Slight, average, and maximum smiles

Intraoral views
- Right and left overjet
- Full arches in occlusion
- Anterior sextants in occlusion
- Right quadrants in occlusion
- Left quadrants in occlusion
- Complete maxillary dentition, occlusal view
- Complete mandibular dentition, occlusal view
- Maxillary right posterior sextant, occlusal view
- Maxillary right posterior sextant, palatal view
- Maxillary anterior sextant, facial view
- Maxillary anterior sextant, incisal view
- Maxillary anterior sextant, palatal view
- Maxillary left posterior sextant, occlusal view
- Maxillary left posterior sextant, palatal view
- Mandibular left posterior sextant, occlusal view
- Mandibular left posterior sextant, lingual view
- Mandibular anterior sextant, facial view
- Mandibular anterior sextant, incisal view
- Mandibular anterior sextant, lingual view
- Mandibular right posterior sextant, occlusal view
- Mandibular right posterior sextant, lingual view

PROSTHETIC

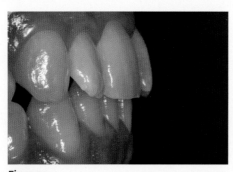

Fig 13-3*a*

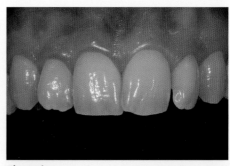

Fig 13-3*b*

Fig 13-3*a*
Right overjet.

Fig 13-3*b*
Maxillary anterior sextant, facial view.

Fig 13-3*c*
Mandibular anterior sextant, facial view.

Fig 13-3*d*
Left overjet.

Fig 13-3*e*
Complete maxillary dentition, occlusal view.

Fig 13-3*f*
Full arches in normal occlusion.

Fig 13-3*g*
Complete mandibular dentition, occlusal view.

Fig 13-3*h*
Maxillary right posterior sextant, occlusal view.

Fig 13-3*i*
Maxillary anterior sextant, incisal view.

Fig 13-3*j*
Maxillary left posterior sextant, occlusal view.

Fig 13-3*k*
Mandibular right posterior sextant, occlusal view.

Fig 13-3*l*
Mandibular anterior sextant, incisal view.

Fig 13-3*m*
Mandibular left posterior sextant, occlusal view.

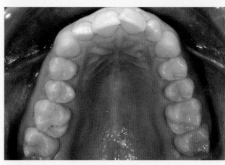

Fig 13-3*e*

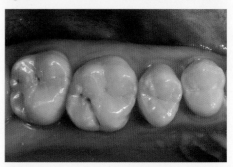

Fig 13-3*h*

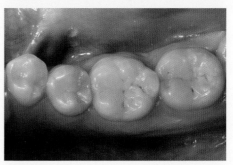

Fig 13-3*k*

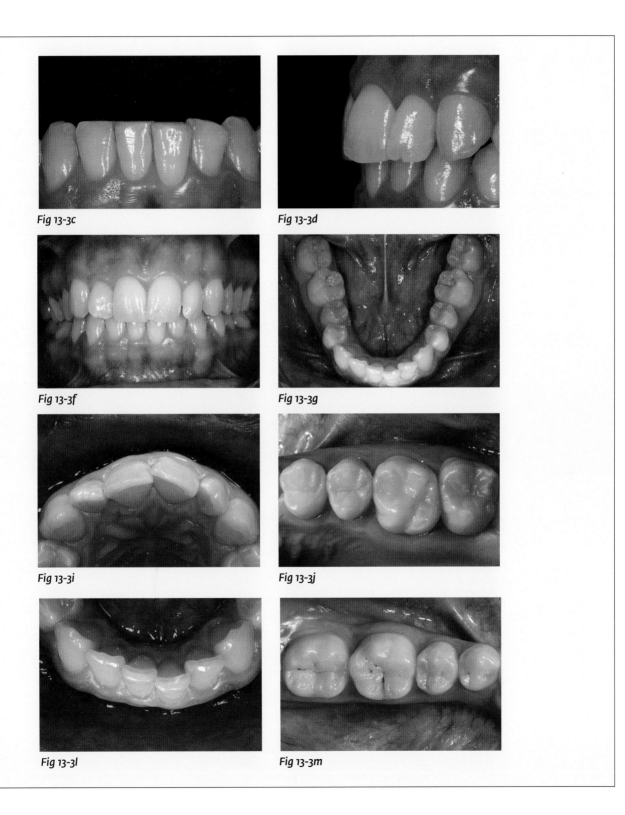

Fig 13-3c

Fig 13-3d

Fig 13-3f

Fig 13-3g

Fig 13-3i

Fig 13-3j

Fig 13-3l

Fig 13-3m

PROSTHETIC

Fig 13-3n
Maxillary right posterior sextant, palatal view.

Fig 13-3o
Maxillary anterior sextant, palatal view.

Fig 13-3p
Maxillary left posterior sextant, palatal view.

Fig 13-3q
Right posterior sextants in occlusion.

Fig 13-3r
Anterior sextants in normal occlusion.

Fig 13-3s
Left posterior sextants in occlusion.

Fig 13-3t
Mandibular right posterior sextant, lingual view.

Fig 13-3u
Mandibular anterior sextant, lingual view.

Fig 13-3v
Mandibular left posterior sextant, lingual view.

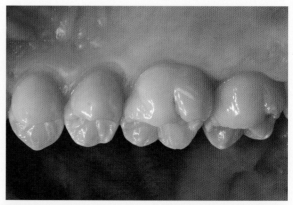

Fig 13-3n

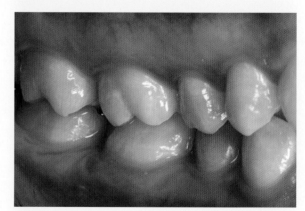

Fig 13-3q

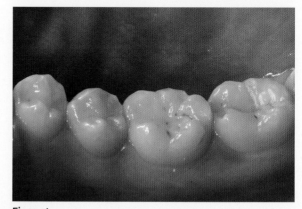

Fig 13-3t

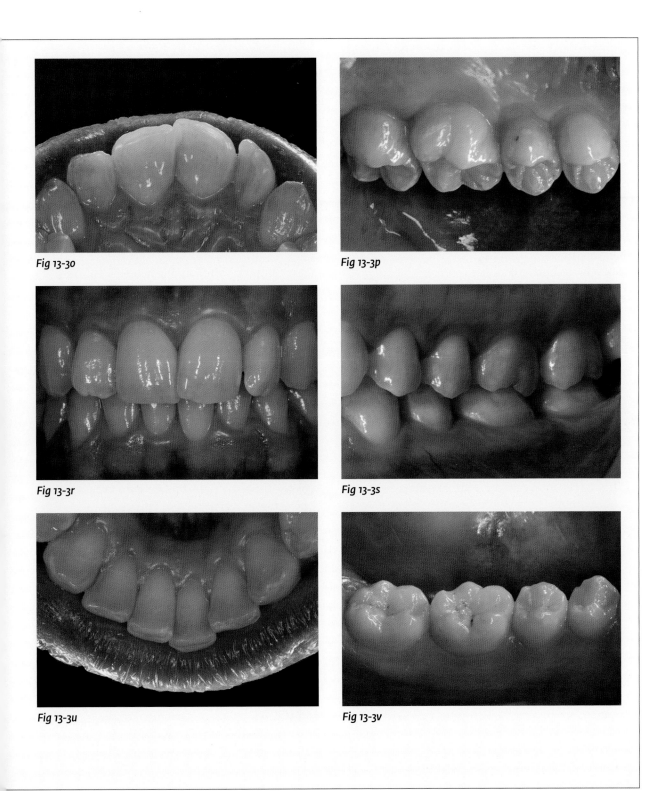

Fig 13-3o

Fig 13-3p

Fig 13-3r

Fig 13-3s

Fig 13-3u

Fig 13-3v

Photographing with rubber dam

In documenting the operative phases of conservative dental treatment, it is necessary to photograph with correctly applied rubber dam.

It is much easier to take photographs, with or without a mirror, with rubber dam in place, because it is not necessary to use cheek retractors, nor is there any possibility of interference from the tongue. The operative field is dry, and the rubber dam material provides a uniform background. However, certain precautions must be taken. First, the clamp used must be intact, preferably new, without any signs of wear or, worse still, adhesive residues.

As noted in chapter 8, the rubber dam clamp can create reflections, which interfere with the functioning of the exposure meter, making the through-the-lens (TTL) function unusable. To circumvent this problem, the clamp can be made opaque with airborne-particle abrasion, or the flash can be set on manual mode.

The use of blue- or green-colored dam sheets is recommended because they do not create visual distractions in the photographs. It is also important to ensure that the dam is reflected into the gingival sulcus to completely isolate the operative field from oral fluids; moreover, the dam must be taut, without any creases.

Following application procedures, a thin adhesive film may remain, which can create a very unpleasant effect if not completely removed. It is advisable to remove any such residues before polymerization, because afterwards it will be difficult to remove the adhesive. It can be removed with a small amount of cotton wool with rubbing alcohol; great care should be taken not to contaminate the prepared tooth surfaces. Alcohol is a solvent for some adhesives,

and contact could prove harmful to the quality of the adhesion of the restoration.

The number and type of photographs to correctly describe operative procedures is a subject of debate. The author suggests showing each operative phase, as if every shot is a single frame in the film of the entire procedure; however, for efficiency, it is a good idea to select only the most relevant steps (Fig 13-4). The following photographic sequence is suggested for a Class 1 composite restoration:

- Pretreatment, prior to application of rubber dam
- Pretreatment, after application of rubber dam
- Removal of previous restoration
- Tooth preparation
- Application of etchant to the enamel surfaces
- Application of etchant to the dentinal surfaces
- Application of the adhesive
- Application of flowable composite resin
- Dentinal buildup with composite resin
- Enamel buildup with composite resin
- Occlusal fissure staining
- Posttreatment, after rubber dam removal and occlusal finishing and polishing

This list of proposed shots represents standard documentation, which is more than adequate for detailed medicolegal purposes, but might prove insufficient in the scope of a conservative dental treatment plan. In summary, the decision of how many and which photographs to take to document the treatment of a patient is always dependent on the final aim of the practitioner.

Fig 13-4a
Pretreatment, prior to application of rubber dam.

Fig 13-4b
Pretreatment, after application of rubber dam.

Fig 13-4c
Removal of previous restoration.

Fig 13-4d
Tooth preparation.

Fig 13-4e
Application of etchant to the enamel surfaces.

Fig 13-4f
Application of etchant to the dentinal surfaces.

Fig 13-4g
Application of the adhesive.

Fig 13-4h
Application of flowable composite resin.

Fig 13-4i
Dentinal buildup with composite resin.

Fig 13-4j
Enamel buildup with composite resin.

Fig 13-4k
Occlusal fissure staining.

Fig 13-4l
Posttreatment, after rubber dam removal and occlusal finishing and polishing.

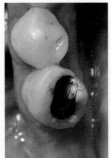

Fig 13-4a

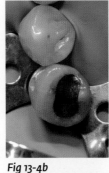

Fig 13-4b

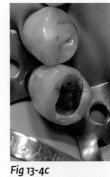

Fig 13-4c

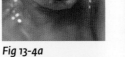

Fig 13-4d

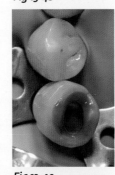

Fig 13-4e

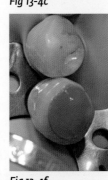

Fig 13-4f

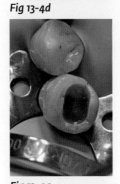

Fig 13-4g

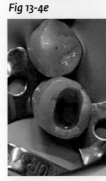

Fig 13-4h

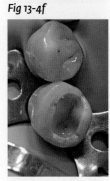

Fig 13-4i

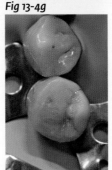

Fig 13-4j

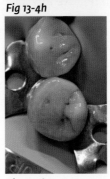

Fig 13-4k

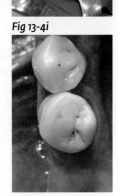

Fig 13-4l

Communication with the Dental Laboratory Technician

Correct communication and a good relationship with the dental laboratory technician is an essential and complex aspect of modern dentistry. It is not advisable to discount this relationship, because the success of prosthetic therapy is dependent on teamwork. Communication between the dentist and the laboratory technician is of fundamental importance when attempting to imitate what nature has created as faithfully as possible.

To accurately reproduce the natural harmony of teeth and their supporting tissues, it is imperative to provide the technician with the greatest amount of data possible, not only of a strictly dental nature (hue, chroma, value, translucency, and characteristics concerning the surface structure), but also those aspects relating to facial expression, harmony, and facial type. The dental technician must be able to faithfully reconstruct, with the aid of photographs, the context in which the teeth are situated and to restore dental harmony in every dimension.

Because images have a communicative power that is extremely useful, it is advisable to provide the technician with several photographs during the course of treatment. Ideally, the patient should visit the laboratory, so that the technician can personally examine the various aspects of tooth color, but often this is not possible because of the distance involved.

Alternatively, a video can be sent to the technician, not for a correct interpretation of color, but to highlight facial expressions, lip movements, and the exposure of teeth and gingiva. A video provides a more realistic and dynamic source of three-dimensional information regarding functioning; it is not static like a photograph, although these remain indispensable. It is desirable that the dentist and the technician should work together toward the selection of the color, adopting a shared procedure. Moreover, the ambient illumination during shade selection should be neutral, without any chromatic dominants present.

Currently, new equipment for the acquisition of color data is being introduced, using groundbreaking instruments such as reflection spectrophotometers. The SpectroShade (Medical High Technologies) is one such instrument; it has been specifically designed for the dental field and accurately measures the hue, chroma, and value of teeth and full-coverage restorations. As discussed in chapter 3, the two methodologies, photography and spectrophotometry, should be considered complementary; the spectrophotometer takes precise measurements for shade selection, while photography is used to obtain and transmit information about a tooth's general shape and surface characteristics (Fig 13-5). It is especially advantageous to take photographs, with color references, at the beginning of the dental appointment to avoid altering the exact perception of color from tooth dehydration during dental procedures.

Fig 13-5a
The porcelain-fused-to-metal crown on the maxillary left lateral incisor does not meet the patient's esthetic requirements.

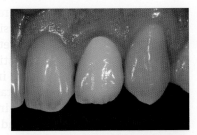

Fig 13-5b
A new all-ceramic crown with zirconia core has been seated.

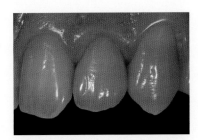

Fig 13-5c
Palatal view of original restoration.

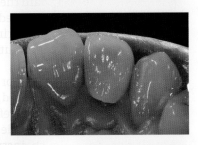

Fig 13-5d
Palatal view of new restoration.

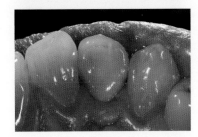

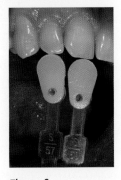

Fig 13-5e
Standard method of shade selection.

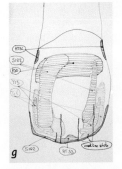

Fig 13-5f
Standard method of enamel shade selection.

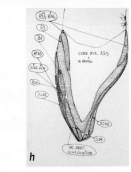

Figs 13-5g and 13-5h
After careful study of photographs, the laboratory technician creates a color map for three-dimensional reconstruction of the tooth shade.

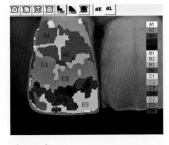

Fig 13-5i
The distribution of color, or digital color mapping, as measured by the SpectroShade spectrophotometer.

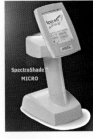

Fig 13-5j
The SpectroShade Micro unit.

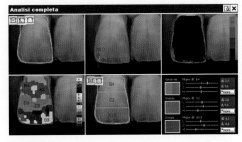

Fig 13-5k
The SpectroShade software performs a complete analysis of the digital color mapping.

Recommended Reading

AHMAD I. **Digital dental photography.** Part 1: An overview. Br Dent J 2009;206:403–407.

AHMAD I. **Digital dental photography.** Part 2: Purposes and uses. Br Dent J 2009;206:459–464.

AHMAD I. **Digital dental photography.** Part 3: Principles of digital photography. Br Dent J 2009;206:517–523.

AHMAD I. **Digital dental photography.** Part 4: Choosing a camera. Br Dent J 2009;206:575–581.

AHMAD I. **Digital dental photography.** Part 5: Lighting. Br Dent J 2009;207:13–18.

AHMAD I. **Digital dental photography.** Part 6: Camera settings. Br Dent J 2009;207:63–69.

AHMAD I. **Digital dental photography.** Part 7: Extra-oral set-ups. Br Dent J 2009;207:103–110.

AHMAD I. **Digital dental photography.** Part 8: Intra-oral set-ups. Br Dent J 2009;207:151–157.

BENGEL W. **Digital photography in the dental practice—An overview (II).** Int J Comput Dent 2000;3:121–132.

BENGEL W. **Mastering Digital Dental Photography.** Chicago: Quintessence, 2006.

BENZ C. **Digital photography: Exposures, editing images, and presentation.** Int J Comput Dent 2003;6:249–281.

BOWERS CM, JOHANSEN RJ. **Photographic evidence protocol: The use of digital imaging methods to rectify angular distortion and create life size reproductions of bite mark evidence.** J Forensic Sci 2002;47:178–185.

CHRISTENSEN GJ. **Important clinical uses for digital photography.** J Am Dent Assoc 2005;136:77–79.

CHU SJ. **Clinical steps to predictable color management in aesthetic restorative dentistry.** Dent Clin North Am 2007;51:473–485.

CHU SJ, DEVIGUS A, RADE P, MIELESZKO AJ. **The Fundamentals of Color: Shade Matching and Communication in Esthetic Dentistry, ed 2.** Chicago: Quintessence, 2011.

CHUMAN TA, HUMMEL SK, BOKMEYER TJ. **Evaluation of working distances at a 1:1 reproduction ratio for seven popular 35-mm dental camera systems.** J Prosthodont 1998;7:91–99.

CLARK EB. **The Clark tooth color system. Parts I and II.** Dent Mag Oral Top 1933;50:139–152,249–258.

ELTER A, CANIKLIOĞLU B, DEĞER S, OZEN J. **The reliability of digital cameras for color selection.** Int J Prosthodont 2005;18:438–440.

FREEHE CL. **Photography in dentistry: Equipment and technique.** Dent Clin North Am 1983;27:3–73.

GOLDSTEIN MB. **Digital photography: Make it your lifeline.** Dent Today 2009;28(5):112–115.

GOLDSTEIN MB. **Digital photography and your laboratory.** Dent Today 2008;27(8):120,122–123.

GOLDSTEIN MB, YOUNG R, BERGMANN R. **Digital photography.** Compend Contin Educ Dent 2003;24:260,264–268,270–273.

GORDON P, WANDER P. **Techniques for dental photography.** Br Dent J 1987;162:307–316.

GRIFFIN JD JR. **Excellence in photography: Heightening dentist-ceramist communication.** Dent Today 2009;28(7):124–127.

HAAK R, SCHIRRA C. **Dental photography in support of patient documentation and communication.** Quintessence Int 2000;31:649–657.

HUFF KD. **Photography: An integral component of oral cancer screening.** Dent Today 2009;28(9):100.

HUTCHINSON I, WILLIAMS P. **Digital cameras.** Br J Orthod 1999;26:326–331.

JARAD FD, RUSSELL MD, MOSS BW. **The use of digital imaging for colour matching and communication in restorative dentistry.** Br Dent J 2005;199:43–49.

KATAOKA S, NISHIMURA Y. **Nature's Morphology.** Chicago: Quintessence, 2002.

LLOP DR. **Technical analysis of clinical digital photographs.** J Calif Dent Assoc 2009;37:199–206.

LOMBARDI RE. **The principles of visual perception and their clinical application to denture esthetics.** J Prosthet Dent 1973;29:358–382.

MAGNE P, BELSER U. **Bonded Porcelain Restorations in the Anterior Dentition: A Biomimetic Approach.** Chicago: Quintessence, 2002.

MASSIRONI D, PASCETTA R, ROMEO G. **Precision in Dental Esthetics: Clinical Procedures.** Chicago: Quintessence, 2005.

MCLAREN EA, CULP L, WHITE S. **The evolution of digital dentistry and the digital dental team.** Dent Today 2008;27(9):112,114,116–117.

MCLAREN EA, TERRY DA. **Photography in dentistry.** J Calif Dent Assoc 2001;29:735–742.

MIYASAKI M. **Photography ensures better lab communications, better restorations.** Dent Today 2001;20(11):96–99.

MUIA P. **The Four Dimensional Tooth Color System.** Chicago: Quintessence, 1982.

MUNSELL AH. **The Munsell Book of Color.** Baltimore: Munsell, 1929.

PAPPEL JE. **Lip retractor for occlusal photography.** J Clin Orthod 1996;30:639.

PERETZ B, KAFFE I, AMIR E. **Digital images obtained with a digital camera are not associated with a loss of critical information—A preliminary study.** Br Dent J 2009;206(5):E9.

POLAN MA. **Digital imaging: It's easier than you think.** Dent Today 2001;20(4):108–110,112–115.

PRAPAYASATOK S, JANHOM A, VEROCHANA K, PRAMOJANEE S. **Digital camera resolution and proximal caries detection.** Dentomaxillofac Radiol 2006;35:253–257.

RUIZ JL. **A systematic approach to dento-facial smile evaluation using digital photography and a new photographic view.** Dent Today 2006;25(4):82–85.

SCHROPP L. **Shade matching assisted by digital photography and computer software.** J Prosthodont 2009;18:235–241.

SHARLAND MR. **An update on digital photography for the general dental practitioner.** Dent Update 2008;35:398–400,402–404.

SHARLAND MR. **Digital imaging for the general dental practitioner: 1. Getting started.** Dent Update 2004;31:266–268,270,272.

SHARLAND MR, BURKE FJ, MCHUGH S, WALMSLEY AD. **Use of dental photography by general dental practitioners in Great Britain.** Dent Update 2004;31:199–202.

SHOREY R, MOORE KE. **Clinical digital photography today: Integral to efficient dental communications.** J Calif Dent Assoc 2009;37:175–177.

SHOREY R, MOORE K. **Clinical digital photography: Implementation of clinical photography for everyday practice.** J Calif Dent Assoc 2009;37:179–183.

SNOW SR. **Assessing and achieving accuracy in digital dental photography.** J Calif Dent Assoc 2009;37:185–191.

SNOW SR. **Dental photography systems: Required features for equipment selection.** Compend Contin Educ Dent 2005;26:309–310,312–314,316.

SNOW SR. **Repeatable alignment—Part 1: Consistent model transfer record accuracy.** Pract Proced Aesthet Dent 2003;15:87–93.

SNOW SR. **Repeatable alignment—Part II: Consistent photographic alignment accuracy.** Pract Proced Aesthet Dent 2003;15:551–557.

SPROULL RC. **Color matching in dentistry. I. The three-dimensional nature of color.** J Prosthet Dent 1973;29:416–424.

SPROULL RC. **Color matching in dentistry. II: Practical applications of the organization of color.** J Prosthet Dent 1973;29:556–566.

STUMPEL LJ 3RD. **Simplifying the correction of the digital image in shade communication.** J Prosthet Dent 2004;92:202–203.

SWIFT EJ JR, QUROZ L, HALL SA. **An introduction to clinical dental photography.** Quintessence Int 1987;18:859–869.

TERRY DA, SNOW SR, MCLAREN EA. **Contemporary dental photography: Selection and application.** Compend Contin Educ Dent 2008;29:432–436,438,440–442.

UBASSY G. **Shape and Color: The Key to Successful Ceramic Restorations.** Berlin: Quintessence, 1993.

WAKOH M, KUROYANAGI K. **Digital imaging modalities for dental practice.** Bull Tokyo Dent Coll 2001;42:1–14.

WANDER PA. **The applications of photography in general practice.** Br Dent J 1987;162:195–201.

WANDER P, GORDON P. **Setting up: Equipment, lighting and accessories.** Br Dent J 1987;162:268–280.

WANDER P, GORDON P. **Specific applications of dental photography.** Br Dent J 1987;162:393–403.

WEISGOLD AS. **It depends on when you take the picture.** Int J Periodontics Restorative Dent 2009;29:241.

WINTER R. **Visualizing the natural dentition.** J Esthet Dent 1993;5:102–117.

ZYMAN P, ETIENNE JM. **Recording and communicating shade with digital photography: Concepts and considerations.** Pract Proced Aesthet Dent 2002;14:49,51,53.

Image Credits

All the photographs in Part 1 were taken by the author, Dr Pasquale Loiacono, and published with kind permission, with the exception of Figs 1-7a and 1-7b, courtesy of Dr Mauro Cabiddu, and Fig 2-19, with kind permission of Dr Domenico Massironi.

The photos in Part 2 were taken by the author, Dr Luca Pascoletti, except for the chapter 10 opener image (p 222) and Figs 10-1 to 10-7 and 10-9; the chapter 11 opener image (p 236) and Figs 11-1 to 11-6, 11-12b, 11-13b, 11-14b, and 11-17; the images related to the positions and accessories in chapter 12; and that in chapter 13 on page 310 were taken by the photographer Alberto Quoco and kindly conceded.

Q~e~